W9-ADB-689

Brain Control

BRAIN CONTROL

A Critical Examination of Brain Stimulation and Psychosurgery

ELLIOT S. VALENSTEIN
University of Michigan
Ann Arbor, Michigan

A WILEY-INTERSCIENCE PUBLICATION

JOHN WILEY & SONS, New York • London • Sydney • Toronto

Copyright © 1973, by John Wiley & Sons, Inc.

All rights reserved. Published simultaneously in Canada.

No part of this book may be reproduced by any means, nor transmitted, nor translated into a machine language without the written permission of the publisher.

Library of Congress Cataloging in Publication Data:

Valenstein, Elliot S
   Brain control.

   "A Wiley-Interscience publication."
   Bibliography: p.
   1. Brain stimulation.   2. Psychosurgery.
I. Title. [DNLM: 1. Brain.   2. Psychosurgery.
WL300 V153b 1974]
QP376.V3   617'.481   73-13687
ISBN 0-471-89784-1

Printed in the United States of America

10 9 8 7 6 5 4 3

Men ought to know that from the brain and from the brain only arise our pleasures, joys, laughter, and jests as well as our sorrows, pains, griefs and tears . . . It is the same thing which makes us mad or delirious, inspires us with dread and fear, whether by night or by day, brings sleeplessness, inopportune mistakes, aimless anxieties, absent mindedness and acts that are contrary to habit. . . .

HIPPOCRATES (c. 400 B.C.)
The Sacred Disease

Foreword

In this time of anguished reappraisal of the human society it is little wonder that the subject of this book, the control of human behavior by electrically stimulating or surgically destroying parts of the brain, has aroused intense public interest and anxiety. Emotions engendered by psychosurgery (perhaps better called psychiatric neurosurgery) have come to run high enough to frustrate meaningful discussions between those who disagree on the use of this practice. On the one hand some view psychosurgery at best as useless, and at worst as a destructive assault on the human spirit, eventually to be used on a large scale to prevent social unrest. On the other hand some consider it defensible in certain cases of otherwise intractable mental disorder and pain.

In the midst of this great and confusing clash of medical, social, legal, and political arguments Dr. Valenstein's book appears not only as a most welcome, fair-minded, critical evaluation, but also as a unique and invaluable store of factual information. In his encompassing survey of the subject, the author, himself a distinguished behavioral physiologist, first reviews the animal experiments whose outcome led to the first attempts to treat mental disorder by brain surgery. He then traces the history of psychosurgery from its earliest beginnings in the middle 1930s through its overly optimistic and, in retrospect, excess-ridden heydays of the 1940s and early 1950s to the generally far more conservative psychosurgical practices of the present time. These historical chapters are remarkable by being at once scholarly and eminently readable even to those who lack prior orientation in the brain sciences. Of greatest general interest, however, are the following chapters in which the author thoughtfully examines the roots of the recent controversy over psychosurgery. Neither of the clashing views escapes his serious criticism, but he nonetheless shows understanding and sympathy both for the social and ethical arguments of psychosurgery's antagonists and for the dilemma confronting the physician required to deal with unmanageable pain or mental disease. An important conclusion that suggests itself from these chapters is that the current conflicts over psychosurgery have their origin not only in the largely pragmatic nature of psychiatric-neurosurgical practices and in the great difficulty of measuring accurately the functional losses associated with their benefits, but also in a surprising absence of legal statutes stating and safeguarding the civil rights of prisoners and other institutionalized human beings. In a final section of his book, the author arrives at some constructive suggestions with respect especially to the ever-haunting problem of guaranteeing maximal consideration for the patient's rights and interests.

No one at present can foresee the future course of psychiatry. Only 40 years ago the idea of a "great sterilizing therapy" for infectious diseases was only a wishful dream, but today's antibiotics have brought it close to fulfillment. Will there ever be a "great normalizing therapy" for mental disorders that will make all current psychiatric treatments, including psychiatric neurosurgery, look like a witch doctor's practices? Even should this come to pass, I believe that this book will retain its value not only as an historical document but also as an example of enlightened analysis of sociomedical problems.

WALLE NAUTA
Massachusetts Institute of Technology

Preface

This book began as a magazine article. It had been apparent to me for some time that most popular accounts of research on the brain presented a very distorted view of reality. The theatrical descriptions of the behavior changes produced by stimulating or destroying specific brain regions seemed to be designed to generate awe rather than convey knowledge. In general, the public was receiving information prepared by writers with little firsthand experience in the field. For obvious reasons, these writers sought out the most dramatic incidents they could find (regardless of how unrepresentative) and then proceeded to let their imaginations run wild—completely unfettered by the restraints that might be imposed by a knowledge of brain physiology. In some cases, the distortions could be attributed, at least in part, to scientists who for their own reasons had exaggerated the implications of their research while displaying the skill of a public relations expert in obtaining the broadest coverage possible.

In the course of compiling material for the article, I became increasingly aware of the extent of the influence of many of the popular articles on brain manipulations. This topic is inherently so dramatic that it has been covered by most communication media including newspapers, magazines, television, motion pictures, science fiction stories, and even serious essays picturing life in the future. Few people have been able to remain uninfluenced by this onslaught and even scientists who possess considerable sophistication in their own fields have often displayed a completely uncritical attitude toward the various popular descriptions of new developments in the brain-behavior field. It is not surprising, therefore, that a great many people have unrealistic fears about authoritarian control that might be gained with the new techniques that have been pictured, while others have equally unrealistic hopes that major social problems could be solved by appropriate applications of our current knowledge of the brain.

In an attempt to provide an adequate antidote for the many distortions that have been promulgated, I found I had written a manuscript that was too long for a magazine article. Either the project had to be abandoned or it had to be extended to sufficient length and scope for a book. I justified the latter course of action on several grounds. First, I felt that the original impetus for the article was sufficient justification for a book. There are many people who would like to obtain a degree of understanding of the present state of this field extending beyond the superficial familiarity required to demonstrate only that one is *au courant*. Among this group of people are some who are involved with ethical issues and questions of legislation and financial subsidies that concern developments in brain research. In a sense, the brain-behavior field tends to bring into sharp focus the many subtle ethical problems that involve the delicate balance between the necessity to conduct experimentation to facilitate progress, the rights of the individual, and the needs of society. As such, this field contains many prototypes of the problems that will have to be faced with increasing frequency in the future.

It has been said that an author should have a clearly defined audience in mind and several writers have even related that they find it a useful device to keep one specific person in mind as they work. There is little doubt that such a technique helps to maintain a consistent and appropriate level of exposition. I have taken the risk of disregarding this advice and have tried to keep several audiences in mind, thereby increasing the possibility of not satisfying any. In addition to the lay audience, this book is aimed at the young professional experimentalist and clinician in such fields as physiological psychology, neurophysiology, neurology, neurosurgery, and psychiatry.

For a number of reasons experimentalists and clinicians have maintained very distinct styles of work and thinking. The clinician is faced with practical problems and usually is not in a position to obtain convincing proof of why a method works. The experimentalist's prime concern is with explanation and therefore he must strive to work under conditions that permit verification of results and conclusions. It is apparent that the latter process is often impossible in a clinical setting. Moreover, most experimentalists have Ph.D.'s rather than medical degrees and they prefer not to place themselves in an environment where there are usually many barriers preventing them from reaching the decision-making levels in the hospital hierarchy. The result has been that the worlds of the clinician and the experimentalist have remained more separate than is ideal. It is not that there is no overlap and that the two approaches do not influence each other, but the degree of interaction leaves much to be desired. Clinicians frequently have only a casual knowledge (restricted to review articles) of data generated in the laboratory, and experimentalists are surprisingly uninformed about evidence very relevant to their own work that could be obtained from the clinic. It may prove to have been completely unrealistic, but I have tried to present material that I judged would be interesting and in some cases useful to the student in related clinical and experimental specialties without losing my lay audience.

In attempting to provide information suitable to both a lay audience and the student pursuing a professional career in science or medicine, it was obvious that certain short-comings were inevitable. To maintain a level of discourse that would be adequate for the lay audience it was necessary to provide physiological explanations and basic facts about the brain that were not necessary (or might even appear condescending) to the scientific audience. This was inevitable, but I concluded that it might not be too great a price to pay if in the process the underlying assumptions of technically sophisticated work could be laid bare and more critically examined as a result.

The documentation style has been influenced by the heterogeneous audience for which the book was intended. I have read or reread great numbers of experimental and clinical reports and have tried to extract the essential arguments and accurately reflect the consensus of the evidence. While much of this resource material has been included in the bibliography, few references are cited in the text. It was hoped that the readability would be enhanced if the text was not encumbered with lengthy scientific citations. The names of the major contributors to this field are sufficiently mentioned in the text so that in most instances the reader who wants documentation will have little difficulty in identifying the relevant reference in the bibliography.

It has been said that if you want new ideas, read old books. Obviously, such a statement has to be qualified, but it does contain an important element of the truth. New books frequently make the same assumptions, whereas older books may actually seem fresh by comparison since they often approach the subject from a different vantage point. Sometimes only older books present the essential arguments and evidence, while contemporary authors may consider such arguments axiomatic. I have spent considerable time in reading some of the older experimental and clinical literature and found that the historical perspective gained better prepared me to understand and evaluate present work. In some instances this happened through an awareness that some new theory was actually a modern statement of an older idea. Often the original observations that had led to the earlier theory had been forgotten, but they were still valuable in speculating about possible causal relationships.

An author of a book of this type is usually indebted to many people and the present author is no exception. This book has benefited from the cooperation of many scientists and clinicians. In almost every instance, any request for more information or clarification has been generously responded to by letters, reprints of publications, prepublication manuscripts, permission to reprint figures, and invitations to visit and talk. I have communicated with hundreds of people throughout a good part of the world and have had an opportunity to talk at length with a good number of these. In spite of the fact that I have disagreed with the conclusions or the reliability of the evidence of some of my colleagues (and I suspect that they were aware of my disagreement in many cases), this never interfered with a willingness to exchange information in a congenial atmosphere. Drs. Stephen Chorover, J. Bradley Powers, and William Uttal generously contributed their time by reading the entire manuscript and offering helpful suggestions of both a scientific and literary nature. In addition, by assuming many of the laboratory responsibilities that were rightly mine, my colleague Brad Powers made it possible for me to have the luxury of writing this book relatively free of interruptions. I am also indebted to the excellent library facilities of the University of Michigan and the research librarians who have been most helpful in obtaining old and, in a few cases, rare articles and books. My secretary, Mrs. Betty Danielson, has maintained her good humor in spite of my obsessional streak, which expressed itself in rapidly modifying the manuscript almost as soon as it was retyped. After Betty left this position (I do not believe it was because of the book), Sandra Johnston took her place and exhibited the same unperturbability in the face of the final surge of changes before the manuscript was taken out of my hands. My wife, Thelma, had many valuable suggestions and she as well as my sons, Paul and Carl, have been more than patient with my need to withdraw from the family and in their own way they have all provided me with the motivation to complete the task without compromising the goal I had set.

ELLIOT S. VALENSTEIN

Ann Arbor, Michigan
July 1973

Contents

Figures

Brain Control

Brain Control: A Modern Myth

A retired engineer maintained that he was being "robotted around" by electrical brain stimulation that forced him to wake up in cold sweats of terror, run around in wild euphoria, or experience overwhelming rages. A recent report in the *Canadian Medical Association Journal* contains a description of a psychiatric patient who "believed his thoughts were recorded and controlled by a small electrical apparatus supposedly introduced by operation in his left ear while he slept." These are not isolated incidents. A survey of psychiatrists among my acquaintances revealed that similar ideas have been expressed with increasing frequency by their patients. Since paranoid symptoms can be sensitive indices of the prevailing fears of a society, it seems important to examine the basis of these fears.

If we reflect about it for a moment, these recent developments should not surprise us. During the past five years there has been an increasing amount of space in newspapers, "picture" magazines, and even the more scholarly monthly periodicals devoted to the new ways of controlling human behavior. This bombardment of accounts, which are usually distorted and always oversimplified and slanted to exaggerate the degree of control possible, could not help but have an impact on our thinking. We have been told that the control that can be gained by these new techniques is so complete, society must immediately face the implications of this awesome power for good and evil before it is too late. Brain stimulation—the direct manipulation of the brain by electrical and chemical probes—has been described as potentially the most diabolic technique for controlling behavior. It is generally portrayed as impossible to resist because it initiates a compelling force from within that cannot be "shut out." The following quotation is not atypical:

"All the ancient dreams of mastery over man and all the tales of zombies, golems, and Frankensteins involved some magic formula, or ritual, or incantation that would magically yield the key to dominion. But no one could be sure, from the old Greeks down to Mrs. Shelley, either by speculation or vivisection, whether there was any door for which to find that key. . . . This has been changing gradually, as knowledge of the brain has grown and been compounded since the nineteenth century, until today a whole technology exists for physically penetrating and controlling the brain's own mechanisms of control. It is sometimes called 'brain implantation,' which means placing electrical or chemical stimulating devices in strategic brain tissues. . . . These methods have been used experimentally on myriad aspects of animal behavior, and clinically on a growing number of people. . . . The number of activities connected to specific places and processes in the brain and aroused, excited, augmented, inhibited, or suppressed at will by stimulation of the proper site is simply huge. Animals and men can be oriented toward each other with emotions ranging from stark terror or morbidity to passionate affection and sexual desire. . . . Eating, drinking, sleeping, moving of bowels or limbs or organs of sensation gracefully or in spastic comedy, can all be managed on electrical demand by puppeteers whose flawless strings are pulled from miles away by the unseen call of radio and whose puppets made of flesh and blood, look like 'electronic toys,' so little self-direction do they seem to have." (London, 1969)

The extent of the penetration of these ideas into our thinking is more pervasive than we might realize. Although Figure 1 was only intended to be an eye-catcher

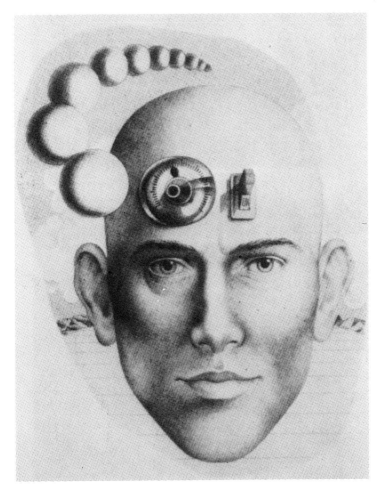

Figure 1. A portion of a magazine advertisement used to attract attention; for many people, however, it represents a view into the future.

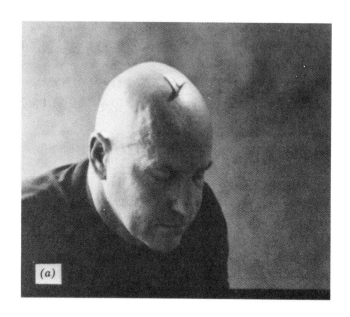

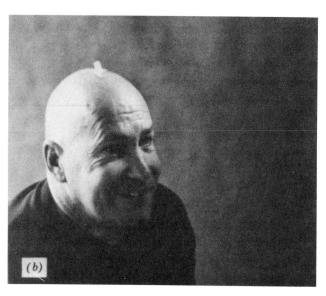

for an advertisement and Figure 2 was to accompany a popular article on brain stimulation, I was amazed at how many college undergraduates thought these were realistic portrayals of what now could be done. There is good reason to suspect that a less sophisticated population might be even more credulous and convinced that we can be electronically controlled.

The publicity given to the topic of human brain stimulation is increasing at a geometric rate. Michael Crichton says about his latest novel, *The Terminal Man*, "I've always wanted to rewrite Frankenstein and this is it." The story describes (in great surgical detail) the process of placing 40 electrodes in the brain for the proposed purpose of regulating a violent patient's behavior by a computer. This novel had been on the "Best Seller List" almost from the date of its publication; prior to this it was serialized in a magazine (*Playboy*) with a large circulation and is scheduled to be made into a movie. It is very likely that many millions of people will be influenced by this story in just a few years.

Taking a different tack, David Rorvik (1969) went so far as to describe a society—not unlike Plato's *Republic* or Aldous Huxley's *Brave New World*—governed by brain stimulation. The ruling class, the "Electroligarchs," transmits the signals that direct the behavior of the other classes, which are "robotized" to varying degrees depending on their number of implanted brain electrodes. The "Electrons," the second rank, would have 50 electrodes implanted in regions that would encourage the development of innovations and new discoveries. The "Positrons" would be the next lower caste and its

---

Figure 2. Turned off *(a)* and turned on *(b)*. The author was amazed at the number of relatively sophisticated people who believed that the model in these pictures actually had some electronic device implanted in his brain (Reprinted from *Psychology Today Magazine*, July 1972. Copyright Communications/Research/Machines, Inc.)

members would have 200 electrodes positioned to assure that they would have maximum dedication to putting the plans into practice, but they might retain minimum personalities. At the lowest level, the "Neutrons," constituting 60 percent of the population, would have 500 implanted electrodes reducing them to the reliability of automatic equipment—"They would, in fact, be completely robotized. They could dig ditches all day and love every minute of it." An *Esquire* article written for shock value and not to be taken seriously, perhaps—but note the title of Karen Waggoner's article in the *Yale Alumni Magazine* (1970), "Psychocivilization or Electroligarchy: Dr. Delgado's Amazing World of ESB".

Although many of these descriptions may be unusually dramatic and in some instances intended only as an exercise in imagination for the purpose of entertainment, such accounts do feed the increasing fear that techniques are available that may soon be capable of completely controlling us. The conclusions are not unrepresentative of those reached in articles that are believed by many to be relatively conservative and reliable science reporting. For example, Boyce Rensberger wrote in *The New York Times* (September 12, 1971) about the scientists who "have been learning to tinker with the brains of animals and men and to manipulate their thoughts and behavior":

"Though their methods are still crude and not always predictable, there can remain little doubt that the next few years will bring a frightening array of refined techniques for making human beings act according to the will of the psychotechnologist."

After learning about the reports that brain stimulation may evoke pleasant or noxious states (see pp. 34–40), some people have begun to speak of "heaven and hell" within the brain. In this vein, Arthur C. Clarke in his

Profiles of the Future (1964) writes:

"Perhaps the most sensational results of this experimentation, which may be fraught with more social consequences than the early work of the nuclear physicists, is the discovery of the so-called pleasure or rewarding centers in the brain. Animals with electrodes implanted in these areas quickly learn to operate the switch controlling the immensely enjoyable electrical stimulus, and develop such an addiction that nothing else interests them. Monkeys have been known to press the reward button three times a second for eighteen hours on end, completely undistracted either by food or sex. There are also pain and punishment areas of the brain; an animal will work with equal singlemindedness to switch off any current fed into these.

"The possibilities here, for good and evil, are so obvious that there is no point in exaggerating or discounting them. Electronic possession of human robots controlled from a central broadcasting station is something that even George Orwell never thought of, but it may be technically possible long before 1984."

The potential of brain manipulations to achieve desirable ends is also expressed by Dr. Kenneth B. Clark in his Presidential Address to the 1971 convention of the American Psychological Association:

". . . we might be on the threshold of that type of scientific biochemical intervention which could stabilize and make dominant the moral and ethical propensities of man and subordinate, if not eliminate, his negative and primitive behavioral tendencies."

Most people have a grossly exaggerated impression of the omnipotence of various brain manipulations, a distorted view of the way specific brain regions are related to behavior, and an uncritical attitude toward suggestions of application of brain technology to social problems. It is easy to understand how this came about. Professional writers are encouraged to provide dramatic accounts that stimulate interest in as large an audience as possible. Unfortunately, this is easiest to accomplish by selecting unrepresentative experimental results, describing them with a minimum of context and qualifications, and ignoring major technical and theoretical obstacles blocking practical applications. While scientists tend to shudder at popular reporting in their own field, there certainly have been cases where they have not been above reproach. Scientists also succumb to the same incentives as other people and there are many examples where the practical implications of preliminary investigations have been exaggerated in an attempt to gain notoriety and increased financial support for their work. The result has been to consistently convey the impression that a wide range of applications to medical and social problems will be possible in the near future. Fears have been generated that brain stimulation will be used to control people while the hope has been fostered that many of those conflicts in society, which are thought to be derived from inherited "aggressive instincts," can be eliminated by brain manipulations. Others have been frightened by what they believe are new developments that are producing a resurgence of psychosurgery—not only as a last resort for treating otherwise incurable psychotics but as a means of behavior control to make people more manageable by destroying their individuality and creativeness.

The purpose of this book is to provide the historical perspective and scientific evidence that places brain manipulations in a more realistic framework. To accomplish this goal it is necessary to review the relevant animal studies and human clinical data and to provide the background necessary to critically evaluate this information.

In a sense, therefore, the ethical and social questions raised by the possibility of human brain manipulations provide a "relevant" framework for discussing a large body of fascinating scientific information concerning the functioning of the brain. It will be apparent that this book was not written for those readers who have no tolerance for uncertainty or those who prefer to be shocked by rather than prepared for future prospects. Much is unknown and many controversies about interpretation of experimental results are unresolved, but familiarity with the issues underlying some of the disputes will provide a closer approximation of the state of our present knowledge.

Large numbers of people have only recently become aware of the techniques for modifying the brain and are consequently of the opinion that these developments are completely new. This unfounded impression of a completely new scientific breakthrough has led to a greatly exaggerated estimate of the clinical and social applications that are likely to appear in the near future. Knowledge of the past history of these techniques and a critical examination of the experimental evidence produced by them is an absolutely essential requirement for extrapolating to the future. Part I of this book presents the historical background and experimental evidence for the discussion of clinical and social applications presented in Part II.

Part I: History and Experimental Evidence

Some Historical Perspective

From the great amount of publicity given to the topic, it would be easy to form the impression that brain stimulation is a completely new development. This is certainly not true at all. Actually, attempts to stimulate the nervous system began shortly before the 1800s just about the time of the origin of neurophysiology as an experimental science. Before it would occur to anyone that it might be possible to stimulate the brain, however, it was necessary to abandon Galen's "hydraulic theory" of the nervous system. Galen had perceived of the nerves as hollow tubes containing fluids that could flow into muscles and make them balloon out and thereby shorten or contract. This view was so generally accepted that when Leeuwenhoek (1632-1723) started to examine nerves with his newly developed microscope he convinced himself that he could see the hollow tubes Galen had described approximately 1500 years earlier.

Toward the end of the eighteenth century a few people began to speculate about the possible role of electricity in bodily functions. Some of the early theories bordered on the mystical. The Austrian physician Friedrich Mesmer (1733–1815), for example, advanced a theory of "animal magnetism" and its relationship to disease that encompassed both Galen's views and the newly emerging interest in electrical phenomena. Mesmer believed that he could direct a "universal energy" into the substance of nerves. This energy, Mesmer thought, had some relation to magnetism. At first he experimented by stroking the bodies of people with metal magnets, but later he thought this was unnecessary to achieve cures and he spoke only of animal magnetism. In his salon in Paris, people sat around in a circle with hands joined or connected by a cord all being linked to Mesmer's famous oak chest, which was said to be magnetized by him. The room was dimly lit and Mesmer—sometimes in a magician's costume—passed around the circle touching some and fixing his glance over others. It was reported that when he fixed his glance on a person and said, "*Dormez!*" the person immediately fell asleep. Clearly, there was much in Mesmer's approach that could be considered a forerunner of hypnotism, and it is very likely that some cures of hysterical symptoms were accomplished.

Many of the practices and paraphernalia used by Mesmer had much in common with spiritualism and he was accused of engaging in magic. Eventually his large and fashionable practice in Paris was curtailed following an investigation by a committee comprised of distinguished scientists appointed by the French Government. Interestingly, Benjamin Franklin was one of the members of this committee, and he apparently concurred with the committee's conclusion that some symptoms were cured, but not by any process related to magnetism. Be that as it may, it is clear that Mesmer's theories were reflecting the attempts at this period in history to try to integrate physical and biological phenomena.

During this same period there was an increasing interest in a more objective examination of electricity as a physical and biological phenomenon. An earlier fascination with the electric eel and the torpedo, an electric ray fish (Figure 3) was revived, and the renowned English physicist Henry

Cavendish constructed an inanimate model of the torpedo out of wood, sheepskin, metal, and 49 glass Leyden jars. Cavendish concluded that "there seems nothing in the phenomenon of the torpedo at all incompatible with electricity," and John Hunter, a fellow English scientist interested in the same phenomenon, wrote: "How far this

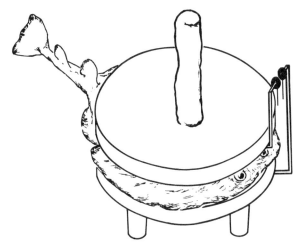

Figure 3. The torpedo, an electric ray fish, as prepared by Carlo Matteucci in 1844 to demonstrate that the shock generated by the fish could cause a spark to bridge a gap. Interest in the torpedo originated much earlier, as indicated by its Greek name, Narke, from which the word narcosis was derived. Scribonius Largus, physician to the Roman Emperor Cladius, wrote in his *Compositions Medicamentorum*: "A chronic and intolerable headache which insistently manifests itself can be eliminated at once if treated by applying a live torpedo fish, black in color, to the site of the pain and leaving it there until the pain stops and the part is swollen. . . . It is necessary to prepare a certain number of these torpedo fish for the benefit . . . is often achieved only after two or three applications." This was repeated by Galen and Pliny the Elder, who also commented on the usefulness of this technique to ease the pain of women during childbirth. The Galvani-Volta controversy about "animal electricity" revived interest in electric fish. Peter Kellaway has written an interesting essay on the part played by electric fish in the early history of bioelectricity and electrotherapy. (Illustration courtesy of the Grass Instrument Company, Quincy, Mass.)

may be connected with the power of the nerves in general, or how far it may lead to an explanation of their operation, time and future discoveries alone can fully determine." There were also several scientists who tried to stimulate nerves and muscles with electricity during the 1770s. It was the great Italian scientists Luigi Galvani and Alessandro Volta, however, who provided the major impetus for the proliferation of experiments on the nervous system that were soon to spring up all over Europe.

The controversy between Galvani and Volta in the 1790s had a tremendous impact on the physiology of the nervous system and on electronic theory. Although the often repeated story of Galvani observing a frog which was attached to a lightning rod twitching in synchrony with distant lightning flashes is true, it does not do justice to the great many systematic experiments performed by· this pioneering scientist. More important in shaping Galvani's thinking was his observation that a frog's muscle contracted when he cranked an electric machine located across the laboratory room and also that a frog suspended from brass hooks would display muscle contractions every time its leg touched an iron plate. The now famous dispute with Volta was over interpretation. Did the electricity reside in the animal or were the contractions caused by an external source of electricity? Galvani wrote:

"I was on the point of deciding that such contractions arose from atmospheric electricity . . . but when I brought an animal into a closed room, placed it on an iron plate, and began to press the hook fixed in the spinal cord against the plate, behold, the same contractions and the same movements. I performed the same experiment over and over, using different metals, at different places, and at different hours and days, with the same result except that the contractions differed according to the metals used; that is, more violent with some, weaker with others."

It is apparent from the preceding quotation that at least initially Galvani did not appreciate that dissimilar metals could produce a "metallic electricity," and Volta, who used this principle to develop a battery, challenged him on this point. Volta maintained that it was only by using heterogenous metal that muscular contractions could be produced. Galvani was forced to perform experiments that did not involve the use of metals, and when he demonstrated contractions by touching a frog's muscle with the cut end of its nerve he was convinced that "animals have a special, independent electricity, deserving the name of animal electricity." The argument persisted after Galvani's death until it was silenced in part by Leopoldo Nobili, who in 1827 measured the electric current in a frog's nerve with his newly constructed galvanometer.

Galvani's demonstrations swept through the scientific community, and a great number of early physiologists began to stimulate animals in spite of the fact that questions about whether nerves actually accomplished their ends by electricity were still disputed. Johannes Müller had postulated the "law of specific energies," which in its essence proposed that no matter how sensory systems are activated they respond in their characteristic fashion:

"For the same cause, such as electricity, can simultaneously affect all sensory organs, since they are all sensitive to it; and yet, every sensory nerve reacts to it differently; one nerve perceives it as light, another hears its sound, another one smells it; another tastes the electricity, and another one feels it as pain and shock."

Although Müller took the position that electricity was an artificial stimulant that had no role in natural excitation, he had provided the justification for its use. Müller's students (duBois-Reymond, Virchow, Schwann, and Helmholtz) dominated German physiology during the middle of the nineteenth century and did not hesitate to use electricity to study the properties of the nervous system. In 1848 duBois-Reymond published a book entitled *Investigations of Animal Electricity*, which sum-

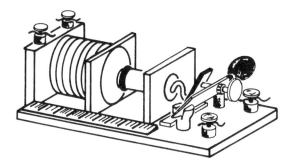

Figure 4. Emil DuBois-Reymond's induction coil stimulator developed about 1848. (Illustration courtesy of the Grass Instrument Company, Quincy, Mass.)

marized many of his experiments that used inductoriums of his own design and static electric generators to stimulate nerves and muscles (see Figure 4). The recognition by the Danish scientist Hans Oersted that electricity and magnetism were interrelated made it possible to develop more sensitive galvanometers and by the 1840s their development had advanced to the point where it was possible to measure many of the electrical changes that accompanied neural activity. Most experiments continued to be conducted on the frog as the tradition inherited from Galvani and Volta persisted well into the nineteenth century.

It is not at all surprising that the newly developed techniques for stimulating nerves and muscles would soon be applied to the brain itself. Several early investigators, including Ernest Weber of Leipzig and Carlo Matteucci, who worked in Florence and Pisa, attempted to stimulate various parts of the brain of living animals, but they used direct *(galvanic)* current for it was not yet known that this stimulus would destroy nerve tissue. In the late 1850s Ivan Sechenov, the "father of Russian physiology," toured European laboratories and after studying for a period under duBois-Reymond he returned to Russia where his lectures on "animal electricity" attracted great attention. L. N. Simonoff, a physiologist in St. Petersburg very much influenced by Sechenov, stimulated the brains of young dogs by using sewing needle electrodes insulated with either melted glass or a resin obtained from wood. Simonoff was searching for "inhibitory centers" in the brains of the dogs as Sechenov had done in frogs. Permanently implanted electrodes were positioned by hand into deep regions of the brain. The whole process of inserting the electrodes through the skin and soft skull of the unanesthetized puppies took less than a minute. Since the skull tended to hold the electrodes relatively fixed in place, it was possible to repeat experiments a number of times on a single puppy over a several week period. Simonoff stimulated the brain with alternating (faradic) current obtained from an inductorium adapted from duBois-Reymond. He even tried chemical stimulation by injecting various stimulants through narrow tubes or cannulae inserted into the ventricles of the brain.

The availability of the skills together with the interest in brain function combined to produce a number of attempts to force the brain to yield its secrets by stimulation of its separate parts. In 1870 Drs. Eduard Hitzig and Gustav Fritsch published the results of their systematic exploration of the cerebral cortex of dogs using electrical stimulation. Their work demonstrated that in a region located in the anterior portion of the cerebral cortex specific movements were elicited by electrical stimulation. They found regions that seemed to control the musculature of the neck, the face, the muscles causing leg flexion, and so forth. The fact that these two investigators lacked sufficient laboratory space did not deter them; much of the experimentation on the dogs was carried out on Frau Hitzig's dressing table in the Hitzig home. Prior to the studies on the dog, Dr. Hitzig, who served as a physician during the Prussian-Danish War (1864), had noted while dressing head wounds of soldiers that irritation of the brain caused twitching on the opposite side of the body.[1] He had followed up these observations in some preliminary experiments on rabbits at duBois-Reymond's Institute before collaborating with Dr. Fritsch.

Among the many investigators who were quick to see the importance of the experimentation of Hitzig and Fritsch was the British neurologist Sir David Ferrier. Ferrier explored the localization of function in many different primates and attempted to extrapolate his experimental results on the monkey to the human brain. During the 1870s he published many of his observations in a journal with the colorful title, *West Riding Lunatic Asylum Medical Report*. Before the beginning of the twentieth century Ferrier's reports would be followed by those of many other investigators who worked on a variety of species including the orangutan, gorilla, and chimpanzee. In addition to his own very many significant contributions, David Ferrier served as an important link in the developing chain of British neurology and physiology. During the 1870s, Ferrier worked with John Hughlings Jackson, who formulated the basic principles of epileptic ("Jacksonian") seizures and who made many contributions to the localization of function within the cerebral cortex. Hughlings Jackson added a considerable degree of sophistication to the problem of localization by postulating a concept of levels of organization of the nervous system wherein most functions were represented at all levels—the lowest consisted of the spinal cord, medulla and pons; the highest was the prefrontal lobes (see pages 300 and 301 for David Ferrier's description of the function of the frontal lobes). During the 1890s, Ferrier worked with Sir Charles Sherrington, who, in addition to describing spinal reflexes and advancing theories about the laws of neural excitation and inhibition, also studied cortical localization in the great apes (see Figure 5).

Perhaps the first account of applying electrical stimulation to the human brain was described in 1874 by Dr. Roberts Bartholow of Cincinnati. Dr. Bartholow, who

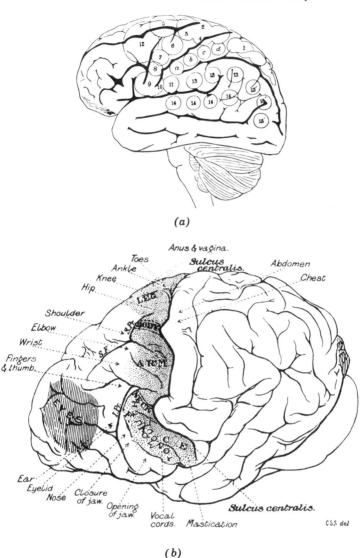

(a)

(b)

Figure 5. *(a)* Lateral view of the human brain from Ferrier (1876), who mapped the cortical function in the monkey brain and then transferred the results to a diagram of the human brain. *(b)* Grünbaum and Sherrington's chart of the function of the chimpanzee cortex as published in 1902. The stippled area represents the motor area. The region marked "eyes" indicates an area from which eye movements could be elicited.

later became well known for his books on practical medical therapeutics, had under his care a woman, Mary Rafferty, a 30 year old, feeble-minded patient with an open ulcer at the posterior portion of the skull. The erosion of the skull was caused by an epithelioma (a cancer) which left a 2-inch hole "where the pulsations of the skull are plainly seen." Dr. Bartholow was able to stimulate the brain with a "Galvano-Faradic Company double cell battery" and with insulated needles about which he wrote: "The needles being insulated to near their points, it was believed that diffusion of the current could be restricted as in the experiments of Fritsch and Hitzig and Ferrier." He was able to elicit some sensations from various parts of the body, and when the strength of the stimulating current was increased

"... in order to develop more decided reactions ... her countenance exhibited great distress, and she began to cry. Very soon the left hand was extended as if in the act of taking hold of some object in front of her; the arm presently was agitated with clonic spasms; her eyes became fixed, with pupils widely dilated; lips were blue, and she frothed at the mouth; her breathing became stertorous; she lost consciousness, and was violent convulsed on the left side. The convulsion lasted five minutes, and was succeeded by coma. She returned to consciousness in twenty minutes from the beginning of the attack, and complained of some weakness and vertigo."

The patient died, presumably not as a result of the stimulation, and an autopsy was performed. Dr. Bartholow wrote: "Although it is obvious that even fine needles cannot be introduced into the cerebral substance of man without doing mischief, yet the fatal result in this case must be attributed to the extension of the epitheliomatous ulceration to the sinus, and the formation of a thrombus." In spite of this somewhat less than auspicious beginning, by the early 1900s electrical stimulation came to be considered an indispensable tool by many of the leading neurosurgeons. Stimulating the brains of lightly anesthetized patients in the operating room became a most important way to localize functions since it was found that physical landmarks were not sufficiently uniform to be completely reliable.

SUBCORTICAL ELECTRODES AND STIMULATION IN UNANESTHETIZED SUBJECTS

One of the most significant advances for those who were to study the role of specific brain regions in more complex behavior was the development of methods to stimulate, fully awake, unrestrained animals over a long period of time. Such "chronic" preparations enabled investigators to observe the effects of brain stimulation on behavior under more natural conditions. Dr. J. R. Ewald's investigations around 1896 may have been the first to involve stimulation of relatively unrestrained animals. Ewald did not write up his results in any detail, but Dr. G. A. Talbert, an American postdoctoral fellow studying in Germany, described the technique and his own extension of Ewald's work in 1900. Since ivory had been investigated for its usefulness in repairing skull damage, Ewald used this material to make a threaded cone that could be screwed into a hole drilled in the skull. Platinum "button" electrodes were positioned on the dog's cortex within the cone and the wires attached to the electrodes were anchored to the cone before being led off to a battery in the experimenter's hand. The dog was led around on a leash and its brain could be stimulated while the animal was engaged in different activities. Other investigators saw the significance of Ewald and Talbert's methods and soon they were adopting their own variations of this basic technique to stimulate a variety of unrestrained animals.

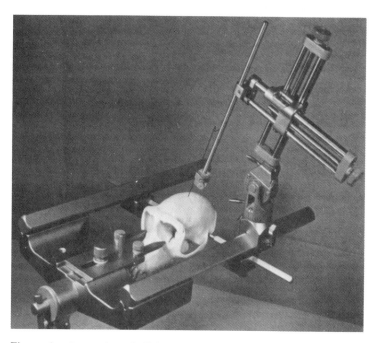

Figure 6. A monkey skull in a stereotaxic instrument. The skull is positioned accurately and held securely by bars inserted in the ear canals, the upper teeth, and the lower ridges of the eye sockets (infraorbital ridges). The carrier holding the electrode wire can be accurately positioned in three planes in accordance with stereotaxic maps of the brain.

Up to the turn of the century, the portion of brain most extensively investigated was the cerebral cortex, primarily because of its accessibility. The development of an instrument in 1908 by the British neurosurgeon and neurophysiologist Dr. Victor Horsley and his associate, R. H. Clarke, made it possible to "direct a protected stimulating and electrolytic needle to any desired part of the brain with very fair accuracy." The Horsley-Clarke stereotaxic device became the model for a great number of instruments which permit the insertion of wires into the depths of the brains of animals and man. Essentially, a stereotaxic instrument positions the head in a fixed plane and, with the aid of three-dimensional anatomical maps (stereotaxic atlases), it is possible to place electrodes through small holes in the skull into almost any sector of the brain. Utilizing the basic principle of the Horsley-Clarke instrument there have probably been developed more than 100 variations of the basic design which are capable of accommodating a great number of different species. Today, there are stereotaxic atlases of the brains of pigeons, mice, gerbils, hamsters, rats, guinea pigs, rab-

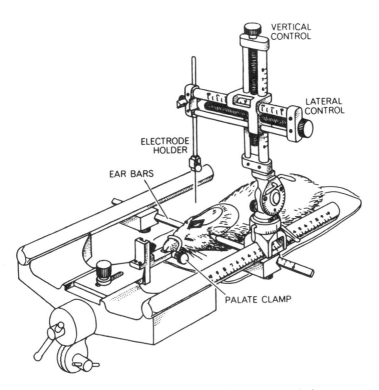

Figure 7. Illustration of a rat positioned in a sterotaxic instrument. (From L. DiCara, "Learning in the Autonomic Nervous System." Copyright January 1970 by *Scientific American, Inc.* All rights reserved.)

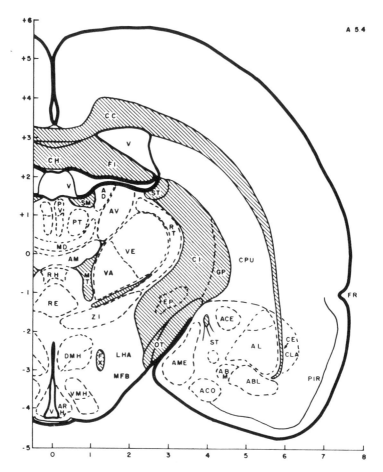

Figure 8.   One of the plates from a stereotaxic map of the rat brain. Pictured is a schematic drawing to scale of one-half of a "frontal" section (a slice approximately perpendicular to the top surface of the brain) with the separate structures identified. The number in the upper right-hand corner indicates the millimeters in front of a plane through the ear canals; numbers on the side and below represent a millimeter scale indicating dorsal-ventral and medial-lateral coordinates. (From J. de Groot, *The Rat Forebrain in Stereotaxic Coordinates*, North-Holland Publishing Co., Amsterdam.)

bits, opossums, cats, dogs, dolphins, many species of monkeys, chimpanzees, and man.

The development of stereotaxic instruments made it possible to investigate the deep portions of the brain beneath the surface. Electrodes could now be inserted with reasonable accuracy into any region of the brain. If the electrodes were insulated except for a small area around the tip, a relatively circumscribed area could be stimulated by using alternating current or destroyed if direct current was applied. This capacity to explore subcortical regions opened up huge avenues for research. Parts of the brain for which literally no function had been known could now be investigated. In the earlier investigations, interest had been centered on the cerebral cortex and the elicitation of movements, but with the capacity to stimulate regions of the brain close to the ventral (bottom) surface of the brain, other responses were observed. After Dr. Ferdinand Winkler of the University of Vienna observed that stimulation of the cat's hypothalamus produced a sweating of the foot pads, Drs. J. Karplus and A. Kreidl of the same university began a very influential series of investigations that were published between 1909 and 1928 under the title *Gehirn und Sympathicus* (The Brain and Sympathetic Responses). These publications emphasized the capacity of hypothalamic stimulation to elicit such reactions of the autonomic nervous system (the portion of the nervous system that innervates the viscera, glands, and certain so-called smooth muscles) as pupillary constriction and dilation, blood pressure and heart rate changes, tearing, and salivation. Some of the reports demonstrated that autonomic responses could be obtained from the frontal regions of the neocortex as well, but only if the hypothalamus was not destroyed. The responses elicited from hypothalamic stimulation, however, were not abolished if the frontal cortex was destroyed. Such observations began to lay the groundwork for the central role of the hypothalamus in regulating those visceral and glandular responses that characterize the presence of emotionality.

STIMULATION AND MOTIVATION

It was the studies of Drs.Walter Rudolph Hess of Switzerland and Stephen W. Ranson of the United States that did much to usher in the present era. Dr. Hess began his investigation in the 1920s and because he worked in Zurich his laboratory was relatively uninterrupted during World War II. In 1949 Hess was awarded the Nobel Prize for his investigations which involved a mapping of the responses elicited by stimulation of approximately 4500 neural sites (principally within the hypothalamus) in about 480 cats. In most of his studies, Hess used fully awake animals, which were restrained only by the connecting cables. At approximately the same time, a group of distinguished anatomists working with Dr. Stephen Ranson at Northwestern University were using a modification of the stereotaxic device of Horsley and Clarke to explore the function of different regions of the hypothalamus and related neural structures.

Many reports from the laboratories of Drs. Ranson and Hess were initially concerned with hypothalamic regulation of isolated responses such as blood pressure and respiratory and cardiac changes as well as pupillary dilation and constriction. Later, an increasing amount of attention was devoted to the pattern of responses involved in such adaptive functions as temperature regulations, defecation, vomiting, and sleep. Toward the end of his investigative career, Hess described the stimulated animal in terms that implied emotional and motivational states such as insatiable hunger (bulimia), flight, defensive reactions, and rage. (Ransom did not stimulate unrestrained animals but he and his associates reported that destruction of discrete areas within the hypothalamus could produce animals that overate and became extremely obese or animals whose sleep patterns or temperature regulation became radically altered.) In Hess' later writings he indicated that he had become convinced that natural states could be induced by hypothalamic stimulation.

"Sherrington long ago showed how easily a decorticated cat may be brought into the state of rage, generally called sham-rage; however, when this state results from stimulation, there is no reason to consider it as different from natural rage."

Dr. Hess' studies of the behavioral and physiological responses that could be elicited by electrical stimulation of the brains of cats led him to conclude that there was an anterior hypothalamic, *trophotropic system* and a middle and posterior hypothalamic, *ergotropic system*. The former was described as a parasympathetic system responsible for restorative and replenishing functions such as sleep and digestion; the latter system was said to regulate the skeletal and vegetative responses involved in vigorous activities such as those displayed during flight or fleeing. In general, such physiological responses as increases in heart rate, blood pressure, and muscle tone, which "aid the organism to greater success in its conflicts with the environment," were elicited by stimulation of the ergotropic zone. In his Nobel Lecture, Dr. Hess pointed out:

"On stimulation within a circumscribed area of the ergotropic (dynamogenic) zone, there regularly occurs a manifest change in mood. Even a formerly good-natured cat turns bad-tempered; it starts to spit and, when approached, launches a well-aimed attack. As the pupils simultaneously dilate widely and the hair bristles, a picture develops such as is shown by the cat if a dog attacks it while it cannot escape . . . functionally, the total behavior of the animal illustrates the fact that, in the part of the diencephalon indicated, a meaningful association of physiological responses takes place, which is related on the one hand to the regulation of internal organs and on the other involves the functions directed outwards towards the environment.''

As will be discussed later, Hess' studies and conclusions have been directly applied to human behavior problems by Dr. Keiji Sano of Tokyo, who labeled his surgical destruction of the posterior medial hypothalamus ''sedative therapy.''

With the exception of a few sporadic reports there was little systematic work in the United States that used brain stimulation to study behavior in relatively unrestrained animals prior to 1950. Dr. Frederick Gibbs of Harvard noted in 1936 that stimulation of a region in the hypothalamus of awake cats produced a ''purring'' reaction, and in 1941 Dr. Jules Masserman of the University of Chicago tried to determine if the stimulation of those portions of the hypothalamus of the cat that seem to elicit rage was producing a true emotion or only the bodily changes associated with emotional states. Although Masserman concluded that only bodily reactions were evoked and the stimulated animals did not experience a true emotion, later investigators were to reach a different conclusion. World War II interrupted almost all basic research in the United States, but shortly after the end of the war a number of investigators working in the behavioral sciences began to use brain stimulation as a means of studying the neural mechanisms regulating behavior.

The use of more sophisticated behavioral tests to evaluate the states elicited by brain stimulation was initiated by people trained in behavior analysis. Physiologists tended to neglect behavioral methods, whereas psychologists considered behavior analysis their "stock in trade." (This distinction between physiologists and psychologists is no longer valid, since many physiologists are now very skilled in the more advanced behavior testing methods and biologically oriented psychologists are often significant contributors to the literature in neuroanatomy and neurophysiology.) In the early 1950s the great potential of brain stimulation was grasped by psychologists, who needed desperately to find

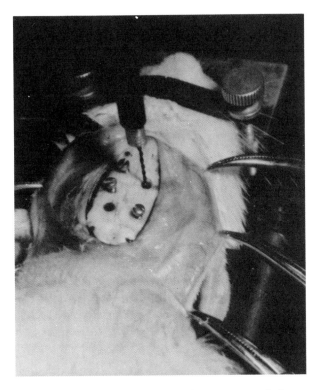

Figure 9. An anesthetized rat positioned in a stereotaxic instrument. The skin and muscles of the head have been retracted to expose the skull. Anchoring screws have been fastened to the skull and an electrode is about to be inserted into the brain through a prepared "burr" hole. An acrylic cement will be applied to bind the electrode pedestal, screws, and skull together.

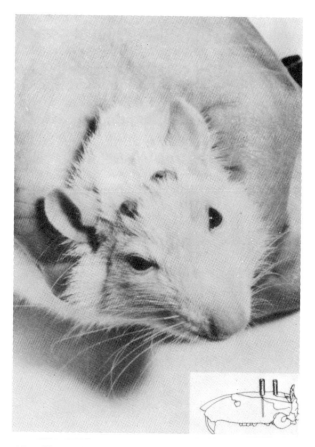

Figure 10. Six weeks after the electrodes were inserted. The skin has healed and the hair has grown back. The insert illustrates a bipolar electrode inserted into the brain and an "indifferent" electrode positioned under a muscle at the back of the skull for monopolar stimulation or recording.

new ways to manipulate and measure their theoretical constructs of motivation and drive. If an animal would eat when some area in its brain was stimulated, it might be possible to manipulate and even to quantify drives such as hunger directly.

Electrode implantation techniques had to be learned by many who had little background in biology and physiology and there was much fumbling and frustration in the beginning. Behavior tests often take a long time and electrodes kept coming loose before the experiments were completed. There were many who thought that it would not be possible to attach electrodes to the thin skulls of animals as small as rats. By the late 1950s, however, a large number of technical articles had appeared which described different electrode assemblies and methods of attaching miniature connectors to the skull. Other reports compared the reaction of brain tissue to various electrode metals and different types of electric current. Like any manual skill, there were numerous little "tricks" that had to be learned and the best materials had to be determined—for example, the type of acrylic cement that would form the most secure bond with the skull. The basic techniques have now become sufficiently routine so that students with no surgical experience can usually become reasonably proficient in the basic techniques after only a few days of instruction and practice (see Figures 9, 10, and 11).

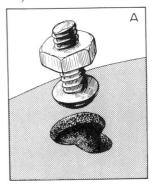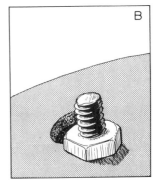

Figure 11.   One technique for firmly attaching various devices to the skull of large animals. A "keyhole" shaped opening in the skull is prepared, which permits a bolt to be slid into place and anchored securely with a nut. The head of the bolt has been ground down to minimize pressure on the brain. Several of these bolts anchored into the skull can provide the support for mounting miniaturized stimulators or transmitters directly on the skull.

When psychologists started to use brain stimulation as an experimental tool they were not concerned mainly with its capacity to activate bodily reflexes. Psychologists tended to concentrate on more holistic behavior patterns such as eating, drinking, and aggression and the mental states that accompanied these responses when they were elicited by brain stimulation. They wanted to know if the animals experienced hunger, thirst, pain, and fear when stimulated. To obtain answers, animals were trained to make some responses to obtain food or to avoid a painful foot shock. It was then determined whether the animal would use these learned responses during brain stimulation. Animals were trained to press a lever, for example, when a warning signal was presented in order to avoid a painful shock. It was known that the animal would try to avoid other unpleasant stimuli, such as a puff of air to its head, by making the same response. By using a variety of such behavior tests it seemed possible to learn something about what the animal experienced during brain stimulation.

REWARDING AND PUNISHING BRAIN CIRCUITS

In the early 1950s, Dr. José Delgado of Yale University noticed that cats stimulated in certain brain areas appeared disturbed and fearful when placed back in the same test chamber in which they had previously been stimulated. In collaboration with a psychologist interested in learning theory, Dr. Neal Miller, and a graduate student, Warren Roberts, it was demonstrated that the cats would escape from and even avoid brain stimulation at these brain sites. If the cats had only been capable of escaping from the stimulation, their responses might have been interpreted as reflexive, but the fact that they elected to use a previously learned response to avoid the stimulation before it was even presented was fairly convincing evidence that some unpleasant emotional state was experienced. To understand the importance of this demonstration it must be appreciated that the evidence available up to this time seemed to indicate that stimulating the brain did not produce any emotional experience in spite of the impression often conveyed by the evoked bodily reactions.

The demonstration that brain stimulation would produce an aversive emotional state capable of motivating an animal to avoid a repetition of the experience opened up many research possibilities for studying the brain mechanisms involved in learning and motivation. Some even speculated that there might be a negative reinforcement system that was activated by all aversive stimuli regardless of their origin and this system was capable of facilitating the learning of any response successful in inhibiting its elevated activity. In addition to any implication for learning theories, the fact that emotional experiences could be evoked by brain stimulation laid the foundation for studying the brain correlates of emotional states and later attempts to alter human moods.

At about the same time as the demonstration that stimulation at some brain sites could evoke an aversive emotional state, investigators at McGill University and the Montreal Neurological Institute were speculating about the possible role of other brain structures in the learning process. It had been demonstrated that destruction of the area of the brainstem known as the reticular formation produced a comatose animal, whereas stimulation of the same area seemed to produce a hyperalert animal. One investigator, Dr. James Olds, was interested in determining if stimulation of the reticular formation could facilitate learning. To test this hypothesis, he planned to stimulate the reticular formation while rats were at some choice points in a maze and then to compare the speed of learning the different parts of the maze. Before the project got very far, however, an accident occurred which led to such a dramatic discovery that the original project was abandoned.

In 1953 the technique for implanting electrodes in rats was very crude and unreliable. Dr. Olds, who had just obtained his Ph.D. degree, was attempting to use the techniques available at McGill University with the aid of a graduate student, Peter Milner, who happened to have had more experience in the relevant surgical and electronic skills. One of the electrodes that was aimed for the reticular formation was accidentally bent during the implantation and ended up a long distance from the intended area—probably in the hypothalamus. (Actually, the brain of this animal was lost, but the results of a great number of later experiments make it likely that the electrode ended up in the hypothalamus or a closely related structure.) Dr. Olds had learned of the work of Drs. Delgado, Miller, and Roberts from a presentation of their results at a scientific meeting. He concluded from this report that if some brain stimulation could elicit aversive reactions, it would be advisable to test for this possibility before beginning the experiment in the maze. Aversive stimulation might interfere with or obscure any influence the stimulation might have on the facilitation of learning. A quick pretest was designed to determine if the stimulation was aversive, but due to the misplaced electrode a very surprising result was obtained. Dr. Olds describes this event in a book edited by the author:[2]

"A rat was free to move around in a fairly large tabletop enclosure (3×3 feet or more). A pair of stimulating wires was planted deep in the brain and insulated except for the cross section of the tip. These were attached to a connector which was held rigidly to the skull, but which penetrated through the scalp to permit attachment of wires from the stimulator. The wires from the stimulator were a pair of fairly light, quite long wires suspended from the ceiling by means of an elastic band which provided no more impediment to movement than a long, loose leash provides for a dog. I applied a brief train of 60 cycle sine wave electric current whenever the animal entered one corner of the enclosure. The animal did not go away and stay away from the corner, but rather came back quickly after a brief sortie which followed the second stimulation. By the third time the electric stimulus had been applied the animal seemed indubitably to be coming back for more."

To quantify the behavior, this animal and many others were placed in a small Skinner box with a large lever. Every time the animal stepped on the lever it received a brief brain stimulation. At first it stepped on the lever accidentally, but if the electrode was in the proper place in the hypothalamus, the animal soon started to press the lever repeatedly. Some of these animals "self-stimulated" by pressing the lever more than 100 times every minute, and they maintained this pace hour after hour.

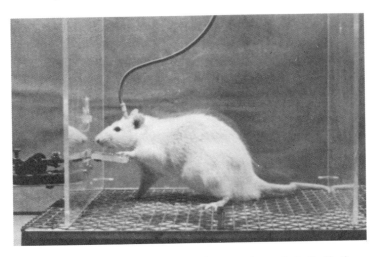

Figure 12. A rat with cable attached to an electrode is "self-stimulating." Every time the rat presses the lever it receives a half-second burst of alternating current in the lateral hypothalamus.

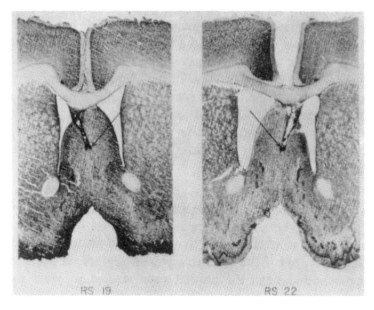

Figure 13. Illustration of the appearance of histologically prepared brain slices used to identify location of electrode tips. The arrows indicate the electrode tips located in the septal area of two different rat brains. Note that it is sometimes possible to see the tips of each wire of the bipolar pair.

In terms of dramatic impact and the amount of theoretical speculation and experimentation generated, no single discovery in the field of brain-behavior interactions can rival the finding that animals could be highly motivated to stimulate certain areas of their own brain. Although many basic questions about "self-stimulation" remain unanswered, a great number of people have speculated that this phenomenon may contain the key to understanding the physiological basis of motivation. Here was a system in the brain that flashed a green light, a signal to continue what was going on. Judging by the animal's behavior, the stimulation was evoking a pleasurable reaction. At least there could be no doubt of the animal's motivation to strive to repeat the experience.

The initial observations have been extended to other animals besides the rat; self-stimulation has been demonstrated in goldfish, pigeons, chickens, rabbits, cats,[3] dogs, guinea pigs, monkeys, dolphins, and as will be described subsequently, even human beings. (Self-stimulation may not be equally compelling in all species, however, but this will be discussed in the next chapter of this book.) The fact that self-stimulation has been obtained from approximately the same anatomical structures in such a variety of species seemed to indicate that a basic mechanism of general evolutionary significance was involved.

Numerous investigators have been captivated by the reports of the rewarding and punishing consequences of brain stimulation. There is now a very large number of scientific papers and doctoral dissertations concerned with one or another of the properties of these neural systems. Originally, most demonstrations of the reinforcement properties of brain stimulation utilized the somewhat stereotyped and repetitive responding involved in lever pressing. There were some people, therefore, who remained unconvinced that the brain stimulation acted as a reward. They argued that the stimulation forced the animals to repeat the response just made; they were really "trapped" rather than rewarded. Indeed, the frenetic way that animals often pressed the levers made this argument seem reasonable. Later, however, it was shown that animals could solve mazes and learn to discriminate between visual patterns if they were rewarded with brain stimulation for making the correct responses. In these and numerous other testing situations, delays were interposed between successive responses and the results left little doubt that the animals were actively seeking out the stimulation. Animals that had not received any brain stimulation for several days have been known to jump from the experimenter's hands into the test chamber, where they would immediately make the responses that had previously been rewarded by brain stimulation.

Other studies, including some that are being pursued at present, have helped to define more precisely the brain structures from which self-stimulation behavior can be obtained. Although a detailed discussion of these anatomical studies would be inappropriate here, it may be helpful to note that "positive sites" tend to be located in the lateral portions of the hypothalamus and the limbic system. (The limbic system, in conjunction with the hypothalamus, appears to play a critical role in emotional reactions; see Figures 24, 25, 26 and page 47.) The anatomical distribution of the punishment system has been studied as well and it also has been located primarily in the hypothalamus and limbic system, but generally in portions that are closer to the midline of the brain.[4] These systems seem to be diffusely located within the hypothalamus and limbic system, since attempts to find a portion of these circuits that could be considered a critical focus by systematically destroying various anatomical areas have met with little success to date. This diffuse and seemingly redundant physical arrangement may serve as a safeguard for the very important function these reward systems play and, in addition, it may make it possible for their influence to be extended to all parts of the nervous system.

THEORETICAL IMPLICATIONS OF THE REWARDING AND PUNISHING CIRCUITS

The presence of these motivationally potent neural systems in the brain have encouraged a revival of hedonistic explanations of behavior. As long ago as 1789, the English philosopher Jeremy Bentham wrote: "Nature has placed mankind under the governance of two sovereign masters, pain and pleasure. It is for them alone to point out what we ought to do, as well as to determine what we shall do." The discovery of the rewarding and punishing neural circuits produced several neurophysiological theories to explain hedonistic behavior. It was not at all surprising that the demonstration of two fundamental motivational systems in the brain would produce theories based on the assumption that the activation of the positive reward system was a common denominator of all pleasurable events, and the common denominator of aversive experiences was the activation of the "punishment" circuit. Relative activity in these two systems might determine which of several possible behaviors is selected. The establishment of abnormal short-circuits between these two systems might even be the basis of masochistic and sadistic behavior.

Simple organisms, living in restricted environments, do not need specialized neural circuits to encourage and discourage new responses. Such animals tend to satisfy their requirements for survival by a number of adaptive reflexes which vary only in reactivity as specific biological needs become stronger or weaker. A structure for siphoning food may be highly responsive or sluggish in its reaction to appropriate stimuli, depending on the elapsed time since the last meal. To a great extent, the fate of these relatively simple organisms is necessarily determined by the benevolence of a restricted environment. The species survives partly because huge numbers are reproduced in a short time, so that even during unfavorable conditions only a small percentage need survive to maintain continuity.

Animals that reproduce only a few of their kind at a time and take a relatively long time to do so cannot afford the risk of being limited to a restricted environment. Should that environment be unfavorable for a period, the whole species might die. Such animals must have the capacity to vary their behavior to be able to adapt to a variety of environments. They must be able to learn rapidly and also to remember the significance of any new response that is tried—which responses should be repeated and which avoided in the future. Under such conditions there is considerable evolutionary pressure placing a premium on behavioral flexibility. It is conceivable that specialized neural circuits have evolved not only to encourage and discourage responses, but to provide a neurophysiological amplification of significant events to stamp them in and facilitate their recall.

It is possible to speculate even further, for the rewarding and punishing neural systems may be involved in other functions in addition to guiding behavior. As published accounts of the verbal reports of patients experiencing brain stimulation began to appear, it became apparent that activation of different parts of these same neural systems could influence mood. Stimulation at some sites produced feelings of elation whereas stimulation at other sites evoked fears, anxieties, and even anger. It is not surprising that knowledge of these results produced speculation that mood and even basic temperament might be regulated by some delicate balance of the two systems.

I have observed, as have others, that stimulation of the positive reward system induces animals to engage in an active exploration of the environment, whereas stimulation of the punishment system usually produces a back-peddling, withdrawal response. Based on a very interesting, albeit highly speculative, extension of these and other related observations, Dr. Jeffrey Gray of Oxford University recently suggested a physiological basis of introversion and extroversion. Dr. Gray argues that introverts have highly reactive punishment systems that constantly cause them to withdraw from the environment; extroverts have relatively insensitive punishment circuits but are highly responsive to positive rewards. Extroverts, therefore, are constantly reaching out to the environment and are not easily rebuffed. Introversion and extroversion may therefore be the result of some conditioned or genetically determined responsiveness of the rewarding and punishing circuits.

The reinforcement systems in the brain may also provide the key to understanding the continuity as well as the disorganization of behavior. If behavior is to be adaptive there must be some coordinating theme; maladaptive behavior is chaotic, disorganized, and seemingly random. Although the continuity of innate behavior may be based on a series of chained reflexes, each responsive to a stimulus produced by the previous response, the cohesiveness of learned behavior seems to be dependent on a shared relationship to a common goal. Anticipation of the goal provides the logical thread connecting a potentially unlimited variety of responses and it also provides the motivation that maintains the progression of the behavior. The concept of anticipation does not presuppose a conscious awarenesss of a goal, but in some manner each response must be evaluated for its appropriateness to some end if behavior is to be purposive rather than random. If a response is very appropriate, it is normally associated with a high level of motivation—the response is expressed vigorously. If the response has a remote connection to the goal, the behavior is expressed lackadaisically. The discovery of a rewarding neural circuit makes it easier to conceive of some physiological mechanism that plays a role in selecting and motivating responses based on a projection of the probability of reward.

There is no reason to limit the concept of goal directedness or purposefulness to overt behavior. Thinking also must maintain direction if a logical connectivity is to be realized. In psychiatric depression both thought processes and behavior are slowed, perhaps because the goals that once were capable of motivating behavior no longer are able to do so. In schizophrenia, as the Swiss psychiatrist Dr. Paul Eugen Bleuler pointed out a number of years ago, there is a fragmentation and thoughts "are not related and directed by any unifying concept of purpose or goal." The disconnected speech pattern ("word salad") of the deteriorated schizophrenic is a striking example of fragmented thought processes.

Dr. Larry Stein of the Wyeth Pharmaceutical Laboratories recently attempted to relate the reward circuit in the brain to psychiatric states such as depression and mania and even to the schizophrenic process. Using self-stimulation performance as an indication of the responsiveness of the reward circuit, Stein was able to demonstrate some engaging parallels between the drugs that cause or alleviate depression in humans and their effect on self-stimulation performance in rats. Drugs that counteract depression usually facilitate self-stimulation. In a bold extension of his laboratory demonstrations, Stein and his collaborator, C. D. Wise, suggested that due to a metabolic abnormality there is a gradual destruction of the reward circuit in schizophrenics with the result that purposive behavior and thought processes cannot be maintained. It is interesting to note in the present context that Dr. Robert Heath of Tulane University indicated in a conversation with the author that schizophrenics with implanted electrodes in rewarding brain sites report very little pleasure produced by stimulation. Although this theory is surrounded by controversy and not without conflicting evidence,[5] the great amount of interest that has been generated will undoubtedly result in the accumulation of much useful information.

BRAIN STIMULATION AND THE ELICITATION OF SPECIFIC BEHAVIOR

Following Dr. Hess' lead, scientists since the 1950s, have provided many examples of brain stimulation triggering drinking, eating, grooming, hoarding, components of maternal behavior such as nest building and retrieving of pups, aggression, and male sexual behavior. In most instances the behavior could be turned on and off, directly correlated with the initiation and termination of the stimulation. Evidence was presented which seemed to indicate that the behavior produced by the stimulation resulted from the activation of natural motivational states rather than the elicitation of reflexes. It was observed, for example, that the stimulation usually did not evoke any response if the appropriate "goal object" was absent. If food was absent, the stimulation did not trigger eating responses. Moreover, animals would perform some learned task to obtain access to the food when stimulated. If an animal is stimulated at a site that normally evokes eating, it may press a lever (or whatever else it has learned) to obtain access to the food.

Dr. John Flynn at Yale University and other investigators as well have shown that a cat which had not displayed any aggressive tendencies toward rats could suddenly be transformed by stimulation into an enraged "Halloween cat" complete with claws unsheathed, hair standing on end, arched back, and hissing. The brain stimulation that elicited such responses was shown by Drs. D. Adams and John Flynn to be aversive to the animals, which escaped from the stimulation if given an opportunity. It is possible, therefore, that the attack response may have been triggered by some component of pain just as foot shock often provokes fighting among animals caged together. Drs. Leopold Hofstatter and Makram Girgis of the Missouri Institute of Psychiatry in St. Louis recently reported that radiostimulation of the lateral hypothalamus of freely moving monkeys may evoke well-directed, aggressive attacks against other animals. According to Drs. Hofstatter and Girgis it was quite clear that the monkeys disliked the stimulation that elicited their own aggressive attacks, since they frequently pulled out the connecting cables and bit at them when the stimulation was turned on.

Potentially more interesting is the finding that stimulation at other brain regions could trigger aggression and even killing without involving pain or aversive stimulation. Stimulation of some hypothalamic regions of the cat, for example, was reported by Dr. Flynn and his collaborators to cause a quiet, predatory "stalking-attack" response. It has been demonstrated in the rat and monkey, as well as the cat, that some stimulation that evokes aggressive responses may produce a positive emotion, so that animals turn the stimulation on themselves—that is, self-stimulate—if given the opportunity. Furthermore, when this stimulation is delivered, a normally peaceful cat demonstrates its motivational state by running to a location where it has learned a rat has been placed. Without the stimulation, this same cat would not be interested in the rat. These observations, based on experiments by Drs. Warren Roberts and Harold Kiess, are particularly significant because they indicate that the stimulation did not just elicit a "killing reflex"—rather, the animal seemed to have been predisposed toward certain types of behavior and it was then motivated to respond in a variety of ways to be able to fulfill this drive. Just as an animal could be motivated to obtain food by stimulating a certain brain region, it seemed that animals could be motivated to attack by a similar manipulation of brain activity, and in both cases the stimulation itself could evoke pleasurable reactions. It is not surprising that such experimental demonstrations have produced considerable speculation that it might be possible to determine the brain areas regulating specific motivational states and those areas responsible for providing the experience of pleasure produced by engaging in behavior relevant to that motivational state.

The trend during the major part of the 1960s was to describe as many behaviors as possible that could be elicited by brain stimulation. As the list of responses that had been elicited grew larger, the potential for controlling behavior and motivation seemed greater and greater. Often there was a rather uncritical acceptance of the significance of these reports, which characteristically claimed to have tapped an anatomical circuit regulating specific motivational states. More recent developments, however, have made it clear that the extrapolations from these initial reports to the possibility of controlling human behavior or even treating clinical problems rested on a very shaky foundation. The critical evaluation of these reports of elicited behavior will be reserved for the chapter on Brain Manipulations and the Control of Specific Behavior.

THE LIMBIC SYSTEM AND EMOTIONALITY

A very significant force in encouraging neurosurgeons to undertake various brain manipulations as a means of treating emotional and behavioral problems was a number of reports of dramatic changes in animal behavior following experimental destruction of parts of the nervous system. Some of the changes actually seemed to radically transform the temperament or personality of the operated animals. These changes were most often seen following destruction of regions either in the limbic system and hypothalamus (see Figures 24, 25, and 26) or in the prefrontal cortical area, which is believed to be part of the same functional circuit. These results provided support for the highly speculative theory proposed by Dr. James Papez in 1937. Papez assembled arguments and clinical data in support of a theory that the limbic system (in conjunction with the hypothalamus) constituted an anatomical circuit regulating emotionality:

"It is proposed that the hypothalamus, the anterior thalamic nuclei, the gyrus cinguli, the hippocampus and their interconnections constitute a harmonious mechanism which may elaborate the functions of central emotion, as well as participate in emotional expression."

The limbic system as a neural circuit regulating emotionality had evolved from the structures that transmitted olfactory information. The relationship was natural as odors are one of the main ways that most mammals learn such vital information as the location of a predator, a prey, or a potential sexual partner. Before 1901, the noted Spanish neurohistologist Santiago Ramón y Cajal had concluded that the hippocampus, a limbic structure that was assumed to be important for olfaction, "had no more than a neighborly relationship" to the olfactory pathway, but it took Papez' theory to give importance to such observations. The distinguished American neuroanatomist Dr. C. Judson Herrick recognized that in addition to subserving the sense of smell the limbic-olfactory system prepared animals for upcoming emergencies. He pointed out that for many mammals the so-called olfactory neural structures are used less for localization than for "the activation or sensitizing of the nervous system as a whole and of certainly appropriately attuned sensori-motor systems in particular, with resulting lowered threshold of excitation for all stimuli and differential reinforcement or inhibition of specific types of responses." In other words, instead of having to maintain a constant state of preparedness, a part of the limbic circuit seems to have been assigned the responsibility of appropriately "tuning" and mobilizing the reactivity of the motor, sensory, endocrine, and visceral systems.

Other observations contributed to the acceptance of Papez' theory. In 1941, Dr. W. F. Allen at the University of Oregon Medical School destroyed extensive portions (but not all) of such important limbic structures as the amygdala and hippocampus and demonstrated that his experimental dogs could still smell. It was also remembered that even in anosmic (without a sense of smell) mammals, such as whale and dolphins, the limbic system is well developed. Apparently this phylogenetically old "smell brain" has taken on an additional function. In 1949 Dr. Paul MacLean elaborated on Papez' theory and suggested that those parts of the limbic system that are common to all mammals represent a "visceral brain" concerned with emotionally laden responses essential to the *preservation of the self* or *preservation of the species.* It is this phylogenetically older part of the brain—in its interaction with the more recently evolved neocortex—that, according to MacLean, contains the key to psychosomatic disease. Presumably, the increased capacity to form associations and to conjure up real and imaginary threats, which developed together with the neocortex, multiplies the possibility of chronically triggering those intense visceral responses that should be reserved for physical emergencies.

In animal experiments regions of the limbic system and hypothalamus were either destroyed electrolytically or aspirated by suction probes attached to vacuum pumps. As a result of destruction of specific regions within the limbic-hypothalamic circuit the behavior of animals was sometimes dramatically changed. Drs. Heinrich Klüver and Paul Bucy reported that ablations of portions of the limbic system in the temporal lobes produced monkeys that, in addition to other changes, became both tame and hypersexual. Later reports by other investigators included descriptions of the transformation of wild, unmanageable beasts into gentle animals that could be fed by hand. Drs. A. Hetherington and Stephen Ranson demonstrated that following destruction of the medial region of the hypothalamus the food consumption of animals increased so markedly that they became extremely obese. In contrast, Drs. Bal Anand and John Brobeck observed that after destruction of a lateral hypothalamic region animals refused food entirely and had to be force-fed to be kept alive. Drs. Joseph Brady and Walle Nauta noted that destruction of the portion of the limbic circuit called the septal area (see Figures 25 and 26) produced a state of rage—called "septal rage"—even in very tame, laboratory rats. As will be discussed later, additonal investigators have made it apparent that it is not always easy to characterize the behavioral changes that follow destruction of discrete neural areas by terms such as aggression and hypersexuality. The changes produced by the brain lesions are more basic and, depending upon many environmental determinants, the mode of expression can vary enormously. The aggressiveness that follows septal lesions, for example, is now believed to be only one manifestation of a basic deficit in ability to inhibit responses. Even when a "septal animal" is punished, it may be relatively unable to stop responding. (The evidence for a "response perseverative tendency" is presented in the reviews by Dr. Robert McCleary and by Dr. Garth Thomas and his collaborators cited in the bibliography.) What should be emphasized in this historical overview, however, is that through much of the 1950s and 1960s the dramatic behavioral changes demonstrated in animal experiments suggested to some psychiatrists and neurosurgeons that the deteriorating psychotic patients in their charge might be helped by appropriate manipulation of what was commonly referred to as the "emotional brain."

ANIMAL EXPERIMENTATION AND CLINICAL APPLICATIONS

Although some readers may doubt that animal experimentation had such a seminal influence on human neurosurgical procedures, the history clearly indicates that the relationship can sometimes be almost frighteningly direct. One example may help to illustrate this point. Dr. Karl Lashley continued his now classic studies of the function of the rat's cerebral cortex in learning and memory at the University of Minnesota. He also encouraged Drs. Heinrich Klüver and Carlyle Jacobsen to pursue similar interests in animals more closely related to man. In the 1920s he introduced Klüver to experimentation on monkeys and a few years later, in the same old building at the University of Minnesota, Lashley also encouraged Jacobsen to study the function of the frontal cortex in these animals. Klüver's work on the temporal lobes in collaboration with Bucy has already been mentioned briefly. These studies, which were conducted at the University of Chicago, were destined (as will be described later) to have a great influence on the development of ideas about the functioning of the limbic system and the regulation of emotions in animals and man. It is Jacobsen's studies that provide one of the most dramatic examples of the direct and immediate influence that animal experimentation may have on the treatment of human problems.

Jacobsen did most of his work during the 1930s in the Yale University laboratory of Professor John F. Fulton. The description of the modification of behavior following surgical destruction of the prefrontal area of the cerebral cortex of monkeys and chimpanzes had a direct and profound influence on the development of psychosurgical procedures. The highly developed cerebral cortex is the main distinguishing characteristic of the human brain, and the prefrontal area in particular had for some time fascinated physiologists. Most of the cortical regions were known to play roles either in processing a particular type of sensory information or in controlling the movement of skeletal muscles. The prefrontal region stood out as a so-called silent area and was therefore suspected of mediating higher functions. Hitzig, for example, wrote that "the store of ideas is to be sought for in all parts of the cortex, or rather, in all parts of the brain; but I hold that abstract thought must of necessity require particular organs and those I find in the frontal brain." This idea persisted and a number of late nineteenth century physiologists contributed observations that supported the belief that the prefrontal area played a special role in higher thought processes (see quotations by Ferrier and Bianchi on pages 300–301). The early observations were not based on the results of objective behavior tests. Jacobsen and Fulton and their collaborators undertook what turned out to be a classic investigation of the prefrontal area. In their study chimpanzees and other primates were tested using a delayed response procedure. This test involves attracting an animal's attention so that it can observe food being placed under one of several cups, but a grill prevents the animal from grabbing the food. An opaque screen is then lowered in front of the animal so that the cups cannot be seen and after some time the grill and the opaque screen are raised, permitting the animal access to the cup of its choice. The number of errors an animal makes in choosing the correct cup after different delay intervals can thus be obtained. Normally a chimpanzee can perform quite well even following delays of several minutes, but the behavior of one chimp, Becky, was very unusual prior to destruction of her prefrontal cortex. Jacobsen and his collaborators describe her "neurosis" in the experimental situation:

"In the normal phase, this animal was extremely eager to work and apparently well motivated; but this subject was highly emotional and profoundly upset whenever she made an error. Violent temper tantrums after a mistake were not infrequent occurrences. She observed closely loading of the cup with food, and often wimpered softly as the cup was placed over the food. If the experimenter lowered or started to lower the *opaque door* to exclude the animal's view of the cups, she immediately flew into a temper tantrum, rolled on the floor, defecated and urinated. After a few such reactions during the training period, the animal would make no further responses. . . .

"When this animal was rendered a bilateral (frontal) preparation, a profound change occurred. The chimpanzee offered its usual friendly greeting, and eagerly ran from its living quarters to the transfer cage, and in turn went properly to the experimental cage. The usual procedure of baiting the cup and lowering the opaque screen was followed. But the chimpanzee did not show any excitement and sat quietly before the door or walked around the cage. Given an opportunity to choose between the cups it did so with its customary eagerness and alacrity. However, if the animal made a mistake, it showed no evidence of emotional disturbance but quietly awaited the loading of the cups for the next trial. . . . It was as if the animal had joined the 'happiness cult of the Elder Micheaux'." (Jacobsen. Wolf, and Jackson, 1935, p. 9-10).

These postoperative changes displayed by Becky, which were reported in the summer of 1935 at the Second International Neurology Congress in London, encouraged the Portuguese neuropsychiatrist Dr. Egas Moniz to attempt to treat severe mental disorders by prefrontal lobotomy.[6] Fulton described this event and wrote that after Jacobsen's presentation "Dr. Moniz arose and asked if frontal-lobe removal prevents the development of experimental neuroses in animals and eliminates frustrational behavior, why would it not be feasible to relieve anxiety states in man by surgical means?" Fulton was a little shocked by the suggestion, because he thought Moniz had in mind that complete removal of a large portion of the prefrontal area in humans as had been done in the chimpanzees. According to Drs. Walter Freeman and James Watts, who were personal friends of Moniz and dedicated their book, *Psychosurgery*, to him:

"He [Moniz] compared in his own mind the querulous, the deluded, the agitated and the obsessed with these apes of Fulton and Jacobsen, and later sought out Fulton and asked him about the possibility of applying such an operation to human sufferers. This was too much for Fulton, but Egas Moniz marshalled his forces and finally persuaded Almeida Lima to operate upon certain patients who had proven refractory to other methods of treatment."

The first operation was performed in Lisbon on November 12, 1935. Alcohol injections into the subcortical fibers were used for the destruction, but by the end of December of the same year incisions were made with a leucotome, a small cutting apparatus especially designed for the purpose. Six cores were cut out of the frontal cortex on each side (Figure 38). In Moniz' monograph describing the results with his first 20 patients, he reported that all had survived, seven were considered recovered, and seven were said to be improved. Best results were claimed to have been obtained with agitated depressed patients, whereas the schizophrenics were not significantly changed. The total number of cases operated on under the supervision of Moniz was only about 100 since he was in favor of waiting for long-term results before proceeding on a large scale and also because he was made a hemiplegic as a result of an assault by a lobotomized patient, which left him with a bullet in his spine. Moniz retired in 1944 and in 1949 he shared the Nobel Prize in Physiology and Medicine with Walter Hess "for his discovery of the therapeutic value of prefrontal leucotomy in certain psychoses."

In September 1936 Drs. Walter Freeman and James Watts of George Washington University in Washington, D. C., introduced the lobotomy technique in the United States. They had been in correspondence with Moniz, and Watts had spent a year in New Haven where he was familiar with the striking behavior changes being displayed by Jacobsen's chimpanzees after removal of the frontal area. Watts and Freeman modified the Moniz "core" operation, which they regarded as inadequate, and developed their *precision method,* a procedure involving the use of skull landmarks to sever predetermined areas of the frontal lobes and the underlying fiber connections (see

Figure 39). By 1950, Freeman and Watts had operated on over 1000 patients. The rate picked up during the next five years before it started to decline, and Freeman later indicated that he had performed, or supervised, various prefrontal operations on over 3500 people.

As will be discussed in more detail in a later chapter, surgical techniques evolved and a large number of neurosurgeons throughout the world performed frontal lobe operations on psychiatric patients. It is difficult to obtain accurate figures of the total number of prefrontal lobotomies of one type or another performed around the world, but estimates of the number in the United States alone are in the order of 40,000. One of the main factors that contributed to the upsurge of psychosurgery in the United States as well as elsewhere was the number of returning veterans at the end of World War II who were psychiatrically disabled. Faced with the demand from relatives for rapid and drastic treatment, an insufficient number of trained psychiatrists, and little in the way of psychoactive drugs, authorities in the Veterans Administration accepted the optimistic reports on prefrontal lobotomy and encouraged its use.[7]

By the late 1950s, availability of a variety of psychoactive drugs and the many reports of undesirable side effects resulting from the operations produced a sharp decline in psychosurgery. (More recently, as described in the chapter on Psychosurgery, new so-called fractional psychosurgical procedures have been reintroduced but on a very much smaller scale than occurred during the peak period between 1945 and 1955.) The undesirable side effects that were observed included intellectual deterioration reflected in a lack of planning ability or foresight. These deficits, however, were not evident in IQ test scores, which were generally reported to be unchanged or even elevated, the latter because of the increased cooperativeness of patients during the tests. Personality changes that were observed included the appearance of inappropriate behavior (sometimes viewed as a lowering of moral standards), a lack of planning, and often a general blunting of emotional responsiveness. The postoperative appearance of epileptic seizures and other symptoms of neurological trauma were also not uncommon. A comprehensive evaluation of psychosurgery is presented later, but to offer a more balanced first approximation, it would have to be noted that many neurosurgeons and psychiatrists have consistently emphasized that the reports of intellectual and personality deterioration following psychosurgery were not representative and they could never be found on objective tests. Moreover, they claimed that there was a high percentage of patients with very poor prognosis whose postoperative condition dramatically improved to the point where they were able to make a good adjustment and lead productive lives.

Although there was a rapid decline in the amount of psychosurgery performed after the mid-1950s, there were still great numbers of psychiatric patients that were not being helped by the available psychiatric or pharmacological techniques. This tended to sustain interest in exploring the therapeutic value of other types of brain operations. Interest developed in searching for more selective methods that might produce the presumed benefits of the former operations without any of the deleterious consequences. One such approach was related to the development of the skills for inserting electrodes into structures deep within the human brain. Dr. Robert Clarke (of Horsley and Clarke fame) had suggested in 1920 that stereotaxic methods might be useful in human neurosurgery and even earlier, in his 1912 British patent, he wrote:

"This invention relates to what may be termed stereotaxic surgical apparatus for use in performing operations within the cranium of living human beings ... [it] is designed to enable a so-called probe ... to reach with absolute precision and by the shortest path, any pre-determined point within the cranium through a comparatively small opening in the wall of the latter, the primary object being to obviate the necessity of extensively laying open or partially dissecting the head and removing considerable portions of the cranial contents in order to gain access to the exact spot whereat the actual operation is required to be carried out."

It was not until 1947, however, that the first application of a stereotaxic instrument for humans was introduced by Drs. Ernest Spiegel and Henry Wycis of Temple University for the purpose of destroying selected areas of the brain for the treatment of intractable pain. In initiating human "stereoencephalotomy," Spiegel and Wycis introduced some important changes in the determination of brain coordinates. Horsley and Clarke had used skull landmarks for reference points, but Spiegel and Wycis suggested the use of a number of reference points within the brain such as the pineal gland and the cerebral ventricles, which could be visualized with the aid of X-rays. Spiegel and Wycis were also the first to use a stereotaxic instrument for psychosurgery and they reported, as early as 1949, that they had destroyed the dorsomedial thalamic nucleus in psychotic patients. (The dorsomedial nucleus is believed to play a key role in the anatomical and functional reciprocity between the prefrontal cortex and the limbic-hypothalamic circuit.) Shortly afterward, Dr. Lars Leksell of Sweden also described a stereotaxic device for humans. There are now a number of different human models available all based in part on the original Horsley-Clarke instrument but supplemented by X-ray visualization of the cerebral ventricles and other landmarks in the brain (see Figures 33 and 35). These skills made it possible to explore the therapeutic potential of destroying a part of almost every brain structure that animal experimentation implicated in the regulation of emotion. Electrodes could be inserted with a minimum of trauma into brain regions that were previously considered inaccessible and electrolytic destruction of neural tissue could be restricted to the region surrounding the uninsulated tip of the electrode.

Dr. Spiegel has published the results of a survey among the members of the International Society for Research in Stereoencephalotomy. He reported that 26,000 stereotaxic operations were performed up to 1965 and an additional 12,000 were estimated to have been done during the 3-year period between 1965 and 1968. These operations, which were designed to relieve some symptoms by producing circumscribed subcortical lesions, can be grouped into four categories based upon their goal:

1. To seek relief from emotional and behavioral disturbances (aggression, hyperkinesis, and psychotic behavior) by destroying selected areas of the limbic-hypothalamic circuit such as the dorsomedial or anterior thalamic nuclei, the amygdala, the posterior hypothalamus, the cingulum, and the pathways to the frontal lobes (see Figures 24, 25 and 26 for location of these structures),

2. To try to relieve pain by destruction of neural areas believed to be mediating the emotional components of pain,

3. To reduce motor and postural disturbances (tremors, choreatic-athetotic movements, and spasticity),

4. To reduce convulsive discharge by destroying epileptogenic foci or by interrupting the pathways conducting the abnormal electrical impulses.

All of these applications will be discussed in more detail in later chapters.

The development of human stereotaxic technique also made it possible to explore the clinical utility of stimulating neural tissue. Stimulation of and recording from subcortical structures was undertaken as both a diagnostic and a therapeutic procedure. As a diagnostic technique it has been used to help locate abnormal scar tissue in the brain or to better localize some area considered to be a good target for psychosurgery. In the early 1950s, Dr. Magnus Peterson and his collaborators at the Mayo Clinic, for example, implanted electrodes in the frontal lobe region in the hope that monitoring electrical activity would make it possible to destroy more restricted areas and thereby reduce the undesirable side effects of the more extensive surgical procedures.

At the same time, Dr. Robert Heath of Tulane University explored the therapeutic possibilities of electrically (and later chemically) stimulating the septal area and other regions of the limbic-hypothalamic circuit. He had been the chief psychiatrist on the team at Columbia University that undertook an extensive study (Columbia-Greystone Project) of the effects of topectomy, a prefrontal psychosurgical operation (see page 312). The study provided little basis for enthusiastic support of this procedure, even though it was concluded that some patients may have benefited. Those interested in a biological approach to psychiatry needed some other techniques. In the foreword to his 1954 book, *Studies in Schizophrenia,* Heath wrote;

"Several of us who had been previously concerned with problems centering about frontal lobe operations had developed similar feelings concerning that work. We felt first that the beneficial changes that were being obtained were minimal and that there was always something in the way of undesirable effects. Even when patients were considered to be benefited by the procedure, the changes could not be definitely related to the one piece of brain that had been removed. We therefore decided that it might be fruitful to study the results of altering the organism without destroying cortical tissue. Our immediate aim, then, was to determine what could be done by altering circuits within the intact person."

In initiating the exploration of stimulation of structures in the depths of the human brain, Heath was influenced by the animal experiments which seemed to reveal neural circuits that had general facilitatory or inhibitory effects on many physiological processes. Heath started to implant electrodes in humans because of the evidence that stimulation of particular neural areas in animals increased general activity and hormonal responses and he hoped that such bodily changes might lead to an improvement of mental and emotional status. The experimentation with implanted electrodes in humans was initiated before there was any evidence from animal studies that brain stimulation might evoke pleasurable sensations. Later, as will be discussed, this was to become an important part of the rationale for continuing the human stimulation studies.

During a discussion with the present author, Heath indicated that while still at Columbia University he had observed significant changes in emotional behavior following destruction of the brain region called the septal area (see Figures 25 and 26). Postoperatively, one of his three experimental cats became irritable while the other two became so catatonic that they displayed so-called waxy flexibility, manifested by a tendency to hold any posture in which they were placed. Other experiments suggested that destruction of brain tissue in this area also reduced endocrine reactions such as the response of the adrenal cortex to stress. There also existed some biochemical evidence that schizophrenics showed less responsiveness to stress. In his writings Heath presented a loosely formulated, theoretical framework that attempted to integrate these experimental and clinical observations with some psychiatric speculations on the roots of schizophrenia. He argued that inhibitory and facilitatory circuits acting on higher cortical centers of the brain form the basis of hedonic experience—that is, the sensation of pleasure and pain. The psychiatrist Dr. Sandor Rado had suggested that it was this hedonic reaction which was particularly deficient in schizophrenia. Combining these bits and pieces of theory and observations, Dr. Heath was encouraged in 1950 to implant an electrode in the septal area of a schizophrenic patient. In his 1954 book, Dr. Heath wrote:

"On the basis of clinical observations we assumed that the over-all effect in schizophrenia was one of cortical impairment. We therefore reasoned that if the subcortex was functioning abnormally as a result of cortical firing, then electrical stimulation to the basal part of the septal region might stir it into more normal activity, thus facilitating cortical activity and bringing the individual out of the sleep-like state of reverie and helping him to make a better interpretation of reality."

Once stimulation of subcortical structures was tried on humans, it was noted that some patients reported an improvement of mood or mental attitude. It was hoped such effects might initiate beneficial changes that would persist, if not permanently, at least long enough for more conventional psychotherapeutic methods to start to be effective. Techniques for electrical and chemical stimulation of the brain have become more sophisticated and the range of suggested application has been greatly extended. These possible applications, some realistic and others pure fantasy, will be discussed in detail in the following chapters.

We are living in a period of such rapid change that the average person today believes that almost anything is possible and, as a result, science fiction descriptions of the future are often accepted as realistic predictions based on firsthand knowledge of the subject matter. Actually, the accounts of brain stimulation read by most people are typically written by free-lance writers or imaginative social scientists, who have had no direct experience with the techniques involved and are often very uninformed about even basic brain physiology. Nevertheless, the possibility of controlling the moods and behavior, if not the thoughts of individuals by remotely controlled electronic devices has such obvious dramatic possibilities that the topic is virtually irresistible to those with a more speculative bent. Usually such people have a very unrealistic conception of the significance of most of the dramatic observations that they delight in describing. Their accounts often emphasize the new developments in brain electrodes and miniature transmitters and receivers—so small they can be attached to the skull—and therefore easy (especially with the long hair styles in vogue) to conceal without difficulty. Is it surprising that it might occur to some people, who may have only a borderline psychiatric adjustment, that they or their neighbors down the street have had brain electrodes surreptitiously implanted?

In addition to possible medical applications, interest in brain manipulations has also been derived from a concern with social problems. Governmental agencies, whether on the national or international level, have been continuously frustrated in their efforts to combat crime and prevent wars. In recent years, there have been numerous suggestions that human conflict might be reflecting some inherited aggressive tendencies that are built into our biological endowment. It was not surprising, therefore, that the demonstrations that aggression could be evoked by brain stimulation, even in normally peaceful animals, would produce speculation that it might be possible to eliminate aggression by manipulating the brain. This possibility will be evaluated after some necessary background information is presented.

Another factor contributing to the present concern about human brain stimulation is the fear that this technique can and perhaps will be used to control people as individuals or in groups. Although this may not be considered very likely by those who critically evaluate such suggestions, there is little doubt that a substantial number of people believe that brain stimulation technique has advanced close to that level of sophistication where soon it will be possible to create a class of human robots. It has been suggested by some that either the movements of people might be completely determined by remotely programmed brain stimulation or their capacity to resist could be effectively eliminated by the administration of powerful rewards and punishments delivered directly to the brain. The following chapters consider such fears and hopes in the context of the available scientific evidence and the state of our present knowledge.

Brain Stimulation: Can It Produce a Population of Slaves or Robots?

If one thinks in terms of the strategy of an invading army, it is generally recognized that the capture of the main command post can be decisive. Similarly, if one is inclined to consider the possibility of completely dominating another individual, it would be logical to think of gaining control over some very central aspect of that person. What could be more central to a person than the brain? The reports of new technical developments for brain stimulation (including the possibility of remotely controlled stimulation), therefore, has led to a concern that it will be used as the basis of an "electroligarchy" where people could be virtually enslaved by controlling them from within their own brains.

To start with the conclusion first, there is actually little foundation for the belief that brain stimulation could be used as a political weapon. The fact that this possibility has been raised repeatedly in the popular media, however, justifies a critical examination of the evidence and the underlying logic. Perhaps a more important justification is that a discussion of the topic provides an interesting framework for presenting information necessary for a more serious consideration of a number of suggested medical and social applications of various brain manipulations. The present chapter evaluates the possibility that brain stimulation can be used as a means of dominating individuals either by evoking irresistible sensations of pleasure or by directly controlling their movements. The following chapter discusses the significance of the many reports that brain stimulation can control such motivational states as those underlying hunger, thirst, sexual appetite, fear or anxiety, and aggression.

It has been suggested repeatedly that stimulation of some brain areas produces such extreme pleasure that complete control over individuals could be gained by a Machiavellian utilization of this ultimate, and therefore irresistible, sensation. The filtered reports of evoked pleasurable sensations have especially captured the imagination of those who have written about the potential of brain stimulation as a means of dominating others. In Larry Nivens' science fiction story *"Death by Ecstasy"* the commonly accepted portrayal of the omnipotence of rewarding brain stimulation has been woven into the plot. The story takes place in the year 2123 and Owen Jennison's body has just been discovered under conditions that appear to indicate a suicide, but the death actually was the result of a carefully planned murder:

"Owen Jennison sat grinning in a water stained silk dressing gown. . . . A month's growth of untended beard covered half his face. A small black cylinder protruded from the top of his head. An electric cord trailed from the top of the cylinder and ran to a small wall socket.

"The cylinder was a droud, a current addict's transformer. . . .

"It was a standard surgical job. Owen could have had it done anywhere. A hole in his scalp, invisible under the hair, nearly impossible to find even if you knew what you were looking for. Even your best friends wouldn't know, unless they caught you and the droud plugged in. But the tiny hole marked a bigger plug set in the bone of the skull. I touched the ecstasy plug with my imaginary fingertips, then ran them down the hair-fine wire going deep into Owen's brain, down into the pleasure center. . . .

"He had starved to death sitting in that chair. . . .

"Consider the details of the hypothetical murder. Owen Jennison is drugged no doubt—an ecstasy plug is attached—He is tied up and allowed to waken. . . . The killer then plugs Mr. Jennison into a wall. A current trickles through his brain, and Owen Jennison knows pure pleasure for the first time in his life.

"He is left tied up for, let us say three hours. In the first few minutes he would be a hopeless addict. . . .

"No more than three hours by our hypothesis. . . . They would cut the ropes and leave Owen Jennison to starve to death. In the space of a month the evidence of his drugging would vanish, as would any abrasions left by ropes, lumps on his head, mercy needle punctures, and the like. A carefully detailed, well thought out plan, don't you agree?"

This is a science fiction story, but the portrayal of the omnipotence and irresistibility of rewarding brain stimulation does not exaggerate the conviction of many people, who have no firsthand knowledge of the actual results obtained in the laboratory and clinic. What is the evidence?

There can be no doubt that our observations of animals and humans have indicated that brain stimulation can produce very rewarding and pleasant sensations that evoke a desire to repeat the experience. It has been demonstrated many times in laboratories that animals will display a seemingly insatiable desire to operate a switch over and over again to stimulate their own brains if the electrodes have been placed at particular neural sites. Following the initial discovery by James Olds, there were many suggestions that the stimulation was only evoking some type of reflex that forced the animal to repeat its last response, but subsequent experiments by Olds and others have provided convincing evidence that brain stimulation can serve as a very potent reward that shares most of the properties of the more conventional rewards. It is not necessary that animals self-stimulate by repeating the same stereotyped response over and over again, but as described earlier, they can learn new responses, not previously in their repertoire, if they are rewarded by brain stimulation.

In addition to possessing most of the essential properties of more familiar rewards, brain stimulation can be an especially potent reward. It has been reported that under certain conditions rats may starve themselves, take painful foot shocks, neglect their pups—in order to obtain access to rewarding brain stimulation. I once observed a rat self-stimulating for 21 days during which time it operated the switch about 850,000 times—an average of approximately 30 responses per minute for the entire period. The animal with its electrode hooked up was placed in a chamber with a stimulation switch and food and water. The electrode had been placed in a rewarding brain site in the lateral hypothalamus and the animal had many previous opportunities to self-stimulate. After a very brief exploration of the new chamber the rat discovered and started to operate the stimulation switch, receiving a brief (1/2 second) burst of current in the lateral hypothalamus each time the lever was depressed. Although the rat pressed the lever rapidly, it did take breaks to eat, groom, sleep, and occasionally explore its environment. Self-stimulation was clearly the dominant behavior, and it occupied the major portion of its time in the chamber. In fact, after it awakened from sleep the animal was observed to stretch and then to go directly back to the lever. There was no indication that the animal would ever break the pattern, and it was only the fatigue of my associate,

Dr. Bernard Beer, and myself—we were taking turns observing the animal around the clock—that finally forced us to end these observations.

Many examples could be given to illustrate the intensity of the interest in exploring the potential power of brain stimulation during the late 1950s and early 1960s. A Department of Defense contract, for example, was given to the Sandia Corporation to look into this question and a film was made of one particularly striking demonstration. The film depicted electrodes being positioned into the lateral hypothalamus of an army mule. Following recovery after the surgery a brain stimulator was placed in a pack on the animal's back. A prism and a mirror were arranged so that they operated a photocell as long as the animal was oriented directly toward the sun. The photocell in turn programmed the stimulator to deliver brief bursts of electric current to the mule's brain as long as orientation toward the sun was maintained. If the mule deviated from its course, the rewarding brain stimulation stopped until the animal got back "on the beam." The mule marched across a large field in New Mexico and over a hill where one of the members of the project reversed the mirror causing the animal to retrace its steps by keeping the sun at its back. I have performed a similar demonstration for students in my class by asking one of them to place any object, such as a key ring or cigarette lighter, on a large tabletop. By operating a push-button switch, I could deliver rewarding brain stimulation every time a rat moved toward the object. I soon "steered" the rat over to the object and, providing the object was light enough, the animal often could be induced to pick it up with its mouth. Such demonstrations illustrate the capacity of the reinforcement system to guide behavior by providing immediate feedback in a way that is analogous to the game of finding the hidden treasure by being told with each step if you are getting "warmer" or "colder."

The brain stimulation technique is much more effective, however, because it maintains a high motivational level at the same time as it is guiding the behavior.

The army mule demonstration was in line with the prevailing interest at that time in exploring such possibilities as using animals to clear mine fields or to deliver explosives to an assigned target. For example, the Russians have described the training of dogs to carry explosives against German tanks during World War II. After the Soviet *Sputnik* success in 1957 the prevalent attitude in the United States government, and particularly among those in command in the Pentagon, was that the country could not afford to be caught napping again. There was even some concern caused by the absence of any Soviet publications of self-stimulation experiments, which was interpreted as evidence that this topic must have been classified as secret. (This line of thought reflected some of the paranoia of the time. It now seems clear that the Russians did not explore the self-stimulation phenomenon primarily because they were pursuing their own traditions in psychophysiological research—traditions that tended to deemphasize the role of rewards and punishments in learning experiments. In 1961, I demonstrated some self-stimulation techniques at the Institute of Higher Nervous Activity in Moscow and subsequently a few studies from this Institute appeared in the Soviet literature.)

The fact that there exist many demonstrations illustrating that brain stimulation can be a very compelling reward has been interpreted by a number of people to indicate that it is irresistible to the point of self-destructiveness. That this is not true can be seen by behavior of the rat we described which self-stimulated for 21 days. This animal stopped to eat, groom, sleep, and even explore the environment and in fact did not even lose any weight during this three-week period. The belief that animals will starve to death while self-stimulating is derived from popular and misleading accounts of an experiment by Dr. Aryeh Routtenberg. Familiarity with the experimental details, however, would have revealed that the rats that starved while self-stimulating did so only under very special and highly artificial conditions. These animals were allowed only one hour a day to press a pedal for food reward. The "payoff" rate was arranged so that the animals had to work the full hour in order to get an amount of food that barely kept them alive. The rats, therefore, were at the borderline between mere survival and death from starvation when they were offered an opportunity to stimulate their brain during the only hour they had to earn food. Under such conditions some of the animals did not receive enough food to survive. When food and brain stimulation are both available continuously, however, it seems clear that animals will take advantage of the food and maintain their body weight adequately. The exaggerated accounts of the "irresistibility" of rewarding brain stimulation are based on experiments using only rats that were tested under very restricted conditions. It would be a mistake to generalize to other conditions or to other species, especially humans. There are important differences between species in the fervor with which they will stimulate their own rewarding brain areas, and the evidence available from observations of human self-stimulation seems to indicate that the experience is not nearly as compelling as it is in some animals.

Dr. Carl Sem-Jacobsen of Oslo, Norway, believes that "the reasons given by patients for continuing self-stimulation seem as complex as man himself. In man, curiosity is probably the most dominant causative factor in initiating self-stimulation." Sem-Jacobsen has described his patients' reactions: "If a patient feels something he might wonder! Precisely what is the nature of this sensation? What am I feeling? Let me try it once more. Once more. Is it tickling? Is it a real pleasure?" Other motivating factors considered important by Sem-Jacobsen include obedience and the desire to cooperate. Most patients want to be helpful to the examiner and will readily self-stimulate upon the slightest suggestion, even when the stimulus gives an unpleasant or punishing response. Dr. Mary Brazier of the Brain Research Institute at the University of California in Los Angeles described a patient who continued to "self-stimulate" even after the master switch was turned off. Drs. M. P. Bishop, S. Thomas Elder, and Robert Heath of the Tulane Medical School reported a similar observation in two patients who were presumably self-stimulating but "when the current was turned off, both subjects continued to press the lever at essentially the same rate until the experiment was terminated by the experimenter after hundreds of unrewarded responses."

Sem-Jacobsen has expressed the need to be cautious in interpreting the experience a patient may receive from brain stimulation. He writes:

"Pitfalls for the examiner in the interpretation of responses can be pronounced in regard to changes in mood. To illustrate, the author tested a rather withdrawn fifty-year old female patient who responded to a stimulus by smiling. Sometimes she even laughed and seemed to enjoy the stimulation of a certain contact. The striking effect was repeated at irregular intervals and at different times of the day with the patient basically in various moods. The result was always the same. This phenomenon was demonstrated to several colleagues, and all were convinced that the electrode being tested was in a strong, positive 'pleasure region.'

"Because of the patient's uniform reactions in repeated sessions, the author took it for granted that she liked it and discussed the significance of this response in her presence without eliciting any comment from her. Suddenly one day the patient became angry and told us that she was 'fed up' and 'did not enjoy these stimulations at all.' She asked us to stop and refrain from any further stimulation of this contact. She said she 'had had enough!'

"The stimulus did not give the patient any pleasure. Instead it created in some of her pelvic muscles a rhythmic contraction which tickled her and caused the laughter. It was evident that the author had not been stimulating either a "pleasure center," nor a center dealing with sensation. He had simply been stimulating muscles which contracted and caused the tickling and, in turn, forced the patient to smile and laugh."

Dr. Robert Heath has commented that human brain stimulation does not seem able to induce an euphoria comparable to that produced by drugs. The reasons that humans stimulate their own brains are often very surprising. Dr. Heath described one patient, for example, who operated the switch because of a frustration evolving from an attempt to bring into focus a vague memory that had been evoked by the stimulation. Often the responses to stimulation at the same site varied with the emotional and physical conditions of the patient, as Heath indicates:

"When the same stimulus was repeated in the same patient, responses varied. The most intense pleasurable responses occurred in patients stimulated while they were suffering intense pain, whether emotional and reflected by despair, anguish, intense fear or rage, or physical, such as that caused by metastatic carcinoma. The feelings induced by stimulation of pleasure sites obliterated these patients' awareness of physical pain. *Patients who felt well at the time of stimulation, on the other hand, experienced only slight pleasure.*" (Italics added.)

There are no reports of pleasure by patients receiving brain stimulation that suggest that the experience was so irresistible that they could be compelled to "sell their souls" for more of the same. This is not meant to deny that there are some very pleasant experiences evoked by brain stimulation. Among Heath's film records of patients receiving brain stimulation is one striking example: a patient who had just attempted to commit suicide by jumping off the roof suddenly started to smile when the electrode in his septal area was activated. It was difficult for him to verbalize his experience more explicitly than, "I feel good. I don't know why, I just suddenly felt good." Upon further questioning the patient implied that there might have been sexual overtones to his experience as he said: "It's like I had something lined up for Saturday night . . . a girl." Given an opportunity to press a button controlling a portable stimulation unit worn around his belt one patient reported: "When I get mad if I push the button I feel better . . . that's a real good button . . . I would buy one if I could." A woman with intractable pain said during the stimulation: "I'm feeling fine . . . feel like I could clean up the whole hospital." In several instances it has been suspected that a patient reached an orgasm during stimulation. Orgasm may have been experienced as a result of genital sensations evoked by the brain stimulation, but Heath does not belive that genital sensations need be present. The patient generally stops self-stimulating after an orgasm is achieved and there is no reason to believe that the experience in such instances is any more compelling than masturbation. In almost all cases where a very pleasurable experience was reported the patient had been experiencing physical or psychological pain. There is no evidence, however, that brain stimulation produces sensations so pleasurable that they would justify the impression they are irresistible to a patient not in pain.

Recently, Dr. N. P. Bechterewa of the Institute of Experimental Medicine in Leningrad summarized the results that she and her colleagues obtained with implanted electrodes in the human brain. These Soviet physicians have studied the effects of brain stimulation in patients suffering from Parkinson's disease and other brain disorders disrupting bodily movements. Patients were observed over long periods of time and considerable attention was given to the emotional and motivational changes evoked by the stimulation. Bechterewa reports several cases where stimulation of the ventrolateral thalamus or adjacent regions evoked erotic and other pleasant sensations. In one case, that of a 37-year-old woman with postencephalitic Parkinsonism, stimulation evoked very pleasant sexual sensations that led to an orgasm. The patient began to visit the electrophysiology laboratory more frequently, and she initiated conversations with the assistants. She also waited for them in the corridors and the hospital garden and tried to find out when the next stimulation session was due. The patient seemed to be particularly affectionate toward the person on whom the electrical stimulation depended and she displayed dissatisfaction when her requests for additional sessions were not granted.

There can be no doubt that the Soviet experience with brain stimulation confirms the reports of earlier investigators that very pleasant experiences can be evoked by these techniques. Interpretations of these reports can be quite complicated, however, since the areas of the brain from which these pleasurable sensations have been evoked are very extensive. Often the sensations may be secondary to the occurrence of some physiological changes. For example, in the case of the Soviet patient just described, stimulation did not evoke experiences of a sexual nature until her menstrual cycles, which had been interrupted for over eight years, were reinstated presumably by some neuroendocrine consequences of the stimulation. The Soviet investigators are quite explicit in stating their belief that the motivational consequences of the brain stimulation were subject to conscious control. In the patient that was motivated to try to obtain repetitions of the pleasurable sensations evoked by stimulation, behavior was never inappropriate and she took great care to conceal this drive. She frequently tried and was successful in diverting her own attention by becoming involved in reading, listening to music, and helping other patients. This ability to gain control over the emotional states produced by the stimulation was particularly striking in a patient in which stimulation of the ventrolateral and dorsolateral thalamus produced a feeling of unexplainable anxiety and even terror when high current intensities were used. In spite of these reactions, this patient was quite willing to repeat the experience—that is, she suppressed all tendencies to avoid the situation—because she believed that the information obtained would be of diagnostic and therapeutic value.

Quite aside from the lack of evidence of an overwhelming compulsion evoked by brain stimulation in humans, there is no reason to believe that this method of control would be as efficient, or practical, as the great number of physical and psychological tortures and temptations that mankind, in its more malevolent moments, has contrived throughout the ages. None of these methods would require an army of "electrode implanters" (just specifying the requirements in this concrete way exposes the absurdity). Dr. Seymour Kety of Harvard University has reached the same conclusion and has pointed out that "It doesn't make sense. Anyone influential enough to get an entire population to consent to having electrodes placed in his head would already have his goal without firing a single volt."

Even more unlikely is the suggesion that brain stimulation might be used to convert men into machines by direct control over bodily movements. The possibility is worth considering, however, because it helps to dispel the generally oversimplified conception of the relationship between brain stimulation and behavior. As already noted, since 1870 when Eduard Hitzig and Gustav Fritsch stimulated the brains of dogs, it has been known that cells located in specific regions of the cerebral cortex partly control the movement of muscles on the opposite side of the body. These investigations provided valuable information on the localization of function within the cortex, but it has to be recognized that only single muscle contractions or twitches could generally be evoked. (There have been a few recent reports that movement of an entire limb is sometimes seen during stimulation of a part of the cerebral cortex, but such responses are not typical.) The effects of cortical stimulation are so limited because it lacks the normal participation of many regions located in the brain depths, which are responsible for the coordination of muscle activity into larger response patterns.

Contemporary investigators have reported the types of response that are elicited from some subcortical brain regions. These responses are not generally restricted to single muscles but rather involve functionally meaningful patterns of several muscles such as those controlling the diameter of the pupil or flexion of a leg. There are a very few reports of more elaborate response patterns being evoked by brain stimulation. Dr. José Delgado, for example, described a monkey who stopped what it was doing every time it was stimulated in a brain area called the red nucleus, circled to the right, walked on two feet to a pole which it climbed, and then, after descending to the floor, made an aggressive attack on a subordinate monkey. Although it has been reported that such complex sequential responses can be elicited repeatedly in a given animal, there is no known way of predicting what behavior sequence, if any, will be obtained from a given electrode. There are many reasons for doubting that complex sequential responses are directly elicited by stimulation at one neural site. It is likely that the responses are at first partly based on the individual animal's pattern of coping with emotional state such as that induced by the brain stimulation. It moves about, climbs a pole, and attacks another animal. It is quite possible that the exact sequence is maintained because of the so-called superstitious tendency of animals to repeat any responses accidentally occurring at the same time that a positive reward was presented or an aversive stimulus was terminated. It is as though the animal concluded that the way to get rid of the disturbing sensation caused by the brain stimulation is to repeat what it last did just before the stimulation was turned off. Delgado believes that brain stimulation may activate neural mechanisms that serve to coordinate large numbers of small response units or fragments into innate and acquired behavioral sequences. This may be true for certain very basic responses required for survival, but is unlikely to be the case for such arbitrary response sequences as illustrated in his example. Regardless of interpretation, it seems true that although stimulation studies may provide us with some information about the way the brain is organized to control movements, the inability to predict the sequence of responses that will be elicited indicates that this phenomenon will have little, if any, practical applications.

Recently Dr. Lawrence Pinneo and his collaborators at the Stanford Research Institute published accounts of one of the more technically sophisticated approaches to the problem of eliciting movements. These investigators have been exploring the possibility of evoking smooth movements by utilizing computer control over stimulation at multiple brain sites. Pinneo's group has been studying the anatomical loci that control specific movements in animals in the hope of being able to apply this information to help people who have lost control over some parts of their body. At the outset, it was recognized that the movements commonly produced by brain stimulation depended on whether the animal was alert or drowsy, standing or reclining, and many other preconditions. To produce reliable results, several discrete brain sites that would invariably evoke the same movement were required. Over 60 electrodes (the plan is to use up to 240 in the future) were implanted in the cerebellum and brain stem of monkeys and a number of sites were found that would elicit the elementary, fragmented components of responses such as extension and flexion of limbs, grasping and extension of fingers, extension and flexion of the joints (wrist, elbow, shoulder, ankle), opening and closing the mouth, movement of the tongue in and out, and curling or sideways movement of the tail. These responses could be elicited regardless of the state of the animal and seemed to be independent of the animal's will. The reliability of the stimulation effects probably was due to the fact that the brain stem is relatively closer to the final pathway to the muscles, just as there are fewer possibilities to change a train's destination near the end of the line.

The next step was to analyze the natural movements of the monkey. This was accomplished with motion picture film analyzers, which made it possible to examine the contribution of the various elementary fragments to the more complex response patterns. The problem was to combine the elementary movements in the appropriate sequence and intensity to produce smooth movements. It was found that elicited movements were graduated in mechanical strength as a function of the intensity of the stimulating current. A computer program was written which used about six of the electrodes and produced smooth movements by utilizing the appropriate intensity and sequence of stimulation. Pinneo describes his results:

"For example, with six electrodes and a particular program of stimulation, we have had a squirrel monkey reach out to a dish in front of him, pick up a piece of food, and bring it rapidly and smoothly to his mouth. Using exactly the same electrodes, but a different program, the monkey was made to reach up as though climbing a cage. With still another program but the same electrodes, upon programmed stimulation he reached back and scratched the base of his tail. And so on through seemingly endless variations."

To make certain that the responses that seemed to be produced by the stimulation were not influenced by voluntary acts on the part of the animal, the portion of the cerebral cortex that controlled voluntary movements was destroyed. This produced an animal that was incapable of voluntary movement of the muscles under study and in that sense duplicated the symptoms of paralysis following some cerebral strokes. In spite of this paralysis, the stimulation continued to produce the same movements as before.

Pinneo points out that this "artificial stroke" experiment suggests that it may be possible to restore

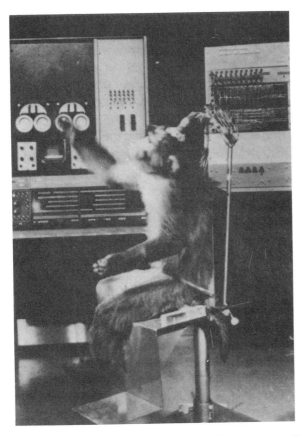

Figure 14. A monkey whose arm movement is being controlled by electrical stimulation delivered to a number of brain sites, each of which regulates a fragment of the total response. The computer controls the intensity and sequence of stimulation. See text for more details. (From L. R. Pinneo, "Experimental Brain Prosthesis for Stroke," *Stroke*, 1972, Vol. 3, Fig. 3. By permission of Dr. Lawrence Pinneo and The American Heart Association, Inc.)

movement to paralyzed muscles by brain stimulation. This may indeed be possible as a *tour de force*, but awareness of the great numbers of technical hurdles that would first have to be surmounted should serve to caution us against overestimating the practical implications of this research. In the first place, the very large number of electrodes that has to be inserted into the brain in order to find the sites that control movements of even one limb constitutes a serious danger. The region of the brain where Pinneo has been inserting electrodes regulates many functions vital to life. In the monkey experiments the number of electrodes that had to be inserted produced suffcient brain damage and edema so that several animals died following the operation.

It is always possible that some system could be developed to stimulate discrete brain sites without implanting huge numbers of electrodes, but no practical method has been devised as yet. Pinneo recognized the dangers inherent in exploring the human brain stem with a great many electrodes and has attempted to develop a system of focusing several electromagnetic energy beams on a specific point within the brain. According to this scheme, which many investigators have thought about although none has found a practical solution, the power density in each of the separate beams could be adjusted to be insufficent to stimulate brain tissue by itself. Stimulation would be possible, therefore, only at the intersection of the several beams as pictured in Figure 15. Unfortunately, it has proven possible for this system to work only at brain depths less than 3 millimeters (approximately .12 inch), which would be insufficient to stimulate critical regions in the human brain. (It has been possible to use the principle of focused ultrasonic beams to destroy tissue in the depths of the brain. See footnote 21.)

Although Pinneo's efforts have provided some important information on the regulation of motor responses, there are many reasons why a practical solution seems unlikely in the foreseeable future, even if the dangers related to multiple electrode insertions into the brain stem are put aside on the grounds that the surgical technique may be improved or that a feasible system for stimulating brain areas without implanting electrodes may be developed. There remain, however, mammoth problems caused by the need to write individual computer programs based on the particular array of fragmented responses obtained from each person's brain and the infinite variety of movements required. Even if this could be accomplished, many other questions would have to be answered. How would the patient specify the movements that were required and learn to transmit appropriate commands to the computer? Would the computer be portable or would it be necessary

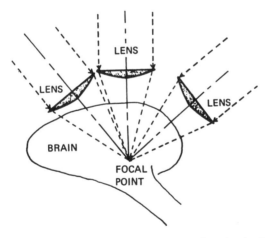

Figure 15. A theoretical scheme for stimulating the brain without inserting electrodes. The power density of each of the separate beams would be below the effective level to stimulate neural tissue. Only at the focal point of all three beams would the power be sufficient to provide effective stimulation. A practical system employing this principle has not yet been developed. See text for details. (From L. R. Pineo, Selective Deep Brain Stimulation with External Electrodes, in Reynolds, D. U., & Sjoberg, A. E., *Neuroelectric Research*, 1971, Fig. 43-7. Courtesy of Charles C. Thomas, Publisher, Springfield, Ill.)

for the patient to be confined to the area where it was located? Considering the dangers inherent in a brain electrode system, it seems much more feasible to utilize one of the more sophisticated prosthetic devices that are currently being developed. Artificial hands have been built which at least theoretically permit objects to be grasped, rotated, held and squeezed, maneuvered, and released on command from muscles still functioning. The "hand" contains sensing devices and a microcomputer that would assume the job of adjusting the intensity of the gripping force and assuring that the held object did not slip out. Although the requirements of the amputee are not necessarily identical to that of the stroke victim, the development of sophisticated prosthetic devices seems to be highly preferable to any program that would involve stimulation of the extremely vital and sensitive brain stem region.

There are numerous other extremely complex control systems that would have to be incorporated into any scheme to help stroke victims by direct stimulation of the brain. The neural control of normal movement involves numerous feedback circuits from the environment as well as from muscles and joints and all of these "data" have to be collated and processed at many brain levels. When our eyes are closed, it is these feedback systems that make it possible to touch our noses or maintain our balance while standing. Our bodies are required to make adjustments rapidly and automatically. The task of reaching out an arm to catch a ball thrown to one side involves not only a very rapid and sensitive series of adjustments based on a changing visual input, but in order to maintain balance, adjustments must also be made to accommodate information from almost everyone of the over 400 skeletal muscles of the body. By using computers, it may be possible to elicit specific responses that could accomplish limited goals under static conditions, but the solution to such a problem is infinitely simpler than that required to program movements that would be able to adapt to rapidly changing environmental conditions.

Further appreciation of the magnitude of the problem can be gained by noting that a muscle contracting against a load must be capable of very rapid compensations for any sudden increase or decrease in the load. It may be necessary to make a great effort to lift a weight, but as soon as inertia is overcome a much smaller muscular effort is required. In the absence of this capacity, movements would swing between inadequate efforts and spastic overshoots. The rapid adjustments are made possible by sensors that are capable of detecting the degree of stretch in the muscle system. The sensors are muscle spindles embedded in an "intrafusal" fiber system that runs parallel to the actual load-carrying muscle fibers. As explained in the legend to Figure 16 the muscle spindles are capable of modifying the excitation level of the motor nerves that control the load-carrying muscle fibers. It would be extremely difficult to design a brain stimulating system for controlling movement that would be sufficiently sensitive to the muscle spindle feedback system to accomplish smooth, graded responses under changing load conditions.

Another approach to the same problem that has seemed particularly seductive to science fiction writers and also to a few scientists involves stimulating areas of the brain with their own characteristic electrical pattern. It is a very tantalizing thought to be able to record the electrical pattern from a specific brain region and then to play back this same pattern through the implanted electrode from which the recording was obtained. The idea would be to record the electrical pattern from critical sites in the nervous system while a person was engaged in a particular activity and then to play it back into the nervous system to reproduce the activity. Superficially, this seems to be an ideal solution to the problem of producing an electric stimulus that duplicates the natural physiological

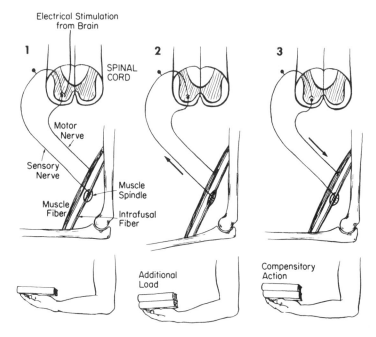

Figure 16. (1) A muscle fiber contracts in response to the activity in its motor nerve. The excitability of the motor nerve is modified by feedback from the muscle spindles in the intrafusal fibers. (2) A sudden unexpected increase in the load causes the nerve fibers in the muscle spindle to stretch and to send additional excitatory impulses (upward arrow) to the motor nerve. (3) The motor nerve increases its activity (downward arrow) and causes the muscle fibers to compensate for the additional load. The adjustment takes less than 1/20 second. (Adapted from P. A. Merton, "How We Control the Contraction of Our Muscles," *Scientific American*, 1972, Vol. 226, pp. 30-37.)

processes. Unfortunately, the glamor of this possibility quickly fades under close scrutiny. The electrical pattern that is recorded is both a distortion and a selection determined by the methods and apparatus used. (A high-fidelity tape recording of the sound of rain on a tin roof does not contain all the information needed to make rain). Even though there may be consistent electrical correlates of certain movements, this does not mean that there is any causal relationship between the electrical pattern in a given brain area and a particular behavioral pattern. There is absolutely no reason to believe that a playback of recorded electrical patterns through a brain electrode will reinstate either a response or, for that matter, any physiological state that was prevalent at the time the pattern was recorded. Although additional arguments may not be needed, it may be useful to point out that it is an illusion to believe that a playback of an electrical pattern duplicates any meaningful physiological response. Recorded electrical patterns of brain waves represent the algebraic sum of the electrical activity of many different individual nerve cells (neurons); the playback does not come close to activating each of the cells with its own idiosyncratic pattern.

Brain stimulation technology should be examined in other contexts besides those related to the very remote possibility that it can be used to control individuals or groups of people. The great number of reports from animal studies and several descriptions of the results produced by human brain stimulation seem to suggest that motivation and emotion can be manipulated in very predictable ways. These reports have prompted numerous people to suggest that brain manipulations of various kinds may contain the solution to many medical and social problems. The next chapter reviews the experimental evidence in greater detail prior to a consideration of practical application in subsequent chapters.

Brain Manipulations and the Control of Specific Behavior

By implanting tiny electrodes in animals' brains, experimenters can send electrical impulses to create specific responses—now making them cringe, now sending them into furious attack, now making them drink, now making them sexually hyperactive.

This quotation from an article by Nicholas N. Kittrie, a Professor of Law at American University, appeared in many newspapers in the United States (for example, *Detroit Sunday News*, March 19, 1972). The facts are not wrong, but as presented they can be very misleading in that they convey a degree of possible control, predictability, and practicality that is not in accord with the evidence. The purpose of the next two chapters is to prepare a more realistic foundation for an evaluation of the medical and social significance of various types of brain manipulation—a topic which will be discussed in the remaining chapters of the book.

It is quite true that animal studies have demonstrated that brain stimulation can initiate eating, drinking, aggression, and many response patterns that are characteristic of a particular species such as carrying objects, retrieving pups, gnawing on pieces of wood, and other natural behaviors. Brain stimulation may also intensify sexual behavior in some animals and produce sleepiness or enhance alertness. Some of these demonstrations are unquestionably very dramatic. Rats that are completely satiated and exhibit no interest in food or water may consume huge quantities of either or both when stimulated. It is possible, for example, to force an animal to eat several times its normal daily amount of food within a short period if brain stimulation is administered during this time. Anyone observing an animal suddenly picking up a pellet of food immediately after the stimulation has been turned on and then continuing to gorge itself until the stimulation has been turned off cannot help but form the impression of a tremendous control that can be exerted by brain stimulation. These first impressions can be very misleading, as can be the extrapolations from these examples to human clinical problems.

A CLOSER EXAMINATION OF THE EVIDENCE

It is one matter to appreciate the value of brain stimulation as a basic research tool that provides a means to learn more about how the brain is organized to carry on its many functions, but is is quite another matter to conclude that we may soon be in a position to manipulate the brain and thereby modify human behavior in a predictable, practical, and desirable manner. One of the main reasons a mere listing of all the behaviors ever evoked by stimulation can be very misleading is that it creates the impression of a greater amount of control and predictability than actually exists. The impression exists that if electrodes are placed in a specific part of the brain, a particular behavior can inevitably be evoked. Those who have participated in this research know that this is definitely not the case. In a large percentage of cases, animals do not display any specific behavior in response to stimulation, even though great care may have been exerted to position the brain electrodes with as much precision as possible. Even in rats, where the behavior is more stereotyped than in monkeys and man, brain stimulation produces very variable results. In my own laboratory, we have provided a large amount of evidence indicating that electrodes that seem to be in the same brain area in different animals often do not produce the same results at all. One rat may start to eat as soon as the electric current is turned on, another may drink, still another may initiate sexual behavior if a cooperative partner is available, and most animals will actively explore their environment—perhaps searching for some "reward" that is not present.

It has frequently been assumed that the anatomical locus for each of the behaviors that can be elicited is discrete and well defined. The evidence does not support this view. Dr. Verne Cox and I recently showed that the neural areas capable of evoking several of the behaviors most frequently studied are much more diffuse than had been implied by many laboratory investigators and certainly than that inferred by writers with only indirect knowledge of the experiments. The elicitation of eating and drinking in the rat can be obtained from very widespread (but not all) areas in the hypothalamus. Others demonstrated that these same behaviors can be evoked from a number of areas outside the hypothalamus. Drs. Bryan Robinson and Mortimer Mishkin made similar observations in the monkey. More recently, in collaboration with Drs. Friedrich Stephan and Irving Zucker at the University of California in Berkeley, I provided evidence that the brain areas which appear to have the capacity to intensify the sexual behavior of male rats are also more diffusely localized than had been suggested in some reports. Although other evidence of this type is available, the important point of this discussion is that the impression that specific behaviors can be reliably manipulated by electrical stimulation of anatomical areas that have been precisely defined is not in accord with the evidence. The experimental data clearly indicate that electrodes that seem to be in the same brain locus in different animals often evoke different behavior, and electrodes located at very different brain sites may evoke the same behavior in a given animal. Such findings reported from stimulation studies conducted in my own laboratory forced me to conclude that some characteristic response tendency of the animal makes a significant contribution to the obtained results and that the behavior that can be elicited by stimulation cannot be predicted accurately from knowledge of the anatomical location of the electrode. Recently Dr. Jaak Panksepp reached a similar conclusion in regard to the elicitation of aggressive responses in rats:

"... the appearance of stimulus-bound quiet attack interacted with the behavioral typology of individual animals. ... animals normally inclined to kill mice were more likely to kill during hypothalamic stimulation than nonkillers. Thus, the electrically elicited response was probably not determined by specific functions of the tissue under the electrode but by the personality of the rat."

The responses that are elicited by brain stimulation in different species also help to round out our understanding of this phenomenon. Dr. Stephen Glickman of the University of California at Berkeley observed that stimulation at many different brain sites frequently elicits a "foot thumping" response from the gerbil. Since "foot thumping" is a characteristic gerbil response when the animal is highly aroused, these observations suggest that the responses elicited by stimulation may *in part* be determined by the prepotent response tendencies of animals rather than the precise anatomical location of the electrode.

Observations that demonstrate the significance of the personality of the subjects in determining the response to brain stimulation have also been reported with humans. At the recently held Third World Congress of Psychosurgery, Dr. Y. Kim of Broughton Hospital in Morganton, North Carolina, presented a paper in collaboration with Dr. W. Umbach of the Free University in Berlin in which the behavior evoked by stimulation of the amygdala nucleus in the temporal lobe (see Figures 25 and 26) of aggressive and nonaggressive patients was reported. These neurosurgeons indicated that amygdala stimulation of aggressive patients increased "aggressiveness and even aggressive acts were provoked, whereas no aggressive reaction was observed in nonviolent cases." It seems evident that it would be an oversimplification to conclude that there is an invariable relationship between stimulation in the amygdala and the elicitation of aggressive behavior.

Another complication that has become apparent is that in spite of the seemingly compelling evidence that satiated animals can be motivated to obtain food when stimulated, recent experiments have cast some serious doubts about their being hungry. There are some puzzling aspects to the behavior evoked by stimulation of animals that demand our attention and should caution us against jumping to the conclusion that we can turn such motivational states as hunger on and off. I have shown in collaboration with Drs. Verne Cox and Jan Kakolewski that in most instances in which one behavior, such as eating, is elicited by stimulation the animal is likely to display several other behaviors when stimulated through the very same electrode even when the intensity of stimulation has not been changed. If the food is removed from the test chamber, the animals are very likely to start drinking or to exhibit some other behavior when stimulated. These observations demonstrate that the behaviors evoked by a given electrode are not only variable, but they cannot be easily related to the same biological need such as food, water, or a mate.

It is frequently overlooked that when Walter Hess spoke of eliciting bulimia (insatiable appetite) by stimulating the hypothalamus, his actual descriptions of the observed behavior raised some questions about the animals' motivation. For example, in 1957 Dr. Hess described the behavior of satiated animals that, prior to hypothalamic stimulation, had refused food:

"Stimulation here produces bulimia. If the animal has previously taken neither milk or meat, it now devours or drinks greedily. *As a matter of fact, the animal may even take into its mouth or gnaw on objects that are unsuitable as food, such as forceps, keys, or sticks* [two photographs were included to illustrate a cat gnawing on a stick and other inedible objects]. . . . Under certain conditions, bulimia induced by electrical stimulation may persist up to an hour. During this period, if an edible or *inedible object* is laid on the table, the cat immediately devours or sinks its teeth into it." (Italics added.)

Furthermore, the stimulated animals often display a degree of inflexibility in their behavior that is not characteristic of a hungry animal. For example, if a rat starts to eat food pellets every time it is stimulated, it usually does not eat the same food if it is ground up into a mash. In contrast, a rat that is known to be hungry (because it has been deprived of food for a day) readily eats the food in either form or any other palatable food. The stimulated rat may leave the new food untouched and eventually it may drink instead of eating. Even if the water the animal has been drinking during stimulation is merely put into a new container, stimulation may no longer evoke drinking.

In many respects the behavior elicited by stimulation seems forced and stereotyped. On several occasions I have observed stimulated animals shoving food into their mouths so rapidly that they choked. One time I neglected to warn a new assistant of this possibility and a stimulated rat scooped food into its mouth so frenetically that it actually asphyxiated itself. It is clear that it is necessary to look beyond the mere fact that stimulation has evoked drinking or eating. If the tests are varied to provide a greater understanding of the motivation behind the behavior, it becomes obvious that it cannot be assumed that the stimulation has duplicated hunger or thirst or any other natural state. One of the reasons animals may change the behavior displayed during the same stimulation is that the state evoked was never clearly hunger, thirst, or sexual appetite.

If studies with relatively homogeneous, inbred animals suggested that there is a great amount of uncontrolled variability in the behavior produced by brain stimulation, we should expect an even greater source of unpredictability in the case of primates and especially humans—and indeed this certainly seems to be true. In monkeys, complex and often very variable behavior may be displayed in response to the same stimulation, depending on the relative social ranking of the animals that are present. Dr. Detlev Ploog of the Max-Planck Institute for Psychiatry in Munich concludes from his brain stimulation studies in socially grouped squirrel monkeys:

". . . one and the same electric stimulus applied at the same brain site in the same animal at different times does not necessarily elicit the same response. Rather, the animals' response depends on the composition and disposition of the group, and on the rank, role, and sex of the stimulated and the interacting animal."

Dr. Bryan Robinson of Florida State University also commented on the difficulty of predicting responses elicited by stimulation of the brains of rhesus monkeys. Dr.

Robinson emphasizes situational determinants as follows:

"One strange fact was that the response of the animal when it was unrestrained and with other monkeys could not be entirely predicted from the response obtained when the animal was confined to a restraining chair. And, the best aggressive responses came from loci which did not produce particularly convincing aggressive behavior in the chair."

SOME ILLUSTRATIVE EXPERIMENTS

A striking example of how easy it is to be misled by the first impression of the behavior that is triggered by brain stimulation occurred in my own laboratory. Dr. Anthony Phillips, who at that time was a graduate student and is now on the staff at the University of British Columbia, had placed electrodes in the so-called lateral hypothalamic reward system of rats. This is a brain area where it is known that rats will be willing to stimulate themselves. After recovery from the surgery, the rats were placed in a rectangular box in which brain stimulation was controlled by two photocell assemblies (see Figure 17). When the animal interrupted the beam on one side it received brain stimulation until the beam at the opposite side of the chamber was interrupted. In a very short time, the animals learned to play the game, running back and forth and turning the stimulation on and off. The first animal we tested in this chamber had previously been observed to eat whenever the brain stimulation was administered. For this reason, we placed food pellets on the side of the test chamber in which brain stimulation was presented. As illustrated in Figure 17, the animal picked up a food pellet and carried it to the opposite side where the animal dropped it as soon as the stimulation was terminated. At first

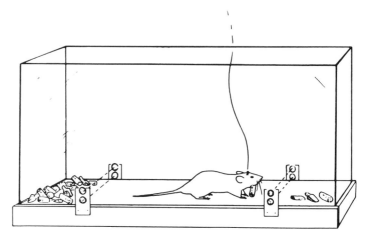

Figure 17. Illustration of a rat carrying a block of wood while receiving hypothalamic stimulation. The rat moves back and forth, receiving brain stimulation on the left side as soon as the photocell beam is interrupted. Upon receiving stimulation the rat picks up an object and carries it to the opposite side. As soon as the rat interrupts the photocell beam on the right side of the test chamber, stimulation is terminated and the object is dropped. See text for an explanation of the relationship between the carrying of objects and brain stimulation.

thought, stimulation seemed to be eliciting the hoarding of food, a behavior that is very common to most rodents. However, when we tested the animal with inedible objects such as pieces of wood and rubber erasers, it carried these objects just as well. In fact, when we placed a rat pup in the test chamber it carried the pup in the same fashion as all of the other objects. Had we observed this behavior first, we would have thought that the stimulation had elicited one aspect of maternal behavior—retrieving of young to the nest site. This tendency to carry objects was so potent under these test conditions that if there was no other object present, the animal occasionally picked up its tail or one of its forelegs and while holding this part of its body in its mouth it struggled back to the oppostie side and "deposited" it on the pile of objects it had been accumulating.

It is fairly obvious that if only food pellets or pups had been placed in the test chamber we might have been convinced that the stimulation was tapping into a maternal behavior or food hoarding neural circuit. Some additional information made it clear that this was not the case. First, *all* of the animals that we tested in this chamber carried objects as long as the electrodes had been placed in an hypothalamic site that produced a positive reward. That is, as long as an animal would self-stimulate, it carried the objects placed in the chamber in spite of the fact that the position of the electrodes varied considerably. Furthermore, if we varied the conditions so that the animal received the *identical* brain stimulation, but independent of its location in the chamber, it stopped carrying objects even when the objects were directly under its nose.

Apparently, for the rat any condition that motivates it to move back and forth and at the same time produces a parallel alternation of arousal and calming is very likely to produce the carrying behavior. It is well known that rats carry objects in situations related to hoarding, nest building, and retrieving of young. They also carry objects that have no utility for them. The pack or "trade" rat, for example, may even leave the object it is carrying in order to pick up an apparently more desirable, shiny object. This transporting of objects by rats is invariably from a more open and vulnerable location that is known to increase their arousal level to a hidden home or nest site that is safer and therefore calming. There is something about the alternation of arousal and calming when it is regularly produced in two different locations that is a potent stimulus for encouraging the rat to carry objects. In spite of our first impressions, it now seems clear that the behavior elicited by the stimulation should not be considered either maternal or hoarding.

Equally important for our understanding of the relationship between brain stimulation and behavior is the fact that object carrying was "situationally dependent." The carrying of objects could only be elicited when the stimulation was delivered under conditions consistent with the environmental arrangements that encourage this behavior. It is also clear that destruction of the neural tissue around any one of the sites that could produce this behavior would not eliminate the carrying of objects or young that is normally displayed under natural conditions. Extensive destruction encompassing all the effective sites might eliminate the carrying behavior under natural conditions, but only because the animal would be severely debilitated. In summary, if we consider the general nature of the motivational state underlying the elicited carrying behavior, the essential role of environmental factors, and the lack of anatomical specificity, the significance of the phenomenon appears quite different from an account stressing only that maternal behavior was elicited reliably from a specific brain site.

The so-called elicitation of male sexual behavior by hypothalamic stimulation is another case that illustrates that many factors have to be considered to understand the relationship between brain stimulation and the behavior it modifies. Dr. Anthony Caggiula showed that if male rats are stimulated intermittently at some sites in the hypothalamus while a receptive female is present, there is a marked tendency for most of the male's copulatory activity to be displayed during the stimulation periods. Commonly, stimulation is delivered to the male's hypothalamus for a three-minute period followed by an equal period without stimulation. Stimulation and non-stimulation periods continue to alternate and it is possible, therefore, to determine the relative amount of sexual activity displayed during the two conditions. It is found that a major portion of the sexual behavior is usually displayed during the periods of stimulation of some brain sites and that the rate of displaying the various components of the sexual act may be speeded up.

A closer examination of the evidence indicates that it may not be correct to conclude from the sexual behavior-stimulation data that a "copulation site" has been located in the brain. There are many reasons why caution should be exercised before this interpretation is accepted. First, the fact that a preponderance of sexual behavior occurs during the stimulation rather than the nonstimulation periods seems to be a by-product of a peculiar property of brain stimulation to inhibit activity during the period immediately following its termination. Even if a rat is in the middle of the act of copulation when brain stimulation is turned off, it is likely to terminate sexual activity for a period of time. The high correlation of sexual activity and stimulation, therefore, may be produced as much by the inhibition that follows the offset of the stimulation than by a facilitation of sexual activity caused by the stimulation.

Another consideration that complicates the interpretation of the reports of sexual facilitation by brain stimulation is related to the fact that it has been known for some time that the sexual behavior of animals, if not also humans, can be facilitated by a variety of influences that produce a general arousal. For example, Dr. Knut Larsson of the University of Göteborg in Sweden showed that merely handling older rats whose sexual capacities had dwindled caused an enhancement of their performance. Drs. Caggiula and Eibergen demonstrated that shocking virgin male rats on the tail in the presence of females increased the sexual behavior of these immature subjects. More recently in a paper with the engaging title "From Dud to Stud" it was reported by Drs. William Crowley, Herbert Popolow, and O. Byron Ward, Jr., that male rats which for some reason did not copulate could be induced to mate by electrical shock to the skin. Once the animals were induced to copulate by the shock they continued to mate on subsequent tests without the shock and were used as reliable studs in the laboratory. Even though not all brain stimulation that seems to arouse an animal enhances sexual behavior, the fact that so many nonspecific treatments such as handling or painful shock can facilitate sexual behavior cautions us against concluding that a specific neural structure regulating sexual performance has been discovered.

The belief that very specific and predictable states can be produced by brain stimulation has been fostered partly by exaggerated descriptions of Dr. Delgado's now famous account of the presumed control of aggression of bulls. For example, Boyce Rensberger wrote in the *New York Times* article referred to earlier:

"Dr. Delgado implanted a radio-controlled electrode deep within the brain of a *brave bull*, a variety bred to respond with a raging charge when it sees any human being. But when Dr. Delgado pressed a button on a transmitter, sending a signal to a battery-powered receiver attached to the bull's horns, an impulse went into the bull's brain and the animal would cease his charge.

"After several stimulations, the bull's naturally aggressive behavior disappeared. It was as placid as Ferdinand."

This interpretation has been accepted by most people, but actually there is no good reason for believing that the stimulation had any direct effect on the bull's aggressive tendencies. An examination of the film record makes it apparent that the charging bull was stopped because as long as the stimulation was on it was forced to turn around in the same direction continuously. After examining the film, any scientist with knowledge in this field could conclude only that the stimulation had been activating a neural pathway controlling movement. According to Delgado, "the result seemed to be a combination of motor effect, forcing the bull to stop and turn to one side, plus behavioral inhibition of the aggressive drive," but actually no evidence was presented to prove that aggressivity had been modified.

Most writers have simply overlooked the major effect on the motor system, preferring the more dramatic interpretation of the stimulation as a pure pacifier, and no one has taken the trouble to correct this impression. Indeed, Delgado's comment that for several minutes following stimulation the bull would "tolerate the presence of investigators in the ring without launching any attack" has strengthened the impression that a significant reduction in aggression had occurred. It is not at all surprising, however, that the confused and frustrated animal displayed a little hesitancy in launching another attack. To conclude from this demonstration that we are close to being able to selectively reduce aggression in the normal human without producing many other effects seems, to put it as diplomatically as possible, very questionable at best (see Figure 18).

Dr. Delgado pioneered the development of many brain stimulation techniques including multiple electrode assemblies and remote "cable-free" stimulation and recording methods, which have been particularly useful in studying behavior in more natural settings. Scientists, therefore, owe him a great debt for the many technical innovations that he and his collaborators have developed. On the other hand, however, his propensity for dramatic, albeit ambiguous, demonstrations has been a constant source of material for those whose purposes are served by exaggerating the omnipotence of brain stimulation. For example, a report from his book, *Physical Control of the Mind*, describes the specific inhibition of aggressive behavior by stimulation of a brain region called the caudate nucleus (see Figure 26):

"When this part of the caudate nucleus is stimulated, the normally ferocious macacus rhesus becomes tranquil,

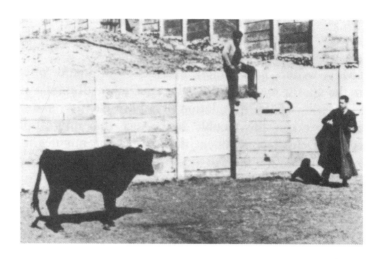

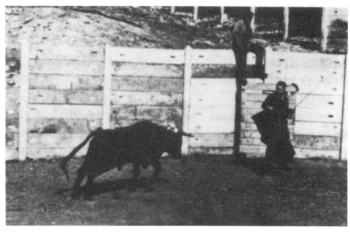

Figure 18. "Brave bulls are dangerous animals which will attack any intruder into the arena. The animal in full charge can be abruptly stopped by radio stimulation of the brain. After several stimulations, there is a lasting inhibition of aggressive behavior." (Reprinted from José M. R. Delgado, *Physical Control of the Mind: Toward a Psychocivilized Society*, Harper & Row, New York, 1969, Fig. 24, pp. 170-171.) See text for an alternative interpretation.

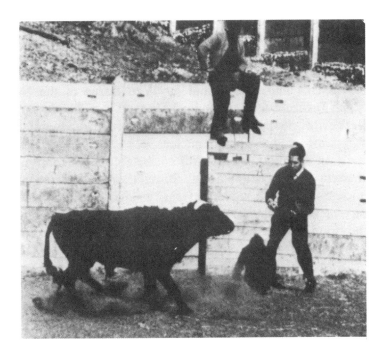

and instead of grabbing, scratching, and biting any approaching object, he sits peacefully and the investigator can safely touch his mouth and pet him. During this time the animal is aware of the environment but has simply lost his usual irritability, showing that violence can be inhibited without making the animal sleepy or depressed. Identification of the cerebral areas responsible for ferocity would make it possible to block their function and diminish undesirable aggressiveness without disturbing general behavior reactivity." (Delgado, 1969.)

The interpretation, which presumes a specific and practical means of inhibiting aggression by caudate nucleus stimulation, would be regarded with the greatest skepticism by most brain physiologists and neurologists. The caudate nucleus is one of several brain structures that are known to play an important role in controlling fine muscular responses. Numerous investigators have reported that stimulation of this structure inhibits movements and produces an "arrest reaction." In man the arrest reaction is characterized by a cessation of voluntary movements and speech, and Dr. Van Buren of the National Institute of Neurological Diseases and Blindness in Bethesda observed this response during electrical stimulation of the caudate nucleus. A patient instructed to continue tapping the table will not be able to do so during caudate nucleus stimulation. Stimulation of the caudate nucleus of man at higher currents produced a stereotyped turning of the head in a direction opposite to the side of the brain stimulated. The patients were also confused for a period after the stimulation and they were often unaware of their behavior during the stimulation. (As suggested previously, it is very likely that this forced head turning and confusion is the explanation of the presumed decreased aggression produced by stimulating the caudate nucleus of the charging bull.)

The role of the caudate nucleus in controlling movement can also be seen by ablation experiments. Destruction of this brain area in animals frequently produces involuntary movements such as those seen in patients suffering from chorea, or St. Vitus dance. Moreover, abnormalities in the caudate nucleus have been reported to be present in some cases of tremor such as seen in Parkinson's disease (see page 198). Delgado, on the other hand, argued that specific parts of the caudate nucleus may control different functions. Whereas one region may inhibit aggression, an area close by is claimed to inhibit appetite:

"At the sight of a banana, the animal usually shows great interest, leaning forward to take the fruit, which he eats voraciously and with evident pleasure. However, his appetite is immediately inhibited as soon as the caudate nucleus is electrically stimulated. Then the monkey looks with some interest at the banana without reaching for it, and may even turn his face away, clearly expressing refusal. During stimulation the animal is well aware of his surroundings, reacting normally to noises, moving objects and threats, but he is just not interested in food. If a monkey is stimulated when his mouth is full of banana, he immediately stops chewing, takes the banana out of his mouth, and throws it away."

Delgado's argument that there may be a number of specific loci in the caudate nucleus cannot be dismissed out of hand, but he has presented no evidence from controlled behavioral studies that his electrodes have tapped into separate centers for the inhibition of aggression, appetite, and other motivational states. Instead he seems to capitalize on every individual effect his electrodes happen to produce and presents little, if any, experimental evidence that his impression of the underlying cause is correct. There is absolutely no reason, for example, to reject the hypothesis that some caudate stimulation may inhibit eating not because it suppresses appetite but rather by disrupting some response related to swallowing. In any case, the idea that manipulation of the caudate nucleus may provide a practical way of controlling aggression would appear to reflect an unrealistic and simplistic view.

In the same book, Delgado reported what he views as a specific effect of electrical stimulation of the brain (ESB) on the maternal behavior of the rhesus monkeys, but it is not too likely that anyone else would find this interpretation convincing. I had an opportunity to observe the behavior of these animals in Dr. Delgado's laboratory and had to conclude that his interpretation is among the most gratuitous in this field. His subjects were two mothers, Rose and Olga, and their respective babies, Roo and Ole. The description by Delgado quoted below requires little comment from the present author:

"Several simple motor effects evoked by ESB (such as head turning or flexion of the arm) did not disrupt mother-infant relations, but when a 10-second radio stimulation was applied to the mesencephalon of Rose, an aggressive attitude was evoked with rapid circling around the cage and self-biting of the hand, leg, or flank. For the next eight to ten minutes, maternal instinct was disrupted and Rose completely lost interest in her baby, ignoring his tender calls and rejecting his attempts to approach her. Little Roo looked rather disoriented and sought refuge and warmth with the other mother, Olga, who accepted both babies without hesitation. About ten minutes after ESB, Rose regained her natural maternal behavior and accepted Roo in her arms. This experiment was repeated several times on different days with similar disruptive results for the mother-infant relation. It should be concluded, therefore, that maternal behavior is somehow dependent on the proper functioning of mesencephalic structures and that short ESB applied in this area is able to block the maternal instinct for a period of several minutes."

It hardly seems necessary to point out that the same stimulation was very likely to disrupt almost any behavior that happened to be going on at the time.

HUMAN RESPONSE TO BRAIN STIMULATION

Considerable light can be shed on the effects of brain stimulation by examining the human evidence, since it is only in these cases that we can obtain verbal reports. Although the most interesting behavior changes in animals have been obtained by stimulating the hypothalamus, humans who have been stimulated in this area have never reported feeling hungry, thirsty, or aggressive, nor have any sexual desires been evoked. In 1940 Dr. J. C. White stimulated various hypothalamic structures in awake humans and failed to evoke any emotional experience, although a number of visceral responses were recorded. The experiences of Dr. Robert Heath's patients were essentially the same: some "abdominal discomfort, feelings of warmth, fullness in the head, pounding heart" were reported, but no clear motivational state was evoked by hypothalamic stimulation. Moreover, even though eating and drinking have been commonly elicited in animals, Dr. Heath indicated to me during a conversation that he has seen no evidence—nor as far as he knew had anyone else—that stimulation at any brain site in humans ever evoked an experience of hunger or thirst.

There is little convincing evidence that human brain stimulation produces a specific and predictable response from the same anatomical structure in different individuals. For example, Delgado described two female patients who, following temporal lobe stimulation, became increasingly "flirtatious" with the therapist. Sem-Jacobsen reported two cases in which stimulation of the "posterior part of the frontal lobe" (a very different location from Delgado's) produced sensations "like a sexual pleasure." Heath reported that stimulation in the septal region evoked a sexual experience and in a very few instances it may have produced an orgasm. In the previous chapter we mentioned that Bechterewa and her colleagues in the Soviet Union reported the evocation of pleasurable sensations and the occurrence of an orgasm during stimulation of the ventrolateral thalamic region. Sexual sensations were evoked, however, in only a very small percentage of the patients, while several other patients presumably stimulated in the same thalamic region experienced very different emotions including anxiety and terror. Other patients stimulated in these same areas do not report any special experience. In some instances, sexual ideation has been an indirect consequence of brain stimulation which produced arousing genital sensations, just as queasy tense feelings, irritability, and even relaxation may be a by-product of bodily pain or changes in blood pressure, heart rate, and other visceral organs. The evidence is not completely conclusive, but it strongly suggests that the contents of the experiences evoked by stimulation are greatly determined by the personal reactions of the patients—reactions which are influenced by their past history and the present setting. The interpretations given by a patient to the state induced by brain stimulation may even be shaped by the content of an interview an hour before stimulation was started.

The emotional states experienced by patients during brain stimulation are usually reported in more general terms such as relaxation, feelings of well being, increased alertness and communicativeness, euphoria, confusion, depression, anxiety, agitation, fear, anger, and rage. There is reasonably good agreement that stimulation of particular brain structures may produce a predictable direction of emotional changes, such as mood elation or depression, but this is clearly not always the case. For example, Heath's patients frequently reported pleasurable reactions from septal stimulation and they often appeared more alert and communicative. Drs. Vernon Mark and Frank Ervin of the Massachusetts General Hospital noted that they were able to elicit positive feelings (usually some dimension of relaxation) from more lateral amygdala placements (a neural structure in the temporal lobe) and unpleasant reactions, such as pain or loss of control, from the more medial areas within this same brain structure. One patient described by these investigators was stimulated in the medial portion of the amygdala; he reported a feeling of "going wild" and said "I'm losing control." When the same patient was stimulated in a region 3 millimeters more lateral he had a sensation of hyperrelaxation, a feeling of "detachment," "just like an injection of Demerol."

Although the general tone of the emotional states induced by the stimulation of a particular brain region may be somewhat predictable, Mark and Ervin noted that the states are expressed as "highly individualized" responses by the patients. Heath reached the same conclusion:

"It has been possible to stimulate each patient several times and in several different regions. The immediate effects differ in many respects, and individual patients have differed somewhat in their responses to the same type of stimulation to the same region at different times. There were, however, some consistent findings in the sphere of affectivity. . . .

"Stimulation to the amygdaloid nucleus resulted in an intense emotional reaction. The nature of the response varied from one stimulation to the next in the same patient, although parameters of stimulation were constant. On some occasions the patient became enraged and attempted to strike out, on other occasions she became fearful and felt an impulse to run."

In another article by Dr. Heath and his collaborators, Drs. Monroe and Mickle, the following conclusion was reached:

"Our studies, as well as the reports in the literature, seemingly suggest that it is impossible to make a one-to-one correlation between stimulation of this nuclear mass [the amygdala] and the behavioral response. Apparently the dynamic physiological-psychological state of the total individual is of the utmost importance in effecting the final response, even though the parameters of stimulation are constant. The same observation has held with our stimulations to other regions, regardless of the type of

stimulation, whether electrical, psychological, or pharmacological."

A similar opinion was expressed by Dr. Van Buren, who
has had considerable experience with electrical stimulation
of the brains of patients:

"Responses of emotional nature have appeared in
reports of depth stimulation in man from time to time.
Fear has been the most common response and has been
reported from stimulation in the amygdaloid region, from
the fornix and from pallidum. It must be noted, however,
that well defined emotional responses to stimulation are
infrequent. . . . We have had difficulty being certain
whether fear actually was the result of stimulation or
whether it was not simply the result of an unusual
sensation experienced under conditions that were alarming
to the patient. In one instance, fearfulness had appeared
from stimulation of electrodes in the depth and on the
cortical surface and practically disappeared as the patient
became accustomed to the procedure of stimulation.
"The curious variability of the responses elicited from
stimulation of the mesial temporal region had attracted
our interest in the study. Since depth electrodes were used
that maintained a constant contact with tissue and the
stimuli were monitored carefully, it led us to the conclusion that the instability must lie primarily in the
neuronal system that was subject to the stimuli."

An impression of precise replicability of the results obtained from brain stimulation has been derived in part
from some of the descriptions of the auditory and visual
hallucinations and memories that have been evoked by
stimulating temporal lobe structures. Dr. Wilder Penfield,
whose studies of epileptic patients at the Montreal Neurological Institute are very well known, stimulated the

brains of awake patients during temporal lobe surgery. This is a standard procedure during such operations, and it is often a great aid to the neurosurgeon in orienting himself within the brain as well as in locating the area of pathology. Penfield reported that temporal lobe stimulation may repeatedly evoke the same memory, sometimes complete in minute details, and that these evoked memories were analogous to tape recording "playbacks" of past, forgotten experiences. Penfield refers to effects of stimulation as "experiential hallucinations" and describes them most picturesquely:

"Let me discuss an experiential hallucination first. During it a patient may hear music, for example. But, if so, he hears a single playing of the music, orchestra, or piano, or voices; and he may be aware of himself as present in the room or hall. He may hear voices, the voices of friends or of strangers. If they seemed familiar to him during the interval of time now being recalled, they are familiar to him now. If they were strange then, they are strange now. He may see the people who were speaking and the piano being played by the man who played it then. He may, on the other hand, see things that he saw in an earlier period without being aware of sound. If he felt fright then, he feels fright now. If he felt a pleasurable admiration then, he feels it now.

"It is a re-creation of those things on which he was focusing his attention in that interval of past time. Now, however, he is conscious of the present as well as the past. It is a little like the double experience of a man who watches a play and yet is conscious of what is going on about him in the audience. The difference is that he discovers himself on the stage of the past as well as in the audience of the present. . . .

"The conclusion is inescapable: there is, stored away in the ganglionic connections of the brain, a permanent record of the stream of consciousness; a record that is much more complete and detailed than the memories that any man can recall by voluntary effort."

The dramatic quality of several of the reports of Penfield's patients during stimulation combined with the speculation (for example, Kubie, 1953) that this phenomenon may represent a neurophysiological confirmation of the psychoanalytic concept of repressed memories has probably resulted in an exaggeration of the importance of these events. Not generally appreciated is the fact that most of the patients' responses evoked by stimulation were very abbreviated and sketchy fragments. The more complete reports by the patients were very few in number and, because they were obtained in a surgical setting, the evidence that the patients were actually reliving a past experience could not be verified. Drs. Paul Fedio and John Van Buren of the National Institute of Neurological Diseases and Stroke in Bethesda, Maryland, have studied perceptual and memory changes during electrical stimulation of the temporal and parietal cortex of patients undergoing a partial temporal lobectomy for the relief of intractable seizures. These investigators report: "We would also like to mention that, in our patients, cortical stimulation did not elicit reports of personal memories or experiential responses like those described by Penfield."

A study by Dr. George Mahl and his collaborators at Yale University helps add some perspective to the interpretation of patients' reports evoked by temporal lobe stimulation. Electrodes were implanted in the brain of a patient and a series of interviews was conducted during which time the patient's brain was stimulated at different neural sites and at different intervals. The use of the interview technique made it possible to reconstruct the origin of many of the responses reported by the patient. There seems to be little doubt that the stimulation can evoke brief hallucinations that often surprised the patient, but these hallucinations were frequently related to the present situation in obvious ways. Even when the hallucinations evoked by the stimulation had been momentary re-enactments of the past, the interview method often revealed that there was an ideational association with the patient's mental content at the moment of stimulation. For example, at one point during the interview when stimulation was suddenly turned on, the word "kerchief" occurred to the patient. One minute before the stimulation the patient had told the interviewer: "I'm all wet—I mean I'm sweating—warm." Later during the interview when the patient complained of sweating and the heat, she requested a handkerchief. At another time, this same patient responded to stimulation by reporting she heard a female voice saying: "I got a baby—sister." The patient had been speaking about her own daughter's desire to have a baby sister or brother. There are also evoked hallucinations that are not as obviously related to the patient's current thoughts, but these probably reflect the fact that temporal lobe stimulation may initiate that kind of dreamlike state which fosters the forming of associations based on a logic (more aptly a psycho-logic) that cannot readily be understood by others. What is remarkable about these evoked hallucinations is not that they represent stored memories unrelated to present thought processes, but rather that the stimulation somehow reinstates an appropriate emotional state which makes these "experiences" extremely vivid and present.

The fact that temporal lobe stimulation often evokes memories that are related to the prevailing thought processes suggests that these memories may not be elicited from the same brain site as reliably as some authors have implied. Indeed, Penfield reported: "If we went back to some point with the lapse of a few seconds or a minute or so, we usually had the same experiential response. If, on the other hand, we waited a little longer time and then went back to the same point, another experience would appear." Similarly, Drs. Adams and Rutkin of the University of California Medical Center in San Francisco recently reported the effects of stimulating temporal lobe structures in 16 patients. Hallucinations or visual images were evoked by stimulation in 30 instances, but they "were never repeated by subsequent stimulation at the same site with the same parameters of stimulation. In other words, a new or different hallucination or visual image was elicited with subsequent stimulation." Furthermore, Drs. Adams and Rutkin reported "that certain images and hallucinations were not derived from memories of real experiences, and at times, recent perceptions, ideas or motives were present in the content of these visual events." In a report on the effects of "deep temporal stimulation in man," Dr. Janice Stevens and her co-investigators at the Massachusetts General Hospital also stressed the variability in the responses elicited from the same implanted electrode. These investigators judged this fact to warrant emphasis as follows: "Subjective changes were elicitable in similar but not identical form repeatedly on the same day, *but often were altered when stimulation was carried out at the same point on different days.*"

It is unrealistic to think that the same stimulation would invariably evoke the same response. Part of the problem is that even among researchers who should know better, there is a tendency to think of the nervous system within too static a framework. It is not realistic to conceive of all nerve cells responding without variation to the same stimulus and being arranged to convey impulses in a fixed direction and sequence. Drs. Kao Liang Chow, David Lindsley, and Morton Gollender showed that the response of a given neuron in the visual pathway to a light stimulus depends on a number of factors that may influence activity in other parts of the nervous system. A flash of light presented to the retina of the left eye may evoke a neuronal response, but this response may be altered by presenting a light stimulus to the right eye, even though the latter stimulus does not produce a detectable response by itself in the neuron under study. Furthermore, the response of the neuron may be conditioned. A light stimulus' capacity to cause the neuron to fire may depend on the presence or absence of a conditioned stimulus (a click or a tone), which prior to the conditioning procedure had no influence on the response of the neuron. If this flexibility is characteristic of a sensory system that has evolved to reflect faithfully the external reality, it is even more applicable to the neuronal circuits that control behavior. All animals above a certain level are capable of learning, and therefore the functional relationships between elements in the nervous system must be capable of being rearranged. It is likely that most nerve cells are involved in many different circuits and the particular circuit which gains priority at any moment depends on a complex interplay of firing and resting (refractory) periods of these cells (see Figure 19).

There is likely to continue to be a significant degree of unpredictability in the responses produced by brain

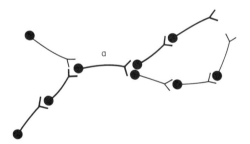

Figure 19.   Neurons forming two pathways. The neuron labeled *a* may be involved in either pathway, depending on the synchronization of its activity with the excitatory or refractory phase of adjacent neurons. This is a very simplified scheme; all the neurons should be shown with potential connections to a number of pathways. The diagram illustrates how the stimulation of a given set of neurons may have different consequences as a function of activity in other parts of the nervous system.

stimulation for the following reasons:

1. Electrodes cannot be positioned with perfect precision because individuals differ in the gross physical dimensions of their brains.[8] Apparently, it does not occur to people that brains differ as much as faces. Furthermore, there is good reason to believe that the microanatomy, that is, the details of the "wiring diagram" of the neuronal circuits of the brain, is variable.

2. The neural circuits responsible for the regulation of different reactions are so closely intertwined that it is almost impossible for electrodes to activate the same configuration of nerve cells in different individuals. Any electrode sufficiently large enough to trigger the number of cells required to produce a behavior change is likely to overlap several of these circuits at the same time.

3. Many different experiments have suggested that stimulation seldom produces a specific "goal-directed" behavior; it produces rather a more general motivational state, which individuals respond to on the basis of their own "personality" and history.

4. The responses to stimulation can be "situationally dependent." There are numerous examples (only a few have been mentioned) that could be provided to illustrate that the responses are influenced by the setting. Responses depend upon who is present, what has just happened, and whether it is a hospital (or laboratory) as contrasted to a life (or field) situation.

5. The responses evoked by stimulation may change over time. This is partly because the responses are "situationally dependent," but, in addition, individuals have the capacity to acquire new associations with the state induced by the stimulation.

CHEMICAL STIMULATION

It has been argued that chemical stimulation may provide a degree of specificity and reliability that cannot be achieved with electrical stimulation. There are many compelling arguments in support of this position. Everyone in this field of inquiry would agree that electricity is a very crude, artificial stimulus that often disrupts neural circuits rather than forcing them to reveal their normal function. Its main advantage is that it can be rapidly turned on and off and conveniently graduated in intensity. In contrast, chemical stimulation may not violate the normal physiology to the same extent since it usually involves drugs that either mimic or antagonize the action of the brain's own chemical transmission system. It is, however, more difficult to turn the effects of chemical stimulation on and off rapidly, and there has to be a constant concern with the possibility that any drug may diffuse over more widespread neural areas than were intended.

To apply drugs to relatively localized areas of the brain, various types of chemitrode have been used in animal research. Most chemitrodes involve a double-barrel (cannula) system where the outer barrel is implanted in the brain and attached to the skull and the inner cannula can be removed and reinserted at will without any additional disturbance of the brain. The inner cannula can be loaded with a drug in crystalline form or drugs in solution can be slowly administered through this cannula into a specific brain region. An arrangement used in our laboratory is depicted in Figure 20. Such an arrangement makes it possible to apply relatively small quantities of drugs to a neural site without many of the undesirable side effects that frequently result from the large doses that have to be injected into the body to achieve adequate levels in the brain. Delgado recently described an experimental transdermal dialytrode that was developed in his laboratory. This device consists of a brain cannula attached to a dialysis bag containing a reservoir of a drug—all of which could be implanted under the skin. The dialysis bag could be adjusted to deliver a prescribed infusion rate of a drug to some brain site in order to accelerate or inhibit neuronal action in that region (see Figure 29).

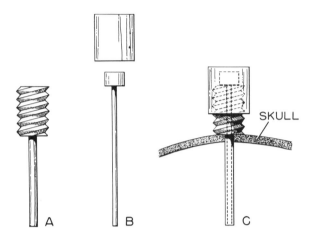

Figure 20. A double-barrel cannula system for administering chemicals in crystal or solution directly to a brain site. Using a stereotaxic instrument, the outer cannula (A) is permanently implanted into (or just above) the target in the brain and attached to the skull. The removable inner cannula (B) may have chemicals inserted into the lumen at the bottom. The crystals will dissolve and diffuse into the brain when the inner cannula is inserted. A flexible tubing may be attached to the top of the inner cannula to permit injection of chemicals in solution. In (C) the inner and outer cannulae are in position and a protective cap has been placed over the top.

It is necessary to consider some basic physiological information to gain perspective on the potential and limitations of chemical stimulation of the brain. Nerve cells communicate with each other by secreting minute amounts of chemical substances, *neurotransmitters*, which either excite or inhibit adjacent cells. Other chemical substances, *antagonists*, are secreted in response to the presence of the neurotransmitters, and these shorten the action of the transmitters by chemically inactivating them or by accelerating the rate of their re-uptake back into the neuron which released them in the first place. The more specific effects of drugs on the brain are exerted by substances that modify the action of only one of the several different neurotransmitters or antagonists. Neural activity can be altered by changing the availability of a neurotransmitter or either mimicking or blocking its action. The amount of a neurotransmitter available can be modified by increasing or decreasing the supply of metabolic precursors (building blocks) or the enzymes necessary for their synthesis. Neurotransmitter action can be blocked by substances that do not have the same physiological consequences, but because they have similar physical properties they may occupy or pre-empt the normal receptor sites.

In a similar manner, drugs may also work by mimicking the action of an antagonist or by increasing or decreasing the amount available. The amount of antagonist present can affect the duration of action of a neurotransmitter. Other drugs may impair the re-uptake of a neurotransmitter, thereby prolonging its action. Some drugs such as barbiturates and alcohol depress the activity of all neurons by altering the characteristics of their semipermeable outer membranes so that the nerve impulse, which ultimately provides the trigger for the release of the neurotransmitter, is more difficult to initiate. (The reader interested in a popular, but more complete, description of the action of drugs on the brain is referred to Ray, 1972, pages 67-75.) It should also be pointed out that in spite of the fact that investigators who administer drugs directly to some brain site generally are most concerned with the effect on neurotransmitter action, drugs may also have significant nonphysiological consequences. Physical properties of drugs such as their acidity, the osmotic pressure they exert, and their capacity to chemically bind (chelate) with various constituents of nerve cells may alter neuronal action without any direct effect on neurotransmitter action.

The observation by Dr. Sebastian Grossman (now at the University of Chicago) that different neurotransmitters administered through the same implanted cannula could

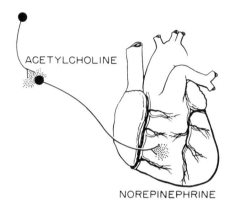

Figure 21. Innervation of the heart by the sympathetic division of the autonomic nervous system. This pathway has two neurons, a pre-synaptic neuron and a postsynaptic neuron, which directly innervates the heart muscle. Note that the postsynaptic neuron is activated by the liberation of acetylcholine from the first neuron, but it liberates nor-epinephrine to accelerate the heart. This example from the peripheral nervous system illustrates that there is no reason to believe a given functional pathway in the brain uses only one neurotransmitter substance.

evoke distinct behaviors suggested that brain circuits which were in close proximity could function inde-pendently because they were coded by their own neu-rotransmitter. He noted that when the neurotransmitter norepinephrine was loaded into the cannula the rat ate, but when acetylcholine was loaded into the same cannula the rat drank. Although it is unquestionably true that chemical stimulation techniques have provided very sig-nificant clues to how the brain may be organized, we are still a long way from being able to control specific be-havior by direct administration of drugs to the brain. Sub-sequent studies, for example, have made it necessary to question the simplified interpretation that drinking is con-trolled by an acetylcholine-based circuit. It has been found that drugs which block drinking induced by acetylcholine do not block the drinking of animals that have been made thirsty by depriving them of water. Moreover, although drinking is elicited by administration of acetylcholine to a great many brain areas in the rat (which incidentally becomes highly aroused in addition to being made thirsty), the same results cannot be obtained in rabbits, guinea pigs, gerbils, cats, or monkeys.

It has to be recognized that whereas there are many different types of behavior, there are only a relatively few neurotransmitters that have been identified. The number of neurotransmitters that have been generally agreed upon is very limited. These are acetylcholine, norepinephrine,

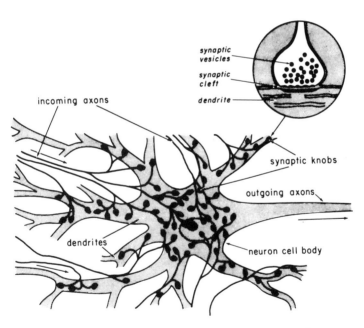

synaptic vesicles

synaptic cleft

incoming axons

dendrite

synaptic knobs

outgoing axons

dendrites

neuron cell body

Figure 22. Illustration of a number of axons originating from many cells terminating at synapses on different parts of a postsynaptic neuron. Axons terminate in synaptic knobs within which are the vesicles containing the neurotransmitter substances (see insert). As explained in the text, the same neurotransmitter may have an inhibitory or excitatory influence on a neuron, depending on whether it acts upon an inhibitory or excitatory receptor site.

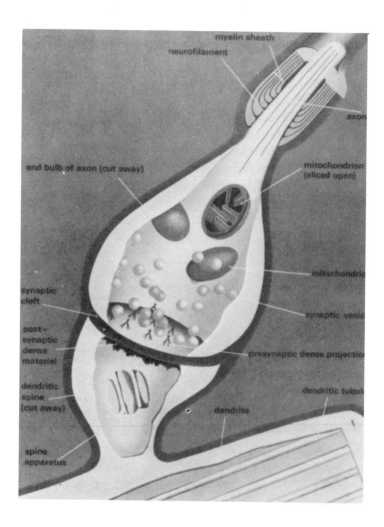

dopamine, serotonin (5HT), glutamic acid, and gamma-amino butyric acid (GABA); their distribution throughout the brain is very widespread, although some regions may have particularly high concentrations of one or another of them. This limited number of neurotransmitters and their lack of confinement to one brain area indicate that the relationship between brain chemistry and behavior cannot be simple. Moreover, it is well known from studies of the peripheral nervous system that a circuit controlling a given physiological function may utilize more than one neurotransmitter substance—a point which adds a further complexity (see Figure 21).

Other new facts about nerve cells accentuate the grossness of our techniques when contrasted with the elegance of the underlying physiology. As illustrated in Figure 22, a single nerve cell may be covered by synaptic knobs (the terminals of the axons) from a great number of connecting nerve cells. The axons may end on an axon (axo-axonic), cell body (axo-somatic), or dendrite (axo-dendritic). Synaptic vesicles within these knobs are the units that contain and release the neurotransmitter substance into the synapse. One of the facts that has recently become apparent from a study by Drs. Daniel Gardner and Eric Kandel is that a single neurotransmitter substance such as acetylcholine may have either an inhibitory or facilitatory action on the receiving (postsynaptic) nerve cell, depending on the part of the cell it acts upon.

Figure 23. A synaptic knob may end on the cell body, dendrite, or axon of another neuron. Illustrated here is an ending on a dendritic spine—one of many projections on the dendrites. Synapses, or functional connections between two cells, are believed to play an excitatory or inhibitory role, depending on the receptor site. When an impulse travels down an axon it induces the spherical vesicles in the synaptic knob to release the stored transmitter substance. The wigwam-like protein fibers probably guide the transmitter though the gap between the two cells where they impinge on the next cell. If sufficient numbers of facilitatory receptor sites are exposed to the transmitter, the receiving nerve fibers fire. The mitochondria illustrated is believed to play a role in supplying the energy for this process. The released transmitter substance is either destroyed by a specific antagonistic enzyme or is reabsorbed rapidly back into the cell of its origin. This process clears the way for the next impulse. (From J. Z. Young (Ed.), *The Explosion of Science, From Molecule to Man*, Crown Publishers, New York, 1969, p. 134.)

Since even the most refined technique for delivering drugs to brain sites—that are still able to influence behavior—may completely bathe a great number of cells, the likelihood of approximating physiological conditions is well beyond our foreseeable capabilities.

Quite aside from the more technical physiological arguments, it is clear that the ratio of the large number of behaviors to the small number of neurotransmitters clearly suggests that each of these is likely to be involved in many behaviors. A drug injected into the body that influences the efficiency of a transmitter system will modify many behaviors and activities in many regions of the brain. A recent report on the results of treating Parkinson's disease (believed to be caused by a deficiency of the neurotransmitter dopamine) with the metabolic precursor L-dopa emphasized this problem. Dr. Frederick K. Goodwin of the National Institutes of Health found evidence of various side effects including confusion, delirium, depression, overactivity, psychosis, paranoia and hypersexual behavior. He concluded that "it is clear that L-dopa does not uniformly produce a specific set of mental changes." Even the direct application of a drug to a localized brain region will have very serious limitations since *there are few areas of the brain that are concerned with the regulation of one and only one behavior and there is no single area in the brain that has complete control over any behavior.*

THE SIGNIFICANCE OF REDUNDANCY IN THE BRAIN

There is probably sufficient redundancy and plasticity in most systems regulating biologically significant behavior to provide safeguards against accidents to any one part of the system. Although a specific behavior may be elicited by stimulation of a particular brain area, it is not correct to conclude that this area is essential to the behavior. Stimulation of the hypothalamus may initiate eating, drinking, or aggression, or it may enhance sexual performance, but in most cases destruction of the neural tissue being stimulated has little or no detectable influence on the same behavior under natural conditions unless the destruction is so extensive that the animal is greatly debilitated and much of its normal behavior is significantly impaired. On this point Hess in 1957 wrote:

"In the analyses of diencephalic functions undertaken by other investigators, some very productive work has been done with ablation and transection methods. The assumption is that it is possible to recognize from the functional *deficit* the contribution that is normally made by the destroyed parts of the brain to the course of total performance. Proceeding with this assumption, we too have made use of destructions, as we have already mentioned, in such a way that stimulation was immediately followed by diathermic coagulation of tissue around the electrode. This step, involving the use of the same electrodes, seemed to us to be most promising, inasmuch as we expected that a comparison of stimulation and destruction effects would provide us with a reciprocal confirmation in the sense of a plus or minus effect. In reality, however, the results were disappointing. Today we know why. Since our procedure aimed for the greatest possible precision, we often produced only correspondingly small foci of coagulation. As is shown by the stimulation study, however, even the best de-marcated "foci" are relatively diffuse . . . an effect is recognizable only if a larger area is affected . . . our findings indicate that the lessening of initiative, which increases with the magnitude of the hypothalamic focus, stands in the foreground. The animal lies about sluggishly."

In other words, destruction of the area around an electrode that elicits a particular behavior has little influence on that behavior unless such an extensive area is destroyed the animal becomes completely debilitated.

Approaching this issue in a different way, Drs. Gaylord Ellison and John Flynn used a specially constructed knife that could be rotated in the brain in order to completely isolate the hypothalamus. In such a preparation there are no remaining functional neural connections in and out of the hypothalamus and all possibilities of communication between this area and the rest of the nervous system are removed unless some humoral substance is capable of bridging the gap created by the knife. Although electrical stimulation of the hypothalamus can trigger aggressive responses, Ellison and Flynn reported that cats in which knife cuts had created "hypothalamic islands" continued to display aggressive reactions when appropriately provoked by external stimulation. It is obvious, therefore, that aggressive behavior would not be eliminated by destruction of the hypothalamic loci that trigger this behavior.

The interpretation of the fact that brain stimulation can evoke a particular behavior can be quite complex. It is usually the case that electrodes at many areas can elicit the same behavior and any or all of these electrodes may be tapping into a complex neural system that ranges over areas of the brain that are located at great distances from the electrode tips. The belief that the neural tissue under the stimulating electrode is essential to the elicited behavior is equivalent to believing that a particular switch is the essence of a light circuit or that all of the beer is contained in the bung of the barrel.

Aggression, Sexuality, and the Temporal Lobe

There has been a heated controversy raging over the question of whether man inherited aggressive instincts from his animal ancestors (for example, see Lorenz, 1966, Kaufman, 1970, and Montagu, 1968). It seems to me that theories based on animal behavior cannot be applied to humans without serious qualifications, since man has not inherited anything from any animal alive today. Man, in common with all living animals, is the result of a long history of separate development and therefore any characteristic originally acquired from some ancient ancestor has been significantly altered during man's unique evolution. Indiscriminate generalizations from the aggressive behavior of black widow spiders, Siamese fighting fish, mice, and even primates can be very misleading. Even the amount of fighting displayed by different nonhuman primates varies considerably, and species could be selected to make any point about man's so-called natural state. Little true light is shed by playing this game as has been effectively argued by Drs. William Hodos and Boyd Campbell (1969).

Similarly, it is also necessary to be skeptical about conclusions regarding man's "natural state" that are derived from observations of any one relatively isolated culture. In this context, Dr. René Dubos makes the interesting observation that the eighteenth-century philosophers accepted the theory of the "noble savage" and man's inherent goodness because of the reports from the early explorers of Tahiti, Hawaii, and Samoa. Had the reports come back from the neighboring Marquesas Island with its ill-tempered cannibals, or the Easter Islands, the concept of man in his native state would have been different. The recently discovered "Stone Age" people, the Tasadays of Mindanao, provide another interesting illustration. As described by Kenneth MacLeish, the Tasadays are extremely peaceful people who have no understanding of the concept of war, do not even hunt and although they have stone axes, these are exclusively tools, not weapons.

William Golding's, *Lord of the Flies*, attempts "to trace the defects of society back to the defects of human nature" by picturing English schoolboys, cast away on a small island, regressing back to a primitive state of meanness and violence. It is, of course, more than possible that Golding's fiction does not reflect human nature, but rather the perversion of English schoolboy values under certain environmental conditions. In a true case, Micronesian children (toddlers to twelve-year olds) marooned on an isolated atoll for several months survived by cooperating and displayed no tendency toward increased violence. Although it cannot be ruled out with absolute certainty, it is highly unlikely that the differences between cultures have a biological basis. What is especially characteristic of man is the great development of his capacity to learn and to thereby acquire very different behavioral propensities, as cultural anthropologists have stressed for some time. Among primitive tribes one can observe a very great range in the amount of aggression displayed.

Studies of animal brains can teach us something about humans, but we must be very careful about the analogies we draw. For example, the situations that involve the greatest destruction and killing among men are those least shared with animals. Warfare is not the result of direct face-to-face threats that evoke innate aggressive reactions. Rather, much of human aggression is the result of more abstract, and therefore acquired motives related to cultural values and economic needs rather than being determined by biological inheritance. In contrast, most examples of killing among animals probably should not be considered aggression since they occur between, rather than within species; moreover, since the animals usually are involved in obtaining food, such attacks are more accurately classified as predatory behavior. Predation and aggression are not necessarily highly correlated. In *The Forest People* Colin Turnbull describes the pygmies of the Ituri forest. These people are extremely efficient hunters, but they are among the most peaceful people known. They rank high as predators but low as aggressors.

Even if for the sake of argument one accepted the theory that man's aggressive impulses are inherited, it would not follow that aggression would be easy to eliminate. The animal experimental evidence, some of which was presented in the previous chapter, indicates that aggression may be very difficult to eliminate selectively. The fact that an aggressive response can be elicited by stimulation of a particular brain area does not mean that aggressive tendencies would be reduced if that area were destroyed. The larger brain ablations that do reduce aggression in animals effect many different types of behavior. Drugs that are partially successful in reducing aggression also modify other functions and usually reduce effectiveness in many areas of activity.

The inseparability of aggression from other behavior may be illustrated by an example. There is a substantial body of evidence in support of the view that, in almost all mammals, the male is more aggressive than the female. With very few exceptions, the incidence of fighting within most mammalian species is much greater among the males. It has also been demonstrated over and over again that the predominantly male hormone androgen plays a very significant role in determining this difference in aggressiveness between the sexes. If males are castrated, particularly if this is done early in life, the amount of aggression displayed is very significantly reduced. The experimental evidence seems very clear on this point and indeed castration has been used for a very long time as a means of making animals more manageable. (Except for those kept intact for breeding purposes, stallions and bulls are almost always castrated.) Castration of humans was practiced by early Assyrians, Chinese, Hindus, Egyptians, Greeks, Persians, and Romans for different reasons, including the control of prisoners, criminals, and slaves. Compulsory castration had been legal up to relatively recent times in several of the United States and it is still practiced under certain conditions in other countries including Switzerland and Denmark. In spite of the fact that most reviews of the human cases conclude that castration leads to a "general pacification" of behavior, we would not expect to have many people seriously suggest that it is a practical means of reducing human aggression on a large scale. The disadvantages of other methods of controlling aggression may be equally severe, but because they may not be as obvious as those produced by castration, they are usually overlooked.

The studies of aggression and brain chemistry also illustrate the difficulty of the task of trying to reduce aggression without interfering with other behavior. There are, for example, a number of investigators who are studying the role of the relationship between neurotransmitter levels in the brain and aggression. Drs. Bruce and Annemarie Welch of the Maryland Psychiatric

Research Center in Baltimore used the aggressive behavior of mice as an experimental model in their studies.
They took advantage of the fact that male mice which
have been isolated for a period have a great tendency to
aggress against and even kill other mice if they are placed
together. The Welches are able to modify this enhanced
tendency toward aggression by pharmacologically interfering with the synthesis of the neurotransmitters
classifed as biogenic amines (norepinephrine, dopamine,
and serotonin), but they concluded that this is accomplished by changing the excitability of the nervous system
to many stimuli. In other words, although aggression can
be reduced by pharmacological treatment, the effects are
not restricted to aggressive behavior—the animals are less
responsive in general and have been described as "neu-
rologically numb." A similar conclusion was reached
following a recent review of the role of neurotransmitters
in aggressive behavior by Dr. Donald Reis of the Cornell
University Medical College. Reis summarizes the
literature as follows:

"There are two broad conclusions to be made. First, it
appears that no single putative transmitter serves as the
unique codon for aggression. Several and possibly all neurotransmitters appear to interact in this complex behavior. . . . Second, the behavioral action of the various
neural transmitters is not uniquely limited to aggression.
Each of these agents has been considered to participate in
other behaviors as well."

There are other complications with pharmacological
manipulations. The effect of any drug can vary enormously in different individuals. Alcohol will put one
person to sleep and make another aggressive, while a third
person may become the "life of the party." Similarly,
amphetamine may be a stimulant for one individual, it
may help a depressed person to get sleep, and it is

prescribed as a means to reduce hyperactivity in others. Dr. Jonathan Cole of the National Institutes of Health commented: "Even if one were only attempting to control the mind of a homogeneous group of psychiatric patients with a drug with which one had considerable experience, the desired effect would not be produced in all patients, and one would not be able to plan specifically that any particular effect would be produced in a particular patient." This variability in response may be caused by differences in sensitivity to drugs. It is well known that a given dose of a drug may be high for one individual and low for another even when body weight is taken into consideration. This factor is only partly responsible for the difference in drug reaction. Equally important is the fact that even when the same physiological change is produced by a drug, the changes in behavior may be very different because of many other response tendencies that influence the manner in which the changes are expressed. A drug that might speed up mental processes could lead to increased productivity in one person while producing an increase in frustration and aggression in another and an exacerbation of anxiety in a third.

It has been argued that much more specific effects could be obtained if pharmacological agents could be applied directly to critical brain sites. The administration through more common routes (mouth and injections) results in the drug affecting many areas and producing numerous "side effects." The hope is that more precise control could be exerted by the direct application of a drug to a discrete brain site. Is there any place in the brain where a drug will have a precise control over aggression? Unfortunately, the answer seems to be clearly, *No!* The brain is simply not organized so that all of one function is localized in one area. As already noted, even though aggressive behavior can be triggered by electrical stimulation of some areas of the hypothalamus, the destruction of these areas does not change the normal aggressive responses of animals to those stimuli which provoke them in natural settings. There is no reason to believe that the results would be any different following chemical manipulations of discrete areas. Furthermore, it is unlikely that the brain is organized into systems that fit our labels. There are probably no neural circuits that are exclusively involved with the regulation of aggression. Responses that are part of aggressive behavior in one setting may be incorporated into sexual behavior under other conditions. For all of these reasons, it has to be considered highly unlikely that a drug modifying neural activity at a specific brain site would be very effective in eliminating aggression and no other behavior.

TEMPORAL LOBE STRUCTURES: SEXUALITY, AGGRESSION, AND OTHER BEHAVIORS

One region of the brain that has been consistently implicated in aggression and sexual behavior is the temporal lobe. Structures lying beneath the cerebral cortex in the temporal lobe, particularly the amygdala and hippocampus, seem to be critically involved in the regulation of emotionality (see Figures 24, 25 and 26). The amygdala and hippocampus are important structures in the limbic system, which, in conjunction with the hypothalamus, form a circuit modulating biologically significant behaviors involved in what one whimsical neurophysiologist referred to as the four F's—feeding, fighting, fleeing, and sexual behavior. There exist a number of reports that stimulation or destruction of this circuit can produce dramatic changes in the expression of emotionality (see pages 47–50).

As long ago as 1937, Drs. Heinrich Klüver and Paul Bucy of the University of Chicago reported striking changes in the behavior of rhesus monkeys following extensive bilateral damage to the temporal lobes. Among

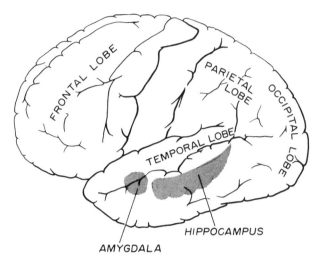

Figure 24. A side view of the human brain illustrating the position of the temporal lobe. The approximate location of the amygadala and hippocampus below the surface of the cerebral cortex in the temporal lobe is indicated.

the changes described were dramatic increases in sexual activity, a pronounced taming, an orality manifested as a compulsive tendency to place objects in the mouth, and a difficulty in recognizing objects presented visually. The monkeys would attempt to copulate with a great variety of inappropriate partners, including members of different species such as the experimenters. Normally rhesus monkeys are difficult to handle in the laboratory; they are usually very aggressive and intimidating, except when a special effort is made to tame them when they are young. Following the temporal lobe operations, the monkeys became much more gentle and could be handled more easily. In one motion picture record of the postoperative behavior, a rhesus monkey is shown sitting peacefully on Dr. Klüver's shoulder, but it soon shifted to a position at the back of his neck where it proceeded to engage in pelvic thrusts of a sexual nature. The compulsive orality has also been recorded in a film depicting a monkey continuously placing objects in its mouth, including a lit cigarette which it quickly threw down after being burned, only to pick it up and place it in its mouth once again.

The dramatic changes in the behavior of the monkeys with temporal lobectomies induced other researchers to pursue these studies further. Drs. Leon Schreiner and Arthur Kling, who were at the Walter Reed Institute of Research in the early 1950s, were able to replicate most of the Klüver-Bucy syndrome in several species by destruction of the amygdala and overlying cortex.[9] In one report, a hypersexual male cat was observed attempting to copu-

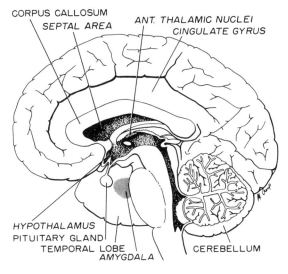

Figure 25. A "sagittal" view of the human brain as it would appear if the brain was sliced in the midline to separate the left and right halves. The structures depicted that are included in the limbic system are the amygdala, septal area, cingulate gyrus, and anterior thalamic nuclei. The amygdala is below the surface and not visible unless some of the cerebral cortex is removed. The hippocampus, which is an important part of the limbic system, cannot be shown in this view (see Figure 24). The hypothalamus, which is located at the base of the brain just above the pituitary gland, has many connections with limbic structures.

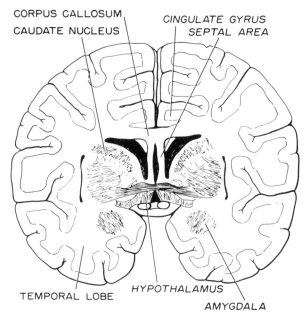

CORPUS CALLOSUM
CAUDATE NUCLEUS
CINGULATE GYRUS
SEPTAL AREA
TEMPORAL LOBE
HYPOTHALAMUS
AMYGDALA

Figure 26.   A "frontal" section (approximately parallel to the face) of the human brain. In this view one can see the position of the septal area and the caudate nucleus.

late with a dog, chicken, and small monkey (see Figure 27). Similar results were reported to have been observed in other animal species.[10] Schreiner and Kling also noted a striking taming effect produced by these brain ablations. The lynx, a wildcat which some regard as untamable, could be fed by hand after surgery. The ill-tempered South American rodent the agouti also became more manageable following this surgical procedure.

Dr. James Woods reported a very striking example of postoperative "taming" in wild Norway (Baltimore sewer) rats. These normally fierce and aggressive rats will kill laboratory mice at the slightest provocation and will escape if given any opportunity at all. It is necessary to handle these animals with heavy gloves to avoid serious injury. Even after many months in the laboratory the aggressiveness of these animals is not diminished. Following amygdalectomy, the majority (31 out of 42) of the wild rats became tame almost immediately and seemed to remain so for long periods. These formerly vicious rats no longer attempted to bite Dr. Woods or kill mice, and they could be carried around for hours in the pocket of his laboratory coat.

Rather than classifying the behavior changes observed after amygdalectomy in categories such as aggression and sexual it should be recognized that the changes observed following temporal lobe operations in animals represent adjustments to more primary deficits produced by the

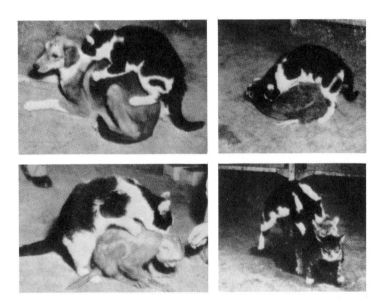

Figure 27. Hypersexuality in a male cat following bilateral destruction of temporal lobe structures. The cat is engaged in sexual mounts including the characteristic "neck bites" with a dog, chicken, and monkey. The lower right photograph illustrates "tandem copulation" among four male preparations. (From L. Schreiner and A. Kling, *Journal of Neurophysiology*, 1953, Vol. 16, p.653.)

brain damage. The results of a number of studies suggest that amygdalectomy often produces a decrease in emotional responsiveness partly reflecting an inability to relate visual information to past experience. The amygdalectomized animal is less able to distinguish the familiar from the novel, and this primary deficit may affect behavior in various ways depending on the particular circumstances. Some of the hypersexuality observed may result from the absence of inhibition that would normally be produced by confrontation with unfamiliar animals or environmental circumstances. Males of most mammalian species do not engage in sexual behavior until they have explored their physical surroundings thoroughly. The male animals with temporal lobe damage seem to require less time to habituate to novelty and as a result engage in sexual behavior even in a strange environment. This tendency may not be the entire explanation of the behavior seen following amygdalectomy, but it certainly exaggerates the impression of hypersexuality. Dr. John Green and his associates at the University of California in Los Angeles observed that even unoperated "Hollywood cats" may appear to be hypersexual under certain conditions. If, for example, unoperated male cats are placed together in a testing arena, where they have been completely habituated and have learned to anticipate sexual opportunity, they often mount each other in a tandem manner much as the operated cats seen in Figure 27. The changes produced by the surgery may have a direct influence on the course of habituation to novel stimuli and only an indirect influence on sexual behavior.

The reduction in aggression following various temporal lobe operations may also be secondary to changes of a much more basic nature. For example, Dr. Pierre Karli of the Institute of Biological Medicine in Strasbourg reported that electrolytic lesions of the amygdala abolished the tendency of aggressive rats to kill mice, but at the same time there was a marked decrease in responsiveness to most stimuli that normally evoke emotional reactions. Drs. D. Caroline and Robert Blanchard of the University of Hawaii recently reported that amygdalectomized rats do not display the normal emotional ("freezing") response to an immobilized cat placed in their cage. In fact, the amygdalectomized rat frequently made contact with the cat and even climbed all over its back.

In other experiments by Dr. Jerome Schwartzbaum, now at the University of Rochester, it was reported that monkeys with damage to portions of the amygdala exhibit little of the "elation" normal monkeys display when surprised by a special food treat. The temporal lobe operated animals are relatively indifferent to changes in the magnitude or quality of the reward and in this respect seem to be emotionally flat. It is almost as though the operated animals do not adequately identify the rewards; therefore they are less responsive to change and to novelty. Most likely for similar reasons, Dr. Bennett Galef found that amygdalectomy reduces the extreme wariness wild rats exhibit to novel foods or even new food containers. Normally wild rats are very slow to try any new food—that is why they are so difficult to poison—but following amygdalectomy this "timidity" is significantly diminished.

The difficulty in predicting an animal's behavior following amygdalectomy is partly related to the fact that the changes may be situationally dependent. For example, Drs. Haldor Rosvold, Karl Pribram, and Allan Mirsky noted that following amygdalectomy, individually caged monkeys often exhibit a decreasing fear toward the human observer, but in a social group they generally become less dominant, although individual animals may become more dominant and aggressive. The observed postoperative changes in the dominance hierarchy seemed to depend more on the previous pattern of social interactions and the length of time the relationships existed than on either the locus or extent of the destroyed tissue.

Somewhat similar conclusions were drawn by Dr. Elzbieta Fonberg of the Nencki Institute in Warsaw. She observed that following amygdalectomy the dogs "seem to be placid and quiet, but at the same time some of them were more irritable and aggressive toward other dogs." Following an additional study Dr. Mirsky hypothesized that the amygdala lesions in monkeys weakened "previously learned connections between complex social stimuli and socioemotional responses." The amygdalectomized monkeys respond directly and fearlessly to the offer of food and seem to have lost their learned fear of humans. In a social situation, other monkeys appear to sense the operated animal's hesitancy and uncertainty, and according to their own pattern of social interaction they may attempt to dominate a previously dominant animal. The operated animals must go through a social relearning process during which they may become more or less dominant, depending on the nature of the animals with which they interact.

Dr. Arthur Kling, who is presently affiliated with the Rutgers Medical School, has continued his interest in the effects of temporal lobe operations by studying monkeys under natural conditions. Field studies of the free-ranging vervet (African green monkey) were conducted along the Zambesi River in Africa several miles from Livingstone in Zambia by Dr. Kling in collaboration with Jane Lancaster and Jerry Benitone. In other investigations, animals were studied on Cayo Santiago (a 39-acre island off the coast of Puerto Rico), where over 900 rhesus monkeys roam freely in seven well-defined social groups. Monkeys whose behavior had been observed in their natural living conditions were trapped in order to perform surgery. Following amygdalectomy the animals were tested in a field laboratory and then released back to their monkey troupe. Several unoperated animals served as controls for the effect of capture, caging, and release. Generally the monkeys were judged postoperatively to be less aggressive and more friendly to the human observers, but after the animals were released a very different impression was formed by members of their troupe. The operated animals responded very inappropriately and acted as though they did not comprehend the significance of gestures from other monkeys. Rather than exhibiting increased friendliness, as they did to their human captors, these operated animals appeared confused and more fearful when returned to their natural group. The complexities of the life in the field seemed too much for them and they were unable to cope successfully. Even when approached in a neutral way by other monkeys, the operated animals responded by escaping from tree to tree. On occasion they responded to a threatening gesture from a very dominant male by displaying outrageous "insubordination"—they attacked and the result was inevitable. In a variety of different situations, all seemingly related to the amygdalectomized animals' difficulty in comprehending communication signals, they all became social isolates. Eventually all the isolated animals died of starvation or were killed by predators.

A similar behavior change was reported by Drs. Leopold Hofstatter and Makram Girgis of the Missouri Institute of Psychiatry in St. Louis. These neuropsychiatrists described the behavior changes seen in amygdalectomized squirrel monkeys. Although these small South American monkeys were not studied in the wild, they could be observed in social observation rooms containing a number of animals. Postoperatively, the amygdalectomized squirrel monkeys became uninterested in social interactions, generally avoiding other monkeys and displaying a tendency to retreat to the highest point in the observation room. Another illustration of the importance of situational factors in determining the postoperative behavior that is expressed can be noted in the fact that neither Kling nor Hofstatter and Girgis observed any of the hypersexuality reported by investigators studying amygdalectomized animals under the more traditional laboratory conditions.

The great variety of ritualized gestures that play such an important role in primate social behavior has been well documented by Dr. Jane Van Lawick-Goodall's classic study of the wild chimpanzee in the Gombe Reserve in Tanzania. Familiarity with the gestures of primates makes it apparent that any animal that lost the capacity to comprehend this form of communication would not be able to live within the group. For example, among the several gestures used by a dominant chimpanzee to reassure a submissive animal that no harm is intended is a pat on the head. The following encounter is described by Dr. Van Lawick-Goodall:

"An adolescent male (Pepe) approached a mature male (Goliath) who was feeding on bananas. Pepe crouched and wimpered, looking at Goliath, and meekly extended his hand. Goliath patted Pepe, and Pepe slowly reached for a banana, but pulled back screaming in fear. Goliath patted him again and finally Pepe gathered a few bananas and hastily retreated."

It has become increasingly clear that it is a mistake to attempt to characterize the changes following these temporal lobe operations by reference to broad and complex behavior categories such as sexuality and aggressivity. Although some of the discrepancies in experimental results might be resolved by more attention to anatomical details and the idiosyncracies of the behavioral situation, it is clear that it will be necessary to describe the deficits in terms of more unitary concepts than sexuality and aggressions. As already noted, there is evidence accumulating that some of the temporal lobe operations produce a deficiency in the animals' ability to respond appropriately to visual stimuli. Consistent with this evidence is information obtained originally by Dr. Kao Chow and later extended by Dr. Mortimer Mishkin and others that the temporal lobe contains a region that is involved in processing visual information. In their initial observations, Klüver and Bucy had noted that their operated animals failed to distinguish between edible and inedible objects and they also observed that the operated monkeys would freely manipulate snakes as though not recognizing them. Normally snakes are very fear provoking for monkeys. Klüver and Bucy labeled this type of postoperative change *psychic blindness*.[11] Other behavioral changes may also be related to this inability to relate visual information to past experience. For example, the postoperative hypersexuality that has been reported was based in part on the observation that animals failed to distinguish between appropriate and inappropriate sexual partners. Dr. Kling noted that amygdalectomized female monkeys that gave birth mishandle their young and behave "as though the infant was a strange object to be mouthed, bitten and tossed around as though it were a rubber ball."

A remarkable demonstration of the changes in behavior that may result from a deficit in visual recognition comes from the studies of Dr. John Downer of University College in London. Downer cut the major fiber bundles that connect one side of the brain to the other. (This includes the corpus callosum and the anterior, posterior, and hippocampal commissures.) Also cut was the optic chiasma, so that visual information received by one eye projected only to the same side of the brain rather than to both sides. An amygdalectomy was then performed only on one side with the consequence that past associations to visual sensations were disconnected only when information was received by one of the eyes. Downer describes the dramatic postoperative behavior of this rhesus monkey:

"Following this operation, the animal appeared to be as wild and intractable as in its preoperative state when observed with both of its eyes open. At the sight of an observer, it would grimace, bare its teeth, and jump to the front of the cage, attempting to bite and claw. Closing the eye projecting to the side of the amygdalectomy did not produce any observable change. However, opening the eye projecting to the side of the amygdalectomy and closing the other eye produced a dramatic change in behavior. The animal then showed no signs of aggression or fear at the sight of human observers and would approach the front of the cage and take proferred raisins quite peacefully. . . .

"This placidity occurred only in response to visual stimuli; touching or prodding the animal's arm would produce a momentary aggressive reaction. The placid response to visual stimuli promptly disappeared when the eye projecting to the side of the amygdalectomy was shut and the other eye opened. These alternations in emotional behavior were observed over a period of three months and appeared to persist without abatement. In effect, it seemed that one could "remove" and "replace" the amygdala, merely by opening and closing the appropriate eyes." (Downer, 1962, pages 99-100)

It should be apparent that the changes that follow amygdalectomy can be very unpredictable and far reaching. Characterizing the total effects of these operations by such phrases as "taming" and "hypersexuality" can be very misleading. Often the observations that have led to the use of such labels were limited to the restricted conditions of the laboratory or hospital. More extensive observations have made it clear that very different and even opposite behavior changes can be expressed under other circumstances. The primary changes produced by these temporal lobe operations in animals may have little to do with the regulation of aggression and sexuality. Certainly the changes can affect behavior that would not be thought of as aggressive or sexual. It would be very surprising indeed if the brain were organized into spatially discrete units that conform to our abstract categorizations of behavior. Armed with this perspective and a few experimental facts, it is now possible to discuss some of the clinical and social ramifications of different brain manipulations.

Part II: Clinical and Social Applications

Therapeutic Applications of Brain Stimulation

ELECTROCONVULSIVE TREATMENT

There are very ancient roots to the belief that massive excitation or exposure to stress may cure the mentally deranged. Many observations illustrated that sudden traumatic events could cure, as well as cause, insanity. It was only natural that attempts would be made to produce the trauma rather than rely on the occurrence of accidents. What was essential was to get the mental patient off "dead center" and somehow force his body and psyche to mobilize its defenses. It was even thought that exposure to snakes or dunking in cold water might be helpful. As the English physician Joseph Mason Cox wrote in his 1804 essay *Practical Observations on Insanity*:

"It is evident that any considerable excitation, some new and violent action provoked in the course of the manic disease, often has the effect of considerably alleviating the mental disorder or of permanently improving it."

Electroshock treatment is a direct descendant of this view.

147

A consideration of electroshock is useful at this juncture not only because it provides an introduction to the topic of implanted electrodes and brain stimulation, but because it also brings into relief some of the difficulty in establishing ethical codes to control experimentation on humans. In the minds of many people, electroshock treatment characterizes most vividly the primitive, if not cruel state of physical approaches to psychiatric problems. To induce convulsions by passing an electric current through the brain conjures up images of "electric chairs" and medieval tortures. In Ken Kesey's novel *One Flew Over the Cuckoo's Nest,* there is a very dramatic representation of electroshock as a device to control and punish patients, having no therapeutic value. The novel may be an effective allegory for attacking authoritarianism, but it certainly does not present electroshock treatment accurately. Very many psychiatrists agree that this treatment can have very beneficial effects on some patients, particularly the severely depressed, and they consider it a valuable psychiatric tool. A challenging thought for those concerned with protecting patients without blocking progress, however, is that even now there is no general agreement on how electroshock works and certainly it would have been very difficult to present a defensible rationale for its use during the initial experimentation. Although it may have been possible to use animals to test the safety of electroshock, it would have been very difficult to test its effectiveness.

Electroshock treatment should be viewed as one of many methods for inducing convulsions or great stress to the nervous system in the hope that it would trigger off a therapeutically useful reaction. Even before electroshock was used, convulsions were induced by injections of insulin and drugs such as metrazol. Inhalation of high concentrations of either nitrogen or carbon dioxide has also been used as a means of producing coma, asphyxia, and radical alterations in the activity of the nervous system. Although a specific physiological mechanism has been claimed for each of these therapeutic methods, they all have a common link to those very early ideas that any stress may have beneficial effects on mental disorders. To induce stress, mental patients in the past were immersed in cold water, injected with smallpox or even horse serum, and subjected to skin wounds or infections produced by various irritants. Somewhat later, but based upon similar reasoning, treatment of psychiatric patients was attempted by introducing malaria, typhoid fever, and other heat-producing agents.

As early as 1785, Dr. W. Oliver published an account of the effects of administering camphor in a case of insanity. Camphor, which is extracted from a particular type of laurel tree, has been used for centuries in China and Japan as a heart stimulant as well as for other medical purposes. In higher doses, camphor has cataleptic (seizure inducing) properties. Dr. Oliver, who was "physician extraordinary to his Royal Highness, the Prince of Wales" had under his care a patient who was despondent, hypochondriacal, "seized with mania . . . and with very few intervals of reason." Apparently some knowledge of the medicinal properties of camphor had reached London at this time, and Dr. Oliver was motivated to give it a trial. The camphor was given by mouth and the patient became very sick and pale and had to be carried to bed. Dr. Oliver's description of the events that followed and his speculations make fascinating reading:

". . . his senses returned to him, and something like a flash of lightning, he said, preceded their return. He now quitted his confinement, and trials were made of his behavior in various companies, at different houses. Parties were formed for him, at his own house; he became natural, easy, polite, and in every respect like himself, and played his game at whist, with great accuracy . . ."

The patient became melancholic again and the camphor treatment was repeated, following which he became "cheerful, rational, and minutely descriptive of all the places he passed through; he ate and drank with appetite." The patient reverted later to a deep depression, but Dr. Oliver concludes:

"It is observable in this case, that both in the year 1781 and 1783, upon the exhibition of camphor in the dose of one scruple[12] each time, a change was worked on the sensorium commune, and that the rational faculties each time returned.

"I cannot help lamenting my not having had an opportunity of repeating this medicine, in the same dose of a scruple; as I think there is good foundation to suppose, that what had effected so considerable a change, might by proper repetition, (the patient's strength admitting of it) render that change permanent."

Apparently interest in the camphor treatment continued for a while; in his 1828 *Commentaries on the Causes, Forms, Symptoms and Treatment, Moral or Medical of Insanity,* Dr. G. Burrows of London wrote: "In a case of insanity in which two scruples [of camphorated oil] were applied, a convulsive seizure was produced, and a complete cure followed." In the 1930s, Dr. Laszlo Meduna, who was working at that time in the Brain Research Institute in Budapest, revised the camphor convulsive treatment. Initially he used intramuscular injections of camphor oil, but it was later found that intravenous injections of metrazol (a soluble component of the synthetic camphor preparation) could produce more reliable convulsions. About the same time, other methods for producing convulsions, such as those induced by the hypoglycemic coma that followed insulin injections, were described by Dr. Manfred Sakel, who began his investigations in Vienna, continued them in Berlin, and after 1936 practiced them in New York. Several other methods for inducing convulsions were tried. For example, during the late 1930s and throughout the 1940s the breathing of high percentages of carbon dioxide was used to induce seizures, which were often accompanied by rich sensory experiences and hallucinations.

Although it has not always been explicitly verbalized, there seems to have been a general acceptance of the idea that a strong challenge or stress to the body elicits a protective physiological reaction that could have a beneficial effect on mental state. There was a recognition, at some level of awareness, that at the root of schizophrenia and also depression was a deficiency in responsiveness—an inability to mobilize energy and defenses to cope with the problems of everyday life. By forcing a reaction to a great physical stress, it is possible that the body's coping responses could be made more responsive in general.[13]

Many of the explicit attempts to explain the mechanisms responsible for the therapeutic value of convulsive therapies involved the *autonomic nervous system.* This part of the nervous system, which regulates the visceral organs, glands, and certain smooth muscles (such as those controlling pupil diameter), is usually divided into a *sympathetic* and *parasympathetic* branch. Sympathetic responses predominate during physical emergency situations and also during less extreme circumstances—when it may be necessary to cope with situations that are perceived as psychological stresses or challenges, such as job interviews and examinations. The parasympathetic branch is internally oriented and dominates during bodily restorative functions such as digestion and sleep. On the basis of this distinction, many of the responses of the viscera and glands are quite predictable—sympathetic discharge results in acceleration of the heart rate, secretion of adrenalin, vascular changes that bring extra blood to the skeletal muscles, mobilization of sugar reserves, and many other physiological reactions. Parasympathetic responses are just the opposite, producing a slowing of the heart and so forth. Even though most responses of the autonomic nervous system involve an organized pattern that combines both sympathetic and parasympathetic components, it may be useful to think of a relative dominance in a given situation or even of a general response tendency of an individual.

Although the autonomic nervous system is heavily represented in parts of the spinal cord and the brain stem, the highest integrating level is believed to occur in the hypothalamus. Dr. Ernest Gellhorn, who studied the physiology of the autonomic nervous system for many years at his University of Minnesota laboratory, proposed the existence of a *hypothalamic tuning,* which produced a predisposition to react with a predominance of either sympathetic or parasympathetic responses. According to this view, the relative dominance of one of these two systems determines much of our psychological and physiological reactions. It predisposes us to respond mentally and bodily in certain ways just as our state when walking alone through a graveyard late at night may determine our response to any stimulus. In general, Gellhorn found sympathetic responses to be regulated in the posterior hypothalamus, whereas parasympathetic responses were controlled by more anterior hypothalamic regions. (These findings closely paralleled those of Walter Hess' division of the hypothalamus into ergotropic and trophotropic regions; see page 29.)

Gellhorn studied individual differences in responsiveness of the systems regulating secretion of adrenalin, blood vessel constriction and dilation, sweating, blood sugar responses, and other reactions regulated by the autonomic nervous system in animals and man. He reported that the responsiveness of the hypothalamic centers controlling sympathetic responses was decreased in schizophrenics. Typical of these findings were reports that schizophrenics did not exhibit the normal responses to cold or that their blood sugar levels did not rise to the same extent as normals during emotional excitement.

Dr. Gellhorn maintained, as have others, that the hypothalamus not only has a so-called "downward discharge" regulating bodily responses, but it also has an "upward discharge" capable of modulating activity in the cerebral cortex. These two discharge pathways were responsible for the consistency between bodily and mental states. The idea that the different convulsive therapies produced a persisting increase in the responsiveness of the sympathetic system—although not necessarily by the same mechanism—was advanced by Dr. Gellhorn and many of the clinicians applying these treatments.

The theoretical ideas we have been describing were generally advanced to explain the therapeutic value of the convulsive treatments, but the initial experimentation generally had much more empirical roots. Dr. H. Steck, who directed a psychiatric institute in Switzerland, noticed, for example, that the insulin he administered to increase the appetite of his patients seemed to improve their mental state. Dr. Manfred Sakel had been experimenting with insulin injections in morphine-addicted patients as a means of decreasing the excitement following the withdrawal of this drug. The hypoglycemic (low blood sugar) state induced by the insulin accidentally reached a level that precipitated a coma:

"I thought first of all, that insulin abolished the phenomena of irritation during abstinence from morphine because the nerve cells were blocked [by the hypoglycemia] and their function quantitatively affected. . . . At this point, as so often happens in such matters, I was helped by chance. By chance I produced deeper hypoglycemic reactions than I had intended. I was able then to observe that such reactions led to much quicker and more substantial alterations in mental states, and could even cause psychotic symptoms to disappear." (1938)

Later, as Sakel became very concerned with the question of priority of discovery, he preferred to describe the origin of the insulin treatment as more planned:

"I started my experiments with the idea that the key to combat mental disease lay in the discovery of a physiological approach to influence the center of the autonomic nervous system, the hypothalamus, which appeared to be the bridge between physiological functions and mental manifestations." (1956)

Since the insulin coma treatment ("Sakel shock treatment") has been almost completely replaced by the more convenient electroshock technique, it would be easy for anyone not familiar with this part of psychiatric history to form the impression that this treatment was a curious, but insignificant, phenomenon. Actually, by 1938 the method had spread throughout all of Europe (including the Soviet Union) as well as Japan, the United States, and Canada. Sakel was asked by the New York Commissioner of Mental Hygiene to teach a six-week full-time course in his technique to 40 staff physicians from mental hospitals throughout the United States and Canada. The technique spread to almost all psychiatric institutions and was used extensively. I can remember that as a student I visited a large ward in the Veterans Hospital in Topeka, Kansas, where 30 patients were writhing and moaning in an insulin coma—like some nightmarish Doré illustration of Hell for Dante's *Divine Comedy*. Despite the negative reaction that might be provoked by such scenes, the results were generally considered to be as therapeutically useful as are those currently obtained with electroshock.

The rationale for the metrazol convulsive treatment developed by Dr. Meduna was based on information suggesting that there was an interaction between the schizophrenic and epileptic processes. Data were presented by several investigators indicating that the correlation of epilepsy and schizophrenia was unusually low and that when they were found together in the same patient the occurrence of an epileptic seizure appeared to reduce the schizophrenic symptoms. Meduna concluded:

"Between schizophrenia and epilepsy there exists a sort of biological antagonism which must be expressed in the pathological course of the two diseases. Without being able to characterize these pathological actions, I feel justified in asserting a priority that these courses are either mutually exclusive or they do, at least to a certain degree, weaken each other in their mutual effects." (1938)

The evidence could hardly be regarded as convincing, since statistics compiled by Hoch (1943, 1961) suggest that the two diseases are independent. Although there is little interest in the question at this time, evidence is still occasionally presented on both sides of this issue. In any case, convulsive treatments have proven most effective in the manic-depressive disorders rather than schizophrenia. At the time, however, the general acceptance of the view that schizophrenia was a progressive and degenerative disease provided considerable justification for undertaking "heroic" efforts to counteract this process. It should not be assumed that Meduna was completely naive about many of the qualifications which all present-day psychiatrists would undoubtedly make. For example, he wrote:

"I am well aware that just as there are several kinds of epilepsy, so also schizophrenia may take numerous forms. . . . I should also like to mention that this treatment of schizophrenia cannot effect a complete cure. For schizophrenia presents a psychic disorder based on a pathophysiological foundation, and, therefore, we must not only influence the biological patterns but must also seek to help the patient along psychological lines."

Dr. Ugo Cerletti, the Italian psychiatrist who is generally acknowledged as having introduced electroshock therapy, had also been concerned with epilepsy. Initially he was interested in developing an animal model of human epilepsy and believed that electric shock might be more convenient than drugs if he was to produce seizures repeatedly in the same subject. There was considerable concern with the safety of this method, since it was commonly believed that hogs were killed by electric current in the slaughterhouse of Rome:

"I went to the slaughterhouse to observe this so-called 'electric slaughtering' and I saw that the hogs were clamped at the temples with big metallic tongs which were hooked up to an electric current. As soon as the hogs were clamped by the tongs, they fell unconscious in the same way as our experimental dogs. During this period of unconsciousness (epileptic coma), the butcher stabbed and bled the animals without difficulty. Therefore, it was not true that the animals were killed by the electric current: the latter was used at the suggestion of the Society for the Prevention of Cruelty to Animals so that the hogs might be killed painlessly."

Up to this time, Cerletti had been avoiding shocking his dogs on the skull and had been attaching his electrodes to different parts of the body, usually the mouth and rectum. He was now encouraged to attach the electrodes directly to the head, to explore the effect of passing the current in different directions and to determine the safe current intensity and duration. It was determined that a few tenths of a second application was harmless, but if the current was of sufficient strength it produced full *tonic-clonic* seizures.[14]

About this time Cerletti became aware of Meduna's theories concerning the possible antagonism between schizophrenia and epilepsy; he now felt his electroshock technique was safe, and he decided to experiment on man. Shortly afterwards the Police Commissioner of Rome sent a man, who was wandering around confused in the train station, to Cerletti for referral. He was diagnosed as schizophrenic because the psychiatric examination revealed the presence of hallucinations, incomprehensible speech studded with neologisms, and inappropriate and paranoid thoughts. The patient was prepared for the electroshock and as soon as the current was applied, his body jolted and stiffened, and he fell back into the bed without losing consciousness and started to sing loudly. It was clear that the voltage was too low, so it was decided to repeat the shock the next day after the patient had some rest. The patient had evidently heard all this for he said clearly: "Not another one! It's deadly!" Since these were the only words that the patient had uttered which were not gibberish, Dr. Cerletti was motivated to try again immediately with higher current:

"We observed the same instantaneous, brief, generalized spasm, and soon after, the onset of the classic epileptic convulsion. We were all breathless during the tonic phase of the attack, and really overwhelmed during the apnea as we watched the cadaverous cyanosis of the patient's face; the apnea of the spontaneous epileptic con-vulsion is always impressive, but at that moment it seemed to all of us painfully endless. Finally, with the first stertorous breathing and the first clonic spasm, the blood flowed better not only in the patient's vessels but also in our own. Thereupon we observed with the most intensely gratifying sensation the characteristic gradual awaking of the patient 'by steps.' He rose to sitting position and looked at us, calm and smiling, as though to inquire what we wanted of him. We asked: 'What happened to you?' He answered: 'I don't know. Maybe I was asleep.' Thus occurred the first electrically produced convulsion in man, which I at once named 'electroshock.' ''

It seemed clear to all of these early investigators, regardless of what other speculations they may have expressed, that these various convulsive therapies were initiating some biochemical changes in the brain. Cerletti, for example, became convinced that electroshock was releasing some "highly vitalizing substances with defensive properties" to which he gave the name acroagonines (*akros*—extreme or supreme; *agon*—struggle or defense). To test his theory, Cerletti obtained a suspension of the homogenate of brains of pigs shocked repeatedly and injected this into psychiatric patients. The patients became somnolent (in one case after three days of treatment, the patient slept for four days) and changes in disposition were reported. None of these results occurred if a suspension of nonshocked pig brains was used. Although little credence is given to this evidence today, several contemporaries of Cerletti reported similar results. Dr. Alves Garcia treated more than 100 psychiatric patients in Rio de Janeiro with a suspension of brains from shocked guinea pigs and reported similar affects on sleep. One psychiatrist claimed favorable results on nonshocked mental patients following injection of serum obtained from patients who had received electroshock. Other investigators used animal recipients as well as donors and claimed that they obtained evidence that injections from repeatedly shocked animals protected recipients against normally fatal diseases such as rabies.

Electroshock treatment, as crude and poorly understood as it is, continues to be used as an effective tool in combating depression. Although the existence of anti-depressant and phenothiazine (major tranquilizers) drugs have narrowed the use of electroconvulsive treatment, there are still cases that respond only to the latter treatment. In severe depression, quick action is important since suicide is often a danger, and if the mental state is not altered the psychiatric problem may become intensified, imagined physical ailments may become real, and the patient's social and economic adjustment may be irreparably damaged. Electroshock, when effective, usually works faster than drugs and is generally considered safe. Following the introduction of short-acting muscle relaxants like succinylcholine, the danger of bone fractures from the clonic-flailing movements has been virtually eliminated. Using succinycholine, the only movements that occur are slow flexions of the plantar surface of the feet during the tonic phase and small movements in the toes, arms, and facial muscles during the clonic phase. For this reason as well as for public relations considerations, the word "shock" is no longer used. The risks are not great and most agree that the morphologic changes in the brains of shocked animals and humans claimed to have been observed in a few reports, if they occur at all, are reversible. There are clear memory losses for the events immediately surrounding the convulsions[15] and with a prolonged treatment series the memory loss commonly extends further and further back in time, so that patients sometimes become thoroughly confused about where they are and even their occupation. Most of the memories return within days or weeks, but some memory gaps persist for six months or longer and there may be permanent loss of recall of events that took place during the period of the treatment. Most clinicians believe, however, that most if not all memories return, but this point has not received the benefit of a large-scale, objective study. The point is difficult to investigate since those treated may be told—in one way or another—about events they cannot recall.

Although we have learned a great number of facts about the nervous system and electroconvulsive treatment since the early speculations on its mode of action, current theories are best classified as educated guesses. Present theories differ from those of the past mostly in detail rather than principles. We now know details about specific neurotransmitters such as their distribution in the brain and the behavior they tend to influence most. The distribution of the transmitter norepinephrine is particularly high in those regions of the limbic-hypothalamic circuit and brain stem that have been implicated in emotion. Drugs that interfere with the synthesis or action of norepinephrine decrease appetite and activity and also interfere with sleep—behaviors that are commonly disturbed in depression. The availability of norepinephrine may also influence the capacity to experience pleasure, as the results of experiments on animal self-stimulation seem to imply (see pages 43–44). A number of investigators have speculated recently that psychiatric depression may result from some deficiency in the neural circuits dependent on norepinephrine. In fact almost all mood-modifying drugs especially influence neural transmission dependent upon norepinephrine, although they may also modify the action of serotonin and dopamine, the other neurotransmitters classified as biogenic amines.

Among other effects that are produced by electroconvulsive treatment is an increase in secretion of epinephrine (adrenalin) and adrenocorticotropic hormone (ACTH). There are complex and only partially understood relationships between ACTH and epinephrine. It has been well established that the secretion of ACTH by the pituitary gland is regulated in the hypothalamus. ACTH stimulates the cortex of the adrenal gland to release adrenal corticoid hormones, which in turn trigger a number of physiological responses adaptive for meeting all types of stress. Among the physiological responses triggered by the adrenal corticoid hormones is the acceleration of the synthesis of epinephrine in another part (the medulla) of the adrenal gland. This may start a reaction that has some of the characteristics of an amplifying feedback loop because epinephrine's action on the hypothalamus results in a further increase in ACTH release. Furthermore, there is evidence that epinephrine may cause a release of norepinephrine. It is generally agreed, for example, that the synthetic substance amphetamine, which is structurally related to epinephrine, does produce a release of norepinephrine at nerve terminals.

The tentative picture that is emerging is that electroconvulsive treatment results in a partially escalating interaction between ACTH and epinephrine that serves to elevate either the production or utilization of those transmitter substances, particularly the biogenic amines, in the neural circuits regulating mood. Much of this story is still controversial and there are many important questions that remain unanswered. One can only guess, for example, why the physiological reactions produced by the treatment should persist long enough to have a meaningful influence on mood. Perhaps there may be one or more substances involved in the synthesis of the biogenic amine that must reach a critical level before the process can become self-sustaining. It is also possible that even a short-term elevation of mood enables the patient to restructure sufficiently the perception of his present situation and future prospects and that this cognitive reorientation has the capacity to generate physiological and psychological changes that may persist. The short-time memory losses and the confusion produced by the treatment may actually create a state of mind that makes it easier to become free of those ideational fixations that interfere with the restructuring of attitudes. In any event, most psychiatrists agree that electroconvulsive treatment may be very helpful in some cases, but they also recognize that the method has to be characterized as nonspecific if not crude. It is generally conceived of as stopgap method useful until that time when we become sophisticated enough to better characterize the physical changes accompanying mental disorders and to apply treatment that is more selective in its action.[16]

DIRECTED BRAIN STIMULATION: IMPLANTED ELECTRODES AND CANNULAE

Although many psychiatrists regard electroconvulsive treatment as a very useful therapeutic technique for some patients, it should not come as a surprise that there are many others who would characterize it as a crude, "electronic shotgun" assault on the entire brain. Obviously, it would be much better if some corrective influence could be applied directly to the brain area that is either responsible for the abnormal behavior or at least capable of counteracting the pathological emotional and cognitive condition of the psychiatric patient. It is this point of view that has encouraged a few investigators to implant electrodes and cannulae in patients and to explore the therapeutic value of applying either an electric current or drugs to specific brain areas.

Considering that the mere thought of having one's brain invaded by probing electrodes or cannulae arouses such strong emotional reactions from most people today, it might seem unlikely that these techniques could ever have an extensive impact on our society. Under appropriate circumstances, however, this attitude could be radically and rapidly changed. Even a casual inspection of history reveals that humans are quite capable of completely accepting customs that at other times were regarded as unnatural, immoral, and even repugnant. We have learned to accept such diverse medical procedures as psychoanalysis, tranquilizers, electroconvulsive therapy, radiation treatment, organ transplants, and cardiac pacemakers. The reports in the popular press describing the accelerating rate of scientific discoveries coupled with the increases in travel have conditioned people to be much more open to novelty and change. The great interest in acupuncture reflects the current readiness to accept "strange" techniques. If placing needles in the body can be accepted, why not acupuncture of the brain? Diagnostic procedures such as heart catheterization, some of which involve greater physical risks than electrode implantation, have been accepted for some time. If brain stimulation could be demonstrated to be safe and beneficial, it is conceivable that it would come to be regarded as routine as the use of tranquilizers and antidepressants.

In spite of the impressions of many people to the contrary, there have not been many attempts to use brain stimulation to induce some beneficial change in the psychiatric state of a patient. (This discounts any application of electrodes for diagnostic purposes such as those used to locate brain structures that might be destroyed in order to alleviate some symptoms. These applications will be discussed in subsequent chapters). It is not surprising that the numbers should be small since the use of brain stimulation to treat mental patients has very few supporters and there are many who vigorously oppose this work on both scientific and ethical grounds. Dr. Robert Heath of Tulane University pioneered this work, but even he has accumulated less than 70 cases. Since most of these cases were studied between 1950 and 1953, the rate of electrode implantation in the Neuropsychiatric Department he heads has actually been decreasing over the last 15 years.

To place these developments in historical perspective it should be recalled that when Heath began this work in 1950, the animal studies that led to the concepts of positive (pleasure) and negative (punishment) rewarding circuits in the brain had not yet been started (see pages 34–40). Heath's work was prompted by a disillusionment with the prefrontal lobotomy procedures and the growing acceptance of the theory that emotionality was regulated by the so-called limbic structures in the brain. Initiating his investigations with patients considered to be hopeless schizophrenics, Heath originally theorized that the core of the disorder was due to an inhibition of certain subcortical brain structures that resulted in a diminished awareness of the environment and a reduced capacity for experiencing emotion. He argued that these subcortical structures, especially the septal region, were responsible for emotional experience and that in schizophrenics the responsiveness of these structures was diminished, perhaps because of some suppressing influence of the neocortex. As described previously, Heath hoped that stimulation of the septal area might precipitate an excitatory reaction that would have beneficial consequences. The evidence implicating the septal area was more suggestive than convincing: it consisted primarily of an impression that the more successful lobotomies occurred in those cases where the brain damage encroached upon the septal area or adjacent structures. Heath also attached importance to some of his early animal experiments in which the destruction of the septal area in cats and monkeys produced some emotional changes. (Some of his animals displayed catatonic posturing following electrolytic lesions while others appeared highly aroused during stimulation of this brain region, a result diametrically opposite to that obtained by most subsequent investigators.) Basically, these animal experiments and the loosely formulated theory of schizophrenia provided the justification to determine whether patients considered to be hopeless schizophrenics could be improved if the neural circuits believed to be critically related to emotional expression were electrically stimulated.

Later, as patients began to report that brain stimulation evoked pleasurable sensations and animal behavior studies provided evidence that there were positive reward or "pleasure circuits" in the brain, other therapeutic possibilities were stressed. Heath's theoretical rationale for utilizing brain stimulation as a therapeutic instrument now emphasizes its potential for activating pleasurable reactions in his patients. In essence, Heath's arguments now seem to rest on the belief that in many psychiatric conditions the basic disorder is related to an *anhedonia,* that is, an inability to experience pleasure and the alerting and energizing influences that normally accompany pleasure. (The central role that Heath affords to pleasure reactions can be noted by his selection of *The Role of Pleasure in Behavior* as a title for one of the books he has edited.) Through the activation of the septal area by electrical stimulation, it was hoped that in some way the neural circuitry underlying the experience of pleasure would regain its normal responsiveness and as a result mood, energy level, and interest in the world would all improve. Recently, this hypothesis has been more explicitly expressed than it was during the period of Heath's initial explorations, as can be noted in his 1971 statement:

"If, we reasoned, the septal region of the schizophrenic patient was indeed functioning abnormally, then electrical stimulation (or perhaps another type of physiological intervention) at this site might correct the aberration and alleviate undesirable signs and symptoms. Specifically, on the basis of findings in *Macaca mulatta* monkeys, we postulated that the patient whose septal region was stimulated should become alert (i.e., come into contact with reality) and his anhedonia should be displaced by a feeling of pleasure."

Over the years, Heath has consistently attributed special significance to the septal area, and he frequently reported that specific electroencephalographic changes in this brain area were correlated with emotional experience. EEG changes consisting of high-amplitude spindling activity are said to appear in the septal area when the patient was experiencing pleasure whether it was produced

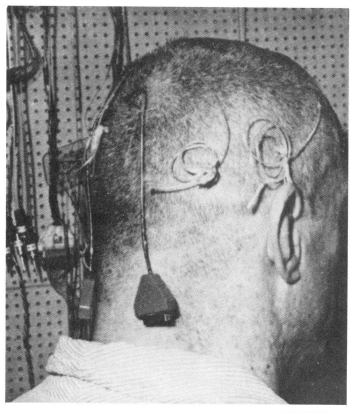

Figure 28. View of a patient's head prepared with deep and surface electrodes and cannulae. Ordinarily, a bandage would be worn around the head. (From R. G. Heath, Depth Recording and Stimulation Studies in Patients, A. Winter (Ed.), *The Surgical Control of Behavior*, 1971, Fig. 2-1. Courtesy of Charles C Thomas, Publisher, Springfield, Ill.)

by sexual orgasm, smoking marihuana, or other causes. Heath also maintains that he has seen "clear-cut physiologic abnormality in the form of spike or slow-wave activity, or both, in the rostral septal region concomitant with psychotic behavior." It is difficult to evaluate these reports since there is little corroborative evidence from other sources and it is well known that one can find support for any hypothesis in the reams of electroencephalographic data unless very careful controls are employed to minimize error due to a selection bias or a subjective interpretation of the records. Most investigators experienced with the electroencephalogram as a research instrument have been very skeptical of Heath's evidence and have argued that the data have not been subjected to sufficient statistical analyses to prove that electrical events in the septal area are uniquely correlated with either psychotic episodes or the experience of pleasure.

As experience with these techniques accumulated, it was noted that following stimulation of the septal area, the general mood of some patients seemed to improve for periods as long as several days. This effect seems to occur most dramatically with patients suffering from the intractable pain that sometimes accompanies terminal metastic carcinoma, but patients experiencing psychological pain caused by anxiety or depression also report the evocation of pleasurable sensations and an elevation in mood that persists beyond the stimulation period. It is said that epileptics also experience a strong pleasure response to septal area stimulation. Possibly of great theoretical significance is Heath's observation that stimulation evokes only a weak pleasure and alerting response of short duration in schizophrenic patients. (See page 173, for example, for a speculative linking of schizophrenia to a degenerated reward circuit in the brain.) This minimal response in schizophrenics convinced Dr. Heath to discontinue this program in these patients since there seem to be no beneficial effects of stimulation if a strong pleasure reaction cannot be evoked.

Those who seek to justify this work believe the observation that brain stimulation may evoke a change in mental alertness and mood that can persist beyond the termination of the stimulus is a very promising psychiatric lead. Heath, for example, has described a patient suffering from narcolepsy who would fall asleep, numerous times throughout the day. Since stimulation kept the patient awake for a period, he was equipped with a portable stimulating unit, which could be used when he felt himself falling asleep. The patient was an entertainer employed part-time in a night club and friends would operate the button on the stimulator if the patient fell asleep too rapidly to stimulate himself. The patient's narcolepsy was very severe; he could change from an alert state into a deep sleep in a matter of a second. In spite of the dramatic aspects of this application of brain stimulation, little evidence has been provided that the patient received very meaningful help. The mental alerting produced by the septal stimulation was not all that the patient experienced. He was also sexually aroused and this produced a "nervous feeling" as he tried unsuccessfully to achieve an orgasm by frantically pushing the button. It seems obvious that if an equivalent effort was expended, a less radical approach to the patient's problem could have been devised which would have provided a means of keeping him awake without involving implanting electrodes in the brain and inducing a state of sexual arousal.

The persisting mood changes that have been reported to be evoked by brain stimulation have prompted much more speculation about therapeutic potential than the very special and limited application to narcolepsy. As indicated earlier, these mood changes can occur in both directions; that is, unpleasant experiences such as anxiety, irritability, and aggressiveness on the one hand and pleasant experiences including relaxation, friendliness, talkativeness, and sexually exciting sensations on the other hand. It is the evocation of pleasant reactions which has been regarded as potentially useful therapeutically. Both Heath and Delgado have implied that a prescribed program of brain stimulation may be useful as an "emotion pacemaker" just as psychoactive drugs may be prescribed for the same purpose. Delgado and a number of his collaborators including Drs. Vernon Mark, William Sweet, and Frank Ervin described intracerebral radio stimulation in completely free patients:

"While the use of cardiac pacemakers is well established in clinical medicine, methodological problems in the development of a similar instrument for cerebral pacemaking are far more difficult because of the requirements of multichanneling, external control of several parameters of stimulation and the far greater functional complexity of the brain in comparison with the heart. These technical problems, however, are soluble, and the possibilty of clinical application should attract the interest of more electric and medical investigators.

"Experimentation in animals has demonstrated the practicality of long term, programmed stimulation of the brain to inhibit episodes of assaultive behavior, to increase or decrease appetite, to modify drives and to modulate intracerebral reactivity. Some of these findings may be applicable to the treatment of cerebral disturbances in man."

Recently Delgado and his collaborators, Drs. Obrador and Martin-Rodriguez, reported the results of stimulating the head of the caudate nucleus of a 35-year-old male with a 10-year history of epilepsy and some neurological evidence of a temporal lobe tumor:

"As shown by direct observation and by analysis of the record, within 30 seconds after application of caudate stimulation there was a significant change in the patient's mood. During controls, he was reserved, his conversation was limited and he was concerned about his illness. After a caudate stimulation, his spontaneous verbalization increased more than twofold and contained expressions of friendliness and euphoric behavior which culminated in jokes and loud singing in a gay *cante jondo* style, accompanied by tapping with his right hand, which lasted for about two minutes. The euphoria continued for about 10 minutes and then the patient gradually reverted to his usual, more reserved attitude. This increase in friendliness was observed following three different stimulation sessions of the caudate, and did not appear when other areas were tested."

Earlier, Drs. Higgins and Delgado had reported a similar change in an ll-year-old epileptic boy, who became significantly more friendly and verbal when stimulated in the temporal lobe region. Heath also described several instances of stimulation producing an improved mood state and mental alertness that persisted beyond the stimulation and indicated that "during the 24 hours following stimulation, improvement was generally maintained." There are several other similar published accounts of persistent changes in mental state. For example, in 1960 Dr. Magnus Peterson of the Rochester State Hospital in Minnesota commented: "In several cases I saw patients who were stimulated at a focus in the frontal medial area. . . . These were patients who were actively disturbed and antagonistic when the stimulation in that area was commenced. After about 15 minutes the patient became quite placid and talked well. That period of calmness might last for a day, or it might last longer."

Both Delgado and Heath have also discussed the use of implanted cannulae to provide chemical stimulation of localized brain areas as a means of changing mood. Heath indicated in several reports that acetylcholine (ACh) consistently produced pleasurable reactions when introduced into the septal area and rage or fear when delivered to the hippocampus. Stimulation of the septal area with ACh produced orgasms in both men and women and repetitive orgasm in the female patient B-5 described below:

"On three occasions, ACh was introduced first through the cannula to activate the hippocampi and then into the septal region of Patient No. B-5. The rage-fear, and sometimes depression, associated with the hippocampal activation was replaced within minutes by intense pleasure as the recordings from the septal area was activated. On other occasions the chemical stimulus was applied to the septal region during periods of spontaneous depression, and again anguish and despair were supplanted within minutes by pleasurable feelings as the electrical recordings changed. Consistently, strong pleasure was associated with sexual feelings, and in most instances the patient experienced spontaneous orgasm with the recording change. This patient, now married to her third husband, had never experienced orgasm before she received chemical stimulation to the brain, but since then has consistently achieved climax during sexual relations."

The possibility of being able to administer drugs at prescribed rates to specific brain structures has been raised by the development of a "dialytrode" by Delgado and his collaborators. The dialytrode consists of a cannula or chemitrode attached to a dialysis bag which can be constructed of different material in order to determine the infusion rate. The entire dialytrode could be implanted under the skin with the tip of the cannula located in a particular brain structure as seen in Figure 29.

Although the phenomenon of evoked mood and mental status changes that last beyond the stimulation period has been sufficiently documented to demonstrate that it can happen, there is no convincing evidence that these changes have ever contributed significantly to any cures. The point can and probably will be argued, but after surveying the literature very carefully I have concluded that no con-

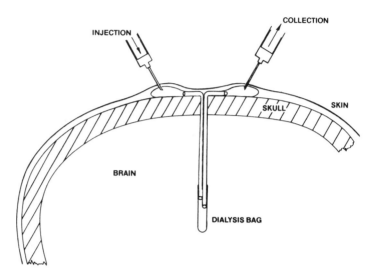

Figure 29. The transdermal dialytrode developed jointly by Dr. José Delgado and the Gulf Environmental Systems Company. The instrument, which has been tested in monkeys, gibbons, and chimpanzees, permits long-term delivery and collection of chemicals to and from the living brain. The dialytrode has been implanted in monkeys for periods of four to six months. Liquid will diffuse out of and into the chemode at a rate determined partly by the characteristics of the porous membrane. There are two silicone rubber reservoirs connected to the chemode. By piercing the scalp with a hypodermic needle, solutions can be added to or withdrawn from the reservoirs. Also, positive or negative pressure can be applied to the reservoirs to modify the rate and direction of the infusion. (Courtesy of Dr. José M. R. Delgado.)

vincing evidence exists. It is possible to form a contrary impression by reading a single optimistic report by one investigator, but a thorough reading of the total record over a number of years has a very sobering influence. For example, in 1954 Monroe and Heath described their psychiatric observations following septal stimulation of their first 20 schizophrenic patients, who were selected for electrode implantation on the basis of a poor prognosis. One patient died five weeks after the operation but of the remaining 19 it was reported that 10 were capable of leaving the hospital and were being followed in the out-patient department for periods ranging from 1 to 16 months. Five patients were judged to have shown "marked improvement," eight others displayed "significant improvement," two "questionable improvement," and four no improvement at all. Considering the prognosis of these schizophrenic patients, the improvement record would have to be considered extremely encouraging if indeed the changes could be attributed to the brain stimulation experience. As Monroe and Heath cautioned, the improvement may have been due in part to the general changes in the rehabilitative procedure. It has been demonstrated frequently that the increased attention and other changes in the hospital routine that an "experimental" patient receives may contribute more to any improvement observed than the manipulations under study. In any case, it would appear that the initial report was much too optimistic. As was indicated earlier, Heath later concluded that septal stimulation is not beneficial to schizophrenics and he no longer considers these patients suitable candidates for electrode implantation.

The possibility that brain stimulation might be helpful in some extreme cases cannot be ruled out; it certainly is conceivable that it might start a patient back on to the road to recovery, but in all probability other types of therapeutic intervention would be required to prevent a relapse. The moods that are evoked by septal stimulation are not pure distillations of happiness that could be indiscriminately programmed in throughout the day. The mood changes almost always include some specific ideas or emotional states. The belief that anyone could adjust in this world if a spontaneous orgasm followed by a detached mental calmness was programmed in at 10, 2, and 6 o'clock seems ludicrous. Nor would a normal adjustment be possible if a person learned to counteract every frustration and minor depression by self-administering an "electric high." The psychological adjustment to such "external" manipulations of emotional states could conceivably produce a psychotic reaction even in a normal person. There is good reason to suspect that brain stimulation, like drugs, would seriously weaken the conception of the "self" as a determiner of one's own destiny.

The reports of pleasurable experiences evoked by septal stimulation encouraged Heath to consider the therapeutic possibilities of a counterconditioning approach to psychiatric problems. Recognizing that inappropriate fear reactions or feelings of repugnance may lie at the root of many neuroses, Heath writes:

"Certainly, most psychodynamic theorists would agree that inappropriate anxiety is the nuclear factor in neurotic behavior. Signs and symptoms represent the inadequate reparative attempts to alleviate the inappropriate anxiety. If those theories are correct, then instantaneous replacement of irrelevant anxiety with positive feelings might provide the key to replacing undesirable behavior with more adaptive patterns."

Elsewhere, Heath says:

"If we could induce pleasure in the phobic neurotic patient when he encounters the objects of his fears, we might be able to correct his maladaptive pattern. Similarly, if the painful repugnant feelings of some homosexuals toward the opposite sex could, in a programmed manner, be converted into pleasurable feelings, their behavior patterns might change. The effects of such physiologic maneuvering, coupled with behavioral programming, are just beginning to be tested in the treatment of patients with pathologic behavior."

Recently Heath and his collaborator, Charles Moan, reported the results of their first attempt to explore the therapeutic potential of septal stimulation in a counter-conditioning program. Their patient was a 24-year-old single male with a long history of psychiatric problems involving suicidal depression, drug addiction, homosexuality, and a number of maladaptive personality characteristics including low frustration tolerance, suspiciousness, anger, and vindictiveness. The patient has had serious adjustment difficulties and has been in and out of psychiatric institutions repeatedly ever since his expulsion from school at age 11.

Since the patient failed to respond to any of the psychiatric treatments provided, it was decided to initiate a therapeutic program that utilized the pleasurable reaction evoked by the implanted electrode in the septal area. Initially the patient was shown a "stag" film picturing heterosexual intercourse and related activities. He was angry and highly resentful over being shown the film and refused to answer any questions. Afterward, the septal electrode was attached to a portable self-stimulation device and the patient was provided with the opportunity to stimulate his own brain while the intensity of the current was varied. This made it possible to determine the preferred stimulation intensity. Following a program of septal stimulation partly controlled by others and partly self-administered, the patient experienced "an almost overwhelming euphoria" and during the following four days there was an improvement in disposition and an increasing interest in the female personnel even though no additional stimulation opportunity was provided. While the patient was in this state, the film was shown again and this time the patient "became sexually aroused, had an erection, and masturbated to orgasm." The patient was willing to talk about his reaction afterward and said he "felt great" and during the next few days he displayed a "preoccupation with sex, and a continued growing interest in women." Encouragement for the developing heterosexual interest was provided and the patient was counseled when he sought advice on sexual techniques and behavior. Periodic septal stimulation seemed to maintain a high level of sexual arousal and the patient expressed a desire for a heterosexual relationship.

At this point in the therapeutic program the cooperation of a 21-year-old prostitute was obtained. She agreed to try to be supportive to the patient after being informed of the circumstances. In a private laboratory prepared for this purpose, the girl talked to the patient while lying next to him and gradually seduced him into heterosexual activity during which time both of them had orgasms. Before this therapeutic program the patient had no active interest in females and he never had any heterosexual relations of any kind. During the next 11 months regular counseling was provided on an outpatient basis. He formed a close, sexual relationship with a girl after leaving the hospital, but the fact that she was married made the situation untenable and they stopped seeing one another. The patient had two homosexual encounters during this period, which were claimed to be only "hustling" when he was out of work and needed money. He asserts that he is motivated to pursue heterosexual activities.

Evaluating the success of the treatment of this patient and determining the contribution of the septal stimulation can only be attempted in a very tentative fashion. Perhaps it should be recalled at the outset that the patient had a number of psychiatric problems involving drug abuse and suicidal depression and unless it is argued that these were all caused by the homosexuality it would appear that the patient could not be considered "cured" in any meaningful sense. Furthermore, the change in sexual orientation, even if it should prove lasting, has not been particularly dramatic, since the patient did not seem to have a strong repugnance toward females and his preference during the homosexual relations was for effeminate males with whom he played the dominant partner during anal intercourse. A more critical question is whether or not the same changes could not have been accomplished without brain stimulation. Although it has been stated that psychiatric treatment had failed up to this point, little information is provided about the nature of the previous treatment. Even though the present therapeutic program has a rationale very similar to that underlying many varieties of behavior modification therapy, desensitization programs for phobic reactions, and the Masters and Johnson approach to sexual impotence, there is no indication that any of these nonsurgical approaches had been explored. None of the behaviorally oriented therapeutic programs involve electrode implantation. Although it is true that in the present case the septal stimulation provided a high base level of sexual arousal that may have been helpful in changing the patient's sexual orientation, it seems very possible that this could have been accomplished by less drastic means. Masturbation, for example, has been used in behavior therapy programs with homosexuals to achieve what has been called "orgasmic reorientation."

In behavior modification programs, rewards and punishments are administered as efficiently as possible to encourage some specific behaviors while discouraging others. In the case described by Moan and Heath, there was no attempt to create a link between the pleasure evoked by stimulation and any specific behavior. The sexual arousal that was created provided a general background against which the psychiatrist could influence the patient's behavior by projecting "stag" films and a cooperative prostitute into the picture. Whether or not more dramatic or lasting behavior changes could have been accomplished if the evoked pleasure reaction had been coupled more directly with specific behavior cannot be answered at present. At this time, however, the more essential question is whether brain stimulation should have been used prior to a thorough exploration of behaviorally oriented programs and whether its therapeutic potential should be considered sufficiently high to justify its use at all as a basis for psychiatric treatment.

BRAIN STIMULATION AS AN INHIBITOR

Very early in the history of physiology the brilliant Russian physiologist Ivan Sechenov (1829–1905) demonstrated that there were regions in the brain of the frog that inhibited spinal reflexes. If these inhibitory brain regions were stimulated when a frog's leg was placed in an acid solution, the reflexive withdrawal of the leg was weakened. If the inhibitory region was destroyed, the reflex response was strengthened. Sechenov's conclusion that inhibition is an *active* physiological process has been supported by many later experiments which showed that the destruction (or suppression by drugs) of some brain regions can produce an exaggerated response as a result of a release from inhibition. The excitable periods that are often seen during the early stages of anesthesia or alcohol intoxication are also believed to be caused by a suppression of inhibitory mechanisms.

It is now generally accepted that there are many neural circuits and perhaps even specific neurotransmitters that function mainly to suppress responses that might otherwise be inappropriately strong. Inhibitory mechanisms may also make it possible to withhold a response long enough to consider alternative courses of action. Most response systems probably have some complementary inhibitory mechanism capable of providing a dampening influence. Brain stimulation can prevent a response by disrupting the neural circuitry underlying its execution, but it may also block a response by activating an inhibitory circuit. Several people have considered the possibility that brain stimulation may under some circumstances produce a desirable effect by activating some specific inhibitory circuits.

Delgado, perhaps more than anyone else, has speculated on the therapeutic applications of the inhibitory action of brain stimulation. He pointed out that brain stimulation can produce three types of inhibitory process: sleep, general motor inhibition, and inhibition of specific behavior categories. Delgado cites an example of stimulation producing sleep: "After 30 seconds of stimulation in the septal area, the animal's [a monkey] eyes started closing, his head lowered, his body relaxed, and he seemed to fall into a natural state of sleep." (Note that Heath reports an alerting effect produced by septal stimulation.) Delgado speculated that such effects might be used to treat chronic insomnia or to establish an unnatural biological rhythm of rest and activity cycles, perhaps one more suitable to space travel. The availability of a number of alternative ways of inducing sleep—from drugs to posthypnotic suggestion—would seem to indicate that there is little incentive to explore the use of brain stimulation in this context. Brain stimulation can also produce a general inhibition or arrest of all bodily movements and Delgado has provided examples of stimulation immobilizing a cat lapping milk so that it became motionless with its tongue out, or "frozen" in the act of climbing between two steps. Other than some contributions to our knowledge of brain function, such general inhibitory effects seem to have little therapeutic value.

It is frequently implied that the potentially most useful inhibitory effects produced by brain stimulation are those that are restricted to one behavior category; the examples provided typically concern the inhibition of food intake, aggressiveness, territoriality, and maternal behavior. Criticism of the evidence that has been claimed to demonstrate the specificity of brain stimulation was presented in some detail in an earlier chapter. The point to be made is that *there is no convincing evidence that stimulation of any brain region specifically activates or inhibits one and only one motivational system.* It may be possible for stimulation to inhibit the movement of specific muscles, or to disrupt a particular sensation, or even to block speech, but these effects involve much more restricted capacities than those utilized in either the arousal or satisfaction of such motivational states as hunger, aggression, and sexuality. The response patterns, sensory capacities, and perhaps even the energy utilized in the arousal and satisfaction of each of the separate motivational states are shared to such an extent that it is highly unlikely that they can be inhibited selectively.

There has been no convincing evidence presented that brain stimulation, or for that matter any brain manipulation, can block aggression or modify moods without altering other types of activities in unpredictable ways. Unfortunately, the attention of most people has been diverted away from this central problem by the bright reflection of new pieces of hardware such as the *stimoceivers,* which permit radio stimulation of the brain and telemetric recording of brain waves. Great interest has been generated by the fact that this device has been so completely miniaturized that it weighs only 70 grams (2.5 ounces) and that it is small enough to conceal under a wig, but little realistic thought has been given to its applications. Delgado describes possible uses of this device as follows:

"A two-way radio communication system could be established between the brain of a subject and a computer. Certain types of neuronal activity related to behavioral disturbances such as anxiety, depression, or rage could be recognized in order to trigger stimulation of specific inhibitory structures. The delivery of brain stimulation on demand to correct cerebral dysfunction represents a new approach to therapeutic feedback. While it is speculative, it is within the realm of possibility according to present knowledge and projected methodology."

The advantage of such a remote communication system is that the electroencephalographic patterns could be recognized by sophisticated electronic detectors in conjunction with computers. The commands for the delivery of stimulation, therefore, could be made contingent upon the occurrence of those EEG patterns that were desirable to inhibit. Moreover, the judgments made by the computer would be automatic and therefore would not require the constant attention of the patient or anyone else. The equipment could be designed to prevent overuse or abuse by the patient, and conceivably the judgments might be more reliable than those made by the patient.

Although the development of miniature stimulators, recorders, receivers, and transmitters can be admired as technical achievements, the practical applications of these devices have never been clearly spelled out. It is certainly true that the monitoring of electrical activity over longer periods of time and more natural conditions may reveal brain abnormalities that would otherwise be missed because they only occur relatively infrequently. A therapeutic stimulation device, however, presents very different considerations. What would we monitor and where would we stimulate? Unless we can answer these questions satisfactorily, Delgado's suggestion is no more realistic than a "magic pill" that would make us good, happy, and productive. It is very likely that if our knowledge of brain physiology becomes sufficiently sophisticated to be able to reliably suppress undesirable moods or to inhibit the development of abnormal neural patterns, we will be able to treat the cause directly rather than relying on the hazards of being permanently locked into some remote control system designed to suppress only symptoms.

Limited applications of inhibitory stimulation might

prove to be useful in instances where there may be some warning in advance. Prior to an epileptic seizure, there is often some preceding aura or other telltale experience that forewarns the subject of the oncoming attack. This is also true in some instances of aggressive outbursts, and there may be a request for help as it is recognized that control is being lost. In such cases the subject might operate the inhibitory device, thus simplifying the process by eliminating most of the gadgetry used to detect and respond to brain signals. This type of system has been tested as a means of combating pain. As will be described in the following section of this chapter, Dr. C. Norman Shealy has attached electrodes to the dorsal column of the spinal cord of patients suffering from severe bodily pain. Patients can turn on a portable stimulator to inhibit the building up of pain as soon as they feel it developing.

In an application of brain stimulation employing a similar principle, Dr. Irving Cooper of St. Barnabas Hospital in New York reported exploratory attempts to use brain stimulation to inhibit the spasticity produced by a stroke. Cooper implanted electrodes in the anterior portion of the cerebellum and led the wires under the skin to a point on the chest. He described a stroke victim suffering from a spastic paralysis for 40 years, who was able to sufficiently reduce his spasticity by periodically turning on the stimulator so that it is now possible for him to walk without a cane. In another application, Cooper recently reported that an epileptic patient was able to block convulsions by activating the stimulator (also attached to an anterior cerebellum electrode) whenever he felt a seizure coming on.

STIMULATION AS A PROSTHESIS

There have been a few interesting attempts to use electrical stimulation to overcome some physical handicap that should be included in this review. The German neurosurgeon Dr. Otfrid Foerster observed that electrical stimulation of the visual portion of the neocortex of humans produced sensations of spots of light called phosphenes that tended to have a fixed position in the visual field depending upon the portion of the cortex that was stimulated. Taking advantage of these observations, Drs. G. S. Brindley and W. S. Lewin of the Institute of Psychiatry in London have been exploring the possibilities of developing a rudimentary visual prosthetic device. Brindley and Lewin permanently implanted 80 electrodes in the visual cortex of a 52-year-old woman who was essentially blind. The electrodes could be stimulated by radio waves emitted from a transmitting coil pressed against the skull. Approximately 50 percent of the 80 electrodes were capable of producing phosphenes, which were reported as being like "a star in the sky" and about the size "of a grain of rice at arm's length." The implanted electrodes and miniaturized receivers have been left in place for several years with no discomfort to the patient, but only 50 percent of the originally functioning electrodes continue to produce phosphene sensations. The spatial distribution of the phosphenes in the visual field did not make it possible to form good representation of the alphabet, but by stimulating eight points together the patient was able to recognize a question mark and a crude representation of the letters "V" and "L." It is at least conceivable that with more implanted electrodes, a blind person might be able to use this system to read and as an aid in getting about in the environment, but many people (including the majority of the blind) have serious reservations about the ultimate practical value of this approach. There are few who believe this method is likely to possess the degree of resolution necessary to produce the subtle details of realistic images.

Other attempts to use neural stimulation as a prosthesis have explored outside the brain itself. Drs. F. Blair Simmons, John Epley, and their collaborators at Stanford University, for example, attempted to produce useful sounds in a deaf person by stimulating the auditory nerve. These investigators permanently implanted six electrodes in the auditory nerve at a position close to one of the malfunctioning ears and led the wires under the skin to a connecting plug that was threaded into the skull. Each electrode produced a characteristic pitch, which could be varied by changing the frequency of stimulation, while the perceived loudness corresponded to the amplitude of the stimulation. However, the pitch that the patient could detect was limited to frequencies below 250 pulses per second and therefore speech could not be understood. Although it might be possible that the patient could learn some code that represented speech, this is quite different from directly perceiving speech or music.

In a recent report Nashold and his colleagues demonstrated that electrical stimulation of the spinal cord of paraplegics at a point below the injury could control the emptying of the bladder. In three of the four patients in whom the electrodes were implanted the patients were able to empty their bladders periodically throughout the day. Most of the side effects produced by spinal cord stimulation such as sweating, increased skin temperature, and penile erection could be controlled by changing the stimulation parameters. It is much too early to evaluate the long-term effectiveness of these techniques, but when considered against the few other alternatives that are available for treatment, they deserve further investigation.

Another prosthetic application of electrical stimulation recently explored led to the development of a device to aid stroke victims in walking. Due to a loss of function of the neural pathway controlling certain reflexes of the foot, patients may suffer from what is called a dropfoot problem. Ordinarily when the heel hits the ground during walking the front of the foot is reflexly lifted up to permit stepping forward without tripping, but in a number of hemiplegic patients who have suffered some cerebral vascular damage this reflex is absent. Following a suggestion by W. T. Liberson and his colleagues that electrical stimulation of the peroneal nerve could be used to lift the leg during walking, members of the Faculty of Electrical Engineering of the University of Ljubljana in Yugoslavia devised a device that stimulates the peroneal nerve every time a switch located in the heel of the shoe is operated. The heel switch transmits a triggering pulse to an antenna-stimulator unit (surgically placed under the skin of the thigh), which then automatically activates the ring electrode placed around a portion of the peroneal nerve. A research team located at the University of Southern California's Rancho Los Amigos Hospital has also utilized a similar technique and such "prosthetic stimulators" have been implanted in 30 patients. Although the device is not yet free of trouble, some successes have been reported.

ELECTRICAL STIMULATION AND RELIEF FROM PAIN

Several reports now demonstrate that electrical stimulation of certain brain areas and parts of the spinal cord may provide relief from pain for periods exceeding the duration of the stimulation. Heath noticed early in his investigations that brain stimulation occasionally produced a prolonged relief from pain. Heath and Dr. Walter Mickle report:

"The group with intractable pain consisted of 6 patients, 4 suffering with far advanced metastatic carcinoma [spreading cancer] who were all on large doses of morphine without gaining relief, and 2 with severe rheumatoid arthritis who were not controlled by the hormonal, i.e., steroid therapies. The effect of stimulating the septal region of these patients is quite startling. They get immediate relief—feel good. The subjects say they feel good. They smile, brighten up, change their facial expressions. As a rule the effect of the stimulation is not long-lasting. It might last for a maximum of two or three days. It is necessary to stimulate the septal region nearly daily, but the effect is immediate (as soon as the current hits). It is a repeatable thing. You can stimulate over and over again. One of the patients with rheumatoid arthritis received a long-lasting effect. He was stimulated a total of 3 times and did not have severe pain from then on. Some discomfort persisted because of osteoporosis, but he had no persistent hot swollen red joints. The second rheumatoid had a lot of contractures; she had not been able to move for quite a time. During the stimulus her joints loosened up and she could pump, like riding a bicycle. However, her effects were of brief duration. They would last for the greater part of the day and then she would have to be restimulated.

"In reply to your question: 'Is it a real relief?' It is certainly different from the freedom of pain you get with lobotomy, i.e., not merely a lack of concern but an apparently real relief of pain. The lobotomy subjects still have pain but don't care about it. Our stimulation patients say they don't have pain and appear to be in excellent contact. We feel it is a disappearance of pain rather than a lack of concern about it."

Dr. A. Gol of the Veteran's Administration Hospital in Houston, Texas, also reported that septal stimulation can produce a dramatic alleviation of pain. Gol implanted an electrode into the septal area of the brain of a 43-year-old male patient who was suffering from severe, intractable pain produced by the terminal stages of metastatic carcinoma. As a result of the pain the patient was in acute distress, continually sweating and groaning. A low level of stimulation was delivered to the septal area during alternate 24-hour periods. No drugs were administered during the three weeks of stimulation. On the days the patient received stimulation, "he was alert and active when awake, talking clearly, fully oriented, cheerful and complaining of no pain at all." Even when questioned, the patient said he had no pain at all. Although the patient was cheerful when stimulated, no specific pleasure sensations were reported. On the alternate days without stimulation, the patient's pain gradually started to return and he began to sweat and become less alert, more drowsy, and exhausted. Apparently septal stimulation does not always alleviate pain; in fact Gol reported that in another case no relief from pain was obtained even though the patient felt more cheerful and alert during stimulation. No pain alleviation was produced by stimulation of the caudate nucleus in four other patients.

Recently, at the International Congress of Psychosurgery held in Cambridge, England (August 1972), Delgado and his collaborators, Drs. S. Obrador and J. Martin-Rodriguez, offered some additional evidence on the alleviation of pain by brain stimulation in a 30-year-old male whose left arm was paralyzed as a result of a car accident. The patient experienced intolerable pain from the paralyzed arm. Since drugs and physical therapy did not help it was decided to try electrical stimulation of the septal area. Electrodes were placed stereotaxically in the septal area and the head of the caudate nucleus and these were connected to a stimulator, which was inserted under the skin on top of the head. One week after surgery, about 10 telestimulations of five seconds duration were delivered to the septal area and "following these excitations, a lasting improvement of the discomfort of the patient was demonstrated, accompanied by a notable decrease in his previous hostility." It was not specified how long the relief of pain persisted beyond the stimulation period, but it was reported that "programmed stimulation" could diminish the otherwise intractable pain of the patient and that the subcutaneously implanted telestimulation device continued to work reliably and to be well tolerated by the patient during the four months that had elapsed following surgery.

A number of years ago, Verne Cox and I performed some animal experiments that involved the almost simultaneous delivery of a rewarding brain stimulus and several types of aversive stimuli. The rewarding stimulus was lateral hypothalamic brain stimulation for which the rats were willing to "self-stimulate." The aversive stimulus was either a painful electric shock to the feet or electrical stimulation at a site in the brain that evoked a very rapid escape response. In either case, however, if the positive hypothalamic stimulation preceded the aversive stimulus by less than a second, the animals behaved as though they were only experiencing a pleasurable sensation. In our situation it was necessary for the two stimuli to be presented within a second of each other in order for the painful experience to be masked. We were stimulating a lateral hypothalamic region, however, not the septal area, and our painful stimulus was a discrete experience, not a sustained, chronic pain. Recently David Mayer and his collaborators reported that focal electrical stimulation of the brainstem of a rat attenuated or blocked the perception of intense pain produced by controlled pressure to the paws or the tail. In that experiment, rats even learned to self-administer an otherwise neutral brainstem stimulation in order to block the perception of a painful stimulus delivered by the experimenters. A few years earlier Dr. David Reynolds of the Stanford Research Institute demonstrated that it was possible to do exploratory surgery, consisting of cutting the abdominal skin and muscles of rats to the extent that permitted visualization of the abdominal cavity and then closing the incision, using only brain stimulation as the analgesic. The animals, which were clearly not paralyzed by the stimulation, struggled if loud noises were presented or if there were sudden movements in their view.

The animal experiments demonstrating analgesia produced by brain stimulation may accomplish this end by modifying the neuronal impulses that signal pain. According to the "gate control" theory of pain proposed by Drs. Ronald Melzak of McGill University and Patrick Wall of University College, London, pain signals are coded by the frequency of firing of the nerves transmitting information from the spinal cord to the brain. The frequency of firing is determined by the proportion of large-diameter A fibers to the number of small C fibers in the sensory nerves that convey information from the body surface to the brain.[17] A fibers normally convey somatic sensations such as touch whereas C fibers, which are less sensitive (higher thresholds), respond to the more intense noxious stimuli. It has been proposed that at the point where these nerves enter the spinal cord there is a "gating mechanism" which operates in such a way that A fibers can inhibit the rate of firing of C fibers. There exist several reports, for example, of increased pain (hyperalgesia) when C fibers have been experimentally or accidentally isolated from the influence of A fibers. Under more natural conditions, any stimulus that increases the activity of A fibers is said to close the "gate" by slowing the transmission rate of C fibers and therefore effectively diminishing the pain signals. This may be the explanation of why it helps to clench one's hands together in the dentist's chair.

Patrick Wall and William Sweet of Harvard speculated that if they could use weak electrical stimulation to selectively activate the low-threshold A fibers, they might be able to reduce pain. They experimented on themselves by inserting needle electrodes through the skin on the face into a branch of the trigeminal nerve. (The trigeminal nerve conveys pain and other sensory information from the face.) Relief from pain could be achieved only during the stimulation period, but encouraged by reports that

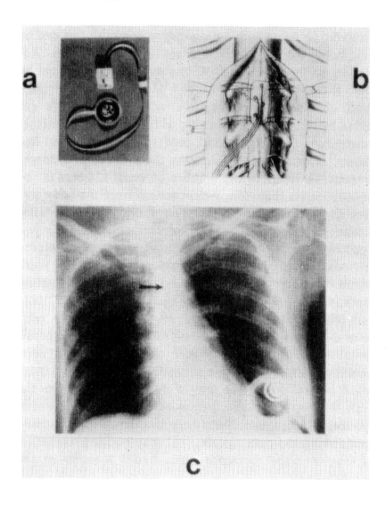

pain after amputation could be relieved by a vibrator applied to the nerves in the stump Wall and Sweet continued
their experimentation on several patients. A woman who
was suffering from severe burning pain of the arm and
sharp bursts in the fingers was equipped with ring electrodes around the ulnar and median nerve in the arm.
Relief of pain and freedom of movement lasted for more
than one-half hour following stimulation.

More recently Dr. C. Norman Shealy of the Pain Rehabilitation Center in La Crosse, Wisconsin, attached electrodes over the dorsal or back part of the spinal cord of patients suffering from the crippling pain caused primarily by ruptured intervertebral disks, but also by cancer of various organs and traumatic nerve injuries. When the discomfort becomes unbearable the patient can obtain relief by turning on the portable dorsal spinal column stimulator. It is presumed, but not proven that relief is obtained by closing the "gate" to pain messages by a massive activation of A fibers. In a few cases where there has been almost continuous pain requiring frequent administration of narcotics, prolonged relief has been obtained by activating the unit for only seven-minute periods, five times daily. Some patients have had such long-term relief that it was necessary for them to use the unit only once or twice a week. In separate studies Dr. Blaine Nashold at the Duke University Medical Center and Dr. Yoshio Hosobuchi and his colleagues at the University of California in San Francisco also reported success with this technique (see Figure 30). Patients have to be carefully selected on a psychiatric basis as well as

Figure 30. (a) System for stimulating dorsal spinal column to alleviate pain. (b) The electrode plate in place over the dorsal column of the spinal cord. Sutures anchor the plate in place and are then used to close the tissue layers. The positioning of the plate is varied with the location of the pain. The dacron mesh electrode is coated with silicon to reduce reaction with the tissues. The plate is connected to a radiofrequency receiver. (c) X-ray view of the receiver implanted under the skin in the chest. An antenna can be seen to the right of the receiver. The connecting wires are under the skin. The patient is instructed how to use a miniature, battery-operated stimulator (not shown) which can transmit pulses of different frequency, duration, and intensity. The effective parameters of stimulation are different for each patient. There have been more than 500 operations since 1967 and a Dorsal Column Study Group has been formed to pool information. (From B. S. Nashold and H. Feldman, "Dorsal Column Stimulation for Control of Pain," *Journal of Neurosurgery*, 1972, Vol. 36, Figs. 1-3.)

preliminary testing of the sensation evoked by spinal cord stimulation. Even then it does not work with all patients, nor does the analgesia always last very long beyond the stimulation period. In addition to uncertainty about the effectiveness in suppressing pain in any individual case it should not be assumed that there is no risk involved in the surgery required to attach electrodes to the spinal cord. The removal of portions of vertebrae necessary to place the electrode on the spinal cord is not a procedure to be taken lightly. Furthermore, accidents can occur as a result of movement of some part of the electrode assembly, and in one case paraplegia was produced by severing of an artery and subsequent damage to the spinal cord.

In other preliminary studies Dr. C. Hunter Sheldon and his colleagues at the Huntington Institute of Applied Medical Research in Pasadena, California, demonstrated that electrical stimulation of the trigeminal nerve produced long-term relief from the recurrent paroxysmal facial pain of trigeminal neuralgia. These investigators implanted electrodes in one branch of the trigeminal nerve in three patients who received relief from the electrical stimulation for varying periods of time. Stimulation was not infallible, however, and in some instances it was ineffective unless drugs were also used. The results on pain suppression by electrical stimulation have been sufficiently encouraging to justify further exploration in cases where relief cannot be otherwise obtained. Intractable pain has required drastic measures such as cutting fiber tracts in the spinal cord that were believed to be primarily carrying pain information. Stimulation systems may be more desirable, but the dangers of these procedures should not be neglected when cases of dramatic success are described.

Although it represents only an educated guess, several pain authorities have speculated that the analgesia produced by acupuncture may also be achieved by increasing the proportion of A fibers activated. As originally proposed, the "gate control" theory was meant to explain pain mechanisms at the spinal cord level. The analgesic effect of acupuncture needles stuck in the face during abdominal surgery and the analgesia produced by brain stimulation as described above suggest that there may be other "gates," perhaps in the thalamus of the brain, that are capable of blocking pain sensations. It is a little humbling as well as amusing to recall the forgotten accounts of electrically induced analgesia that appeared as long ago as the middle of the nineteenth century. W. G. Oliver, a dentist residing in Buffalo, described the successful use of electrical analgesia during dental and medical surgery in 1858. In a refreshingly direct style that is complete with testimonials from satisfied patients and witnessing medical authorities, Oliver wrote:

"During the summer of 1857, the idea crossed my mind that by proper application of an electric current, the pain incidental to Dental operations could be mitigated, if not entirely controlled. I owned a magneto electric machine, and designed to make the experiment with it as soon as I could obtain it from a friend to whom I had lent it. He was a Captain of a vessel and was absent on a voyage. . . . .At length the apparatus was obtained from my friend, and put in order for experiments."[18]

Oliver described the use of the magneto to block the perception of pain initially during extraction of teeth, but later during childbirth, surgical removal of ulcerated tissue from the leg, and amputations. Details of how and where the electrodes should be placed were provided ("the current must be sent in a contrary direction to the normal action of the nerve") for several procedures including an amputation ("When the limb is separated, it is suggested that the wire should be taken from the ankle and attached to the knee while the operation is finished."). After reading Matteucci's 1840 lectures on the electrophysiological characteristics of animals, Oliver concluded that the electricity "has the effect of disarranging, depolarizing or reversing the operation of the nervous force." It is a provocative thought that even though the theory was crude and not specific in any detail, had the techniques been available, the explanation offered by Oliver might have led—over 100 years ago—to the same therapeutic investigations that are now being explored.

Although there is insufficient experience to be able to specify how reliably pain can be alleviated by brain stimulation in humans, the phenomenon seems to be genuine. It is possible that there may be two separate mechanisms involved in these demonstrations of "electrical analgesia." As described previously, in some cases the effect seems to be produced by disrupting or modifying the pattern of neural impulses that are conveying information that will be interpreted as pain. In other cases, the perception of pain may be blocked by activating the positive reward circuits, which may have a built-in capacity to inhibit the interpretation of pain at some higher level in the nervous system. We certainly do not know how this is accomplished, but there are many examples of the perception of pain being greatly influenced by mental attitude, expectancy, and numerous psychological and cultural factors. These examples range from the well-known descriptions of soldiers, who under certain conditions may not complain of pain even though they have severe wounds and are completely conscious, to the report in 1916 by M. Erofeyeva, a student of Pavlov, that dogs stop exhibiting aversive reactions to very painful electric shocks to their legs if the shock serves as a signal (conditioned stimulus) for the presentation of a palatable food.

Chronic pain may partially reflect some persisting neural activity that is interpreted as pain Perhaps stimulation of the positive reward circuit may be able to cancel out the neural substrate of chronic pain for a period of time. At what point one should conclude that more conventional methods are unlikely to provide relief for the patient and to justify the risks of surgery is difficult to decide by formula. It seems apparent though that if a technique could be devised for stimulating selective brain areas from outside the head, without surgery, such a procedure would be tried with much less hesitation. Whether this would be desirable or not would depend on what else besides the experience of pain would be changed.

SUMMARY

There is no doubt that there are now some fascinating reports suggesting that brain (or spinal cord) stimulation may under special circumstances provide significant relief from pain, spasticity, and perhaps epileptic seizures. It is difficult to predict the future usefulness of these techniques, but there is sufficient reason to continue investigations on a limited and cautious scale. The use of electroconvulsive treatment, as crude as it may be, will certainly be continued until some elegant treatment for severe depression has been shown to achieve comparable results. There is, however, very little evidence that stimulation techniques that use implanted electrodes have made a significant contribution to psychiatric problems. There are numerous optimistic predictions of the potential psychiatric usefulness of the ability of brain stimulation to improve mood, increase alertness, and produce sexual orgasms, but the only specific application that has been described is Heath's use of brain stimulation as part of a conditioning program for homosexuality. I have already commented on my serious reservations to this therapeutic approach.

There have been a few demonstrations that brain stimulation may inhibit aggressive outbursts, but no plan has been presented for its practical use in a therapeutic situation. It is possible that stimulation may block aggression by inhibiting the neural activity of some brain foci that triggers aggressive outbursts, or it may reduce aggression by producing a relaxed and pleasant mood. In the first instance, if a single brain site could be determined to be the cause of dangerously aggressive outbursts, it would seem desirable to ablate it rather than to rely on the uncertainties inherent in a lifetime regimen of brain stimulation. The other alternative, that of programming stimulation (chemical or electrical) to be delivered at some rate estimated to be able to maintain a relaxed and calm mood, is theoretically possible. At present, however, there is no way of knowing the consequences of a prolonged and unnatural manipulation of mood. There are good reasons for questioning whether psychological health is possible under conditions where mood changes are programmed by the clock rather than appropriately reflecting the external situation. One person subjected to remote brain stimulation at the Massachusetts General Hospital believes that he is still being "controlled," even though the electrodes have been removed and he is now in Los Angeles. It is true that the patient is said to have been seriously disturbed before any brain stimulation experience, but it would not be too difficult to imagine a situation where external control over emotional states could be a major factor in precipitating a psychotic break. The alternative, giving the patient control over the stimulation system so that mood changes could be self-programmed, runs the danger of producing such a strong dependence on the system that it would be likely to lead to a withdrawal from reality.

Brain Surgery: The Treatment of Movement Disorders and Epilepsy

Parts of the human brain are surgically removed for a number of reasons. For our purpose, perspective may be gained by ordering these reasons along a continuum ranging from those disorders where there are clearly identifiable physical causes such as tumors, blood vessel damage, or traumatic head injuries, to psychosurgery where there is virtually no indication of the physical cause at all. Between are a number of disorders in which there is some experimental or clinical reason for believing that a particular brain structure normally participates in the function that is disturbed, but where there is usually no evidence that the structure is diseased or injured. Nevertheless, it may be possible to alleviate the symptoms by destroying perfectly healthy brain tissue. It is important to consider, even if only briefly, this intermediate category, since both the rationale and surgical techniques have much in common with psychosurgery where the evidence of involvement of a particular brain area may be much more tenuous.

In the intermediate group should be included a variety of motor disorders, which are collectively called *dyski-*

nesias. This category includes Parkinson's disease and other causes of tremors and spasticity as well as involuntary movements such as the jerking or twisting-rhythmical gyrations of the limbs seen in *choreoathetosis* or the swinging movements of the arms seen in *hemiballism.* Some types of epilepsy also belong in this intermediate category. Surgical treatment of temporal lobe epilepsy will be discussed briefly because of the involvement of the same brain area as has been implicated in certain types of aggressive patients and because both disorders share certain episodic characteristics.

MOVEMENT DISORDERS

Since the publication of the "Essay on the Shaking Palsy" by James Parkinson in 1817, numerous reports have implicated the *basal ganglia* in this disease. The basal ganglia occupy a large area in the brain and, although the term is not precisely defined, as a functional system it is said to include such structures as the caudate nucleus, putamen, globus pallidus, red nucleus, and the substantia nigra.[19] These structures are located over a large region, but all have been involved by either pathological or experimental evidence in the modulation of movement. There have been autopsy reports, for example, that described abnormal cell pictures in the substantia nigra and globus pallidus of patients who had Parkinsonism, but pathologists agree that in most cases these structures appear normal.

Movement disorders are believed to result from an unbalanced condition in those basal ganglia circuits that normally excite or inhibit the neural pathways responsible for the innervation of muscles. A decrease in activity in an inhibitory circuit may lead to muscular rigidity, tremors, or several different types of sudden, involuntary movement. The abnormalities in these various structures that are responsible for the changes in the balance of excitation and inhibition may be the result of subtle biochemical alterations in specific structures. Although this is not the entire explanation, there is reasonably good evidence, for example, for the belief that the neurons in the basal ganglia, which utilize the neurotransmitter dopamine, are inhibitory in their function. The basis for the introduction of L-dopa treatments is that this metabolic precursor of dopamine permits patients suffering from Parkinsonism to increase the availability of dopamine in the deficient inhibitory circuits. In this way the inhibitory pathways are facilitated and tremors and some types of spasticity may be reduced.

In 1950, before any of the foregoing information was known, Drs. Spiegel and Wycis announced at a meeting of the American Neurological Association that they had started to treat patients suffering from involuntary movement disorders by electrocoagulation of parts of the brain. With the aid of the human stereotaxic instrument that they had described in 1947, they destroyed parts of the globus pallidus in patients who had seriously disrupting involuntary jerky (chorioform) or slow writhing (athetotic) movements. Soon afterward, in 1952, Dr. Irving Cooper of St. Barnabas Hospital in New York was operating on a Parkinsonian patient when it suddenly became necessary to occlude an artery (anterior choroidal) to stop profuse bleeding. Since this artery had recently been reported to supply the globus pallidus and other structures in the center of the brain that modulated motor activity, Dr. Cooper elected to discontinue the operation he had originally planned in order to determine the consequences of the arterial occlusion. When the patient recovered from the anesthesia that evening the tremors, which had incapacitated him for almost 10 years, were gone. Dr. Cooper followed up this promising lead by purposely occluding the anterior choroidal artery in other patients, but later he developed techniques for destroying portions of the basal ganglia by alcohol injections, electrolytic means, and by a freezing probe.[20]

To answer questions about which brain structures, when destroyed, would provide the most relief, various techniques were developed to suppress or stimulate specific brain structures, enabling researchers to anticipate the effects of destroying that region. In some cases cannulae are implanted in the brain and drugs are used to modify the activity of a particular brain region. Procaine, for example, has been injected into a given brain structure so that the change that takes place when activity in that region is suppressed could be observed, although not always with interpretable results. Cooper developed a unique technique for temporarily suppressing the neural activity in a given region. He designed a double lumen cannula in which one lumen contained a small balloon inserted into the tip. After the cannula was positioned in the brain, a radio-opaque liquid was injected in order to inflate the balloon and make it possible to visualize by means of X-ray (see Figures 31 and 32). The inflated balloon partially blocked neural conduction due to compression, and if properly placed it could ameliorate or relieve tremors and rigidity. The balloon could be left inflated for 24 hours so that the effects of permanent tissue destruction could be estimated before the damage was produced. The balloon could then be deflated and withdrawn and the second lumen in the cannula could be used to inject a destructive chemical agent into the area vacated by the balloon. In more recent work Cooper prefers to use nondestructive cooling to suppress neural activity, rather than the balloon compression technique. Lower temperatures can then be used to destroy the tissue.

Electrical stimulation as used by Dr. Sem-Jacobsen of Oslo has also provided some indication of the functions that are regulated in the region. In cases of Parkinson's disease, tremors and muscle rigidity could be inhibited, modified, or exaggerated by such techniques. Once

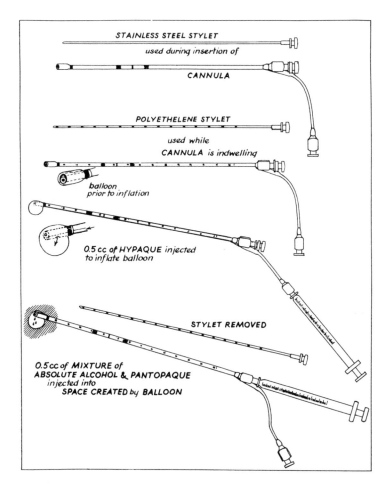

Figure 31.   The double lumened balloon cannula used by Dr. Irving Cooper for destruction of the globus pallidus and parts of the thalamus in the brains of Parkinson patients. (From I. Cooper, *Parkinsonism. Its Medical and Surgical Therapy*, 1961, Fig. 9. Courtesy of Charles C. Thomas, Publisher, Springfield, Ill.)

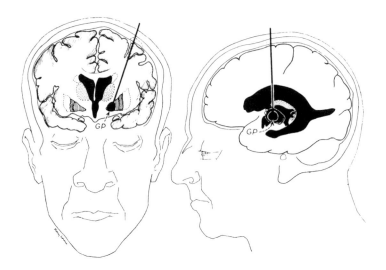

Figure 32.   Diagramatic representation of the balloon cannula in place in the medial portion of the globus pallidus. (From I. Cooper, *Parkinsonism. Its Medical and Surgical Therapy*, 1961, Fig. 28. Courtesy of Charles C. Thomas, Publisher, Springfield, Ill.)

located, the abnormally functioning brain area could be excised by one of several techniques.[21]

As experience with this type of surgery accumulated, Cooper concluded that destruction of different portions of the ventral thalamus produced greater relief of either Parkinson rigidity or tremors or the involuntary movements characteristic of hemiballism. Cooper also reported alleviation of spasticity after destruction of a portion of the pulvinar, a posterior thalamic structure. He described a patient whose hand had been locked in a gnarled, clawlike position, who was able to relax it following localized freezing of the pulvinar, called "cryopulvinectomy." In his nontechnical book *The Victim Is Always the Same*, Cooper describes in detail the history of two young girls suffering from the disfiguring spastic disorder *dystonia musculorium deformans*. Over the past two decades,

procedures were being explored for psychiatric problems concurrently in Europe and the United States. In discussing the factors that led him to the hypothalamic operation, Sano writes:

"At first, however, we were afraid that surgical interference with the hypothalamus might cause such serious autonomic and endocrine disturbances as to endanger life. This is why we made, so to speak, a detour until finally we attempted the hypothalotomy. After we had found the long-term results of the anterior cingulectomy and the thalotomies not altogether satisfactory, we tried fornicotomy and upper mesencephalic reticulotomy."

More recently, Dr. Schvarcz and his colleagues at the University of Buenos Aires have adopted Sano's posterior hypothalamotomy technique. This group has operated on 11 patients, who were subsequently observed for periods between 6 and 48 months. The patients were aggressive either toward others or toward themselves, usually exhibiting very violent and destructive behavior. It is claimed that in all cases extensive psychiatric treatment had failed and the patient's families were unable to cope with them. One patient, who had been in solitary confinement for 12 years because of extremely violent and aggressive behavior, was discharged three months after the operation and is now living with his family. In summary, Schvarcz and his colleagues report that in seven of the 11 cases, there was marked improvement after the operation; aggressive or violent behavior was absent and the patients were adapting socially. In view of Sano's very low-intelligence population, it is interesting that Schvarcz' group claims that the best results were obtained in patients of normal intelligence.

During a visit to Japan I had an opportunity to speak with several of Sano's younger colleagues (Drs. H.

Sekino, I. Hashimoto, and K. Amano) in the Department of Neurosurgery at the University of Tokyo. These neurosurgeons stressed several points in our conversation. First it was emphasized that their surgical procedure was used only with patients exhibiting intractable epilepsy combined with mental retardation, hyperactivity, and a history of violence or destructiveness. They also stressed that in the operation now performed a maximum of 3 millimeters of brain tissue is destroyed and this really at the junction of the anterior border of the reticular arousal system and the posterior hypothalamus and not in the hypothalamus proper. These last points may have been designed to deflect the mounting criticism of many scientists who have expressed their dismay at a procedure that involves destroying tissue in the hypothalamus—a structure generally accepted as a critical coordinator of many endocrine and visceral functions. By emphasizing that the destruction is not in the hypothalamus and that the destroyed area is very small and the patients seriously disturbed, criticisms may be turned aside. They report little change in the basic personality of their patients and indicated that motivation or drive is elevated rather than being depressed postoperatively. At least the ability to stay with one task seems to create the impression of an increase in motivation. They did observe one patient who suffered from confusion and a deficit in recent memory after the operation. It is possible that these deficits were produced by damage to the posterior hypothalamic structure, the mammilary bodies, as this region has been implicated in the Korsakoff alcohol syndrome, which also is associated with a recent memory loss. (The Korsakoff patient is known to make up or confabulate stories in an attempt to cover up the loss of recent memories.) Dr. P. Nádvorník of Comenius University in Czechoslovakia has also adopted Sano's posterior hypothalamic operation and he too observed one instance where mental confusion appeared postoperatively. In general, however, it has to be regarded as quite remarkable that destruction of even small hypothalamic areas does not produce greater deficits in view of the many demonstrations that this area regulates so many important endocrine and autonomic functions.

Recently Dr. Peter Breggin, a Washington psychiatrist, has received a great amount of attention because of his strong views against all forms of psychosurgery. In his zeal to convey the seriousness of the problem, Breggin has given the impression that psychosurgery is undertaken casually and that in some places a child need only be a behavior problem in school to run the risk of being considered a candidate for surgery.[26] Psychosurgeons disagree vigorously on this issue and Sano, for example, observes that it is necessary to understand certain cultural factors to comprehend his patient population. He points out that in Japan family cohesiveness is much greater than in the United States. (The strength of this family cohesiveness is dramatically illustrated by the fact that it is not a rare event, perhaps six cases a year in Tokyo, for an entire family to commit suicide together.) Within this cultural framework, a family will admit to a behavior problem and surrender a child to the hospital only under the most extreme circumstances. The patients who have received these operations generally present convincing evidence of general brain damage and are very severe behavior problems. Part of the problem may be semantic, since the term hyperactive child is misleading and does not convey the seriousness of the disorder. Nevertheless, the neurosurgeons' arguments would be stronger if they were more explicit than they generally are about the exploration of less drastic treatments before neurosurgery is undertaken. For example, it is often stated in the case record that before surgery, drugs were found to be ineffective, but it is rare that the specific drugs, dosages, and duration of administration are presented. This precaution seems especially important in view of Dr. Sadao Hirose's comment that "after the Second World War psychosurgery became a fashion in Japan."

MULTITARGETED OPERATIONS

As already noted, not all the patients considered candidates for surgical treatment of hyperactivity or aggression have demonstrable abnormalities in their brains. Some of the aggressive and hyperactive patients have serious psychiatric problems such as schizophrenia, drug and alcohol addiction, and depression, sometimes with suicidal tendencies. Several neurosurgeons have suggested that such patients can be treated only with destruction of multiple sites in the limbic system. The rationale for selecting the brain sites to be partially destroyed rests partly on the belief that there exists a relatively specific locus for many psychiatric problems. Moreover, it has been argued that a lesion made in one brain structure has to be sufficiently large to be effective and as a result the probability of producing undesirable behavior deficits is increased. Since different brain areas frequently are recommended as candidates for destruction for the same set of symptoms, it has been suggested that multiple small lesions in several neural structures may alleviate the behavior problems without producing such undesirable side effects as apathy, mental impairment, and endocrine disbalance.

The nature of the evidence presented for the specific localization of the different symptoms can be illustrated by a description of a patient of Dr. M. Hunter Brown of the St. John's and Santa Monica Hospitals in California. Brown described a 24-year-old girl with a nine-year history of intermittent depression, suicide attempts, and explosive physical violence against others without external provocations. Following bilateral amygdalectomy, Brown reports the patient's hostility and antisocial behavior were controlled, but the depression remained. Subsequently, destruction of the cingulum (see Figures 25 and 26) was reported to produce "good emotional balance" and the patient returned to work, being employed without problems for the next eight months.

Dr. Y. Kim of the Broughton Hospital in Morganton, North Carolina, and Dr. W. Umbach of the Free University in Berlin report that they combine destruction of the posteroventral hypothalamus and the dorsomedial nucleus of the thalamus in patients displaying aggressive behavior and a compulsive neurosis. Even a casual reading of a number of such cases makes it obvious that a different combination of brain lesions would be used on the same patients depending on the neurosurgeon. Often the prescription of the specific multitargeted brain surgery undertaken seems to have some of the quality of a cooking recipe—each surgeon performing these operations has his own favorite ingredients and variations.

Although several neurosurgeons have expressed concern and fear about the consequences of this multitargeted surgical approach, it has to be regarded as quite remarkable that patients seem to be able to tolerate this extensive damage to their brain. Brown, for example described a 23-year-old male patient who was diagnosed as a chronic schizophrenic with a homicidal and suicidal history. In one operation, Brown destroyed bilaterally a part of the cingulum, a neural region called the substantia innominata (substance without a name) and the amygdala. Following this six-target operation, which Brown ironically abbreviates as a CIA, he reports: "on recovery from his anesthesia he was sane, lucid and appropriate and has remained entirely well. He will reenter college on the west coast this fall." It is much too early to evaluate these claims except to marvel at the remarkable ability of the brain to withstand trauma. This operation may also illustrate the great capacity of the brain to conceal its deficits by solving problems in different ways. Often it requires specially designed tests to reveal the nature of the deficits. It is indeed unfortunate that this type of sophisticated testing is seldom done and that the effects of these operations are so inadequately and subjectively described that readers are usually forced to accept or reject the conclusions on faith or bias.

SOCIAL IMPLICATIONS OF THE DYSCONTROL SYNDROME

A somewhat different slant to the problem of the brain and aggression is presented by Drs. Vernon Mark and Frank Ervin in their book, *Violence and the Brain.* Mark is chief of neurosurgery at Boston City Hospital and Ervin, a psychiatrist and neurologist, is now associated with the Center for the Prevention of Violence of the University of California at Los Angeles. This book has received a great amount of attention because of its thesis that a method for controlling human violence on a large scale may soon be developed. Although Mark and Ervin do not present any new clinical evidence or even a new theoretical framework, their book has served as a catalyst for much heated discussion because they imply that their approach may help to curtail the accelerating incidence of violence. Actually, the one aspect of their approach that is different from that of the other groups we have discussed (most of whom have considerably more experience with this type of surgery) involves the use of remote stimulation and recording electrodes and the emphasis on discrete abnormal brain foci, referred to as "brain triggers of violence." These brain triggers are not always evident; they may be missed during a routine scalp electroencephalographic examination.[27] Implanted electrodes and the remote stimulation and recording techniques that have been developed in Delgado's laboratory make it possible to study the patient's brain continuously and under more natural conditions thus increasing the probability of detecting the abnormal brain foci that trigger episodic rage.

In their book, Mark and Ervin describe a set of symptoms which together constitute a behavior constellation they label the *dyscontrol syndrome:*

"We found that these violent people usually had four characteristic symptoms (which were not, however, always present at the same time): (1) a history of physical assault, especially wife and child beating; (2) the symptom of pathological intoxication—that is, drinking even a small amount of alcohol triggers acts of senseless brutality; (3) a history of impulsive sexual behavior, at times including sexual assaults; and (4) a history (in those who drove cars) of many traffic violations and serious automobile accidents." (Mark and Ervin, 1970, page 126)

In some percentage (but it is not clear how high the percentage is) of the people whose behavior seems to conform to the description of the *dyscontrol syndrome,* the standard electroencephalographic (EEG) recordings from the scalp may suggest a triggering focus located in some area deep in the brain—commonly, according to Mark and Ervin, in the temporal lobes, particularly the amygdala area. Electrical recordings from implanted electrodes in this area are used to help locate the pathological brain tissue more precisely. It is claimed that further anatomical verification can be obtained by noting the location of abnormal electrical patterns triggered by those "significant environmental stimuli" which in the past characteristically precipitated the assaultive outbursts. In one patient, for example, a baby's cry had a high probability of triggering an explosive reaction; here a discrete brain area should be sought that responds whenever a record of the baby's cry is played. It is also said that additional confirmation of the brain trigger can be obtained by precipitating a violent outburst by electrically stimulating a discrete brain area. Instances have been reported where stimulation produced outbursts of rage and assaultive behavior that seemed very similar to the patient's spontaneous, episodic violence. Finally, after locating the discrete trouble spot it can be removed, and the abnormal behavior will be eliminated.

The foregoing arguments sound so logical that unless one has some experience with these techniques the arguments may be found to be irresistible. What could be more elegant than using sophisticated stimulation and recording techniques to locate the trouble spot in the brain and then eliminating it by destroying a very discrete amount of abnormal tissue? Presumably, because the tissue destroyed would be only minimal, there need be no adverse side effects. How far short the actual results are from this idealized version will be discussed after illustrating the type of patient that comes closest to conforming to the pattern described by Mark and Ervin.

At the time of surgery, Julia was 21 years old. She is the daughter of a professional man, and following a childhood episode of encephalitis there has been a history of epileptic seizures, usually consisting of lapses of consciousness, staring, lip smacking, and chewing. After some seizures, she would panic and run great distances. Sometimes these "racing spells" ended up in dangerous neighborhoods where she would come out of her fugue-like state feeling alone and confused. Because of this, Julia had developed the habit of carrying a knife for protection. On 12 different occasions she assaulted people without apparent provocation. The most serious incident occurred when she was 18. While attending a movie with her parents she realized she was going to have another of her "racing spells" and told her parents she would wait for them in the lounge. Mark and Ervin have described what took place afterwards:

"When she got to the lounge, she looked in the mirror and perceived the left side of her face and trunk (including the left arm) as shriveled, disfigured, and 'evil.' At the same time, she noticed a drawing sensation in her face and hands. Just then another girl entered the lounge and inadvertently bumped against Julia's left arm and hand. Julia, in a panic struck quickly with her knife, penetrating the other girl's heart and then screamed loudly. Fortunately, help arrived in time to save the life of her victim." (pages 97–98)

Another serious incident occurred after Julia was sent to a mental hospital. While her nurse was writing a report, Julia cried out "I feel another spell coming on, please help me." The nurse said she would be with her in a minute, but Julia grabbed a pair of scissors out of the nurse's pocket and drove them into the woman's chest. Fortunately, the nurse recovered.

The EEG record obtained from electrodes implanted in Julia's brain revealed an abnormal discharge from the posterior amygdala in the right temporal lobe. Stimulation of this area when Julia was playing the guitar caused her to stop singing and to stare blankly. A "cascade of abnormal spikelike epileptic brainwaves" was then recorded and she suddenly swung her guitar powerfully, narrowly missing her psychiatrist and smashing the guitar against the wall. A destructive lesion was made in the right amygdala. It is too early to judge the effectiveness of this operation, but it was noted that she had two mild rage episodes during the first postoperative year and none in the second. However, Julia still had epileptic seizures and her psychotic episodes continued, perhaps because she had "generalized brain disease and multiple areas of epileptic activity." Even if her rage attacks do not return—and this would be a risky prediction, as will be seen from the results obtained with other patients—Julia is still a very sick person who is not likely to be able to function in an unprotected environment.

It seems to be generally agreed that amygdala lesions are unlikely to improve psychotic thought processes. What is the likelihood that stimulation and recording technique, using depth electrodes, can locate specific abnormal brain foci that trigger violence? The data obtained from animal and human brain stimulation studies suggest that it may be much more difficult to locate such foci than one might conclude from the presentation by Mark and Ervin. In an earlier study, for example, William Chapman, who also worked at the Massachusetts General Hospital, concludes:

"Some of the clinical features of temporal lobe epilepsy may be reproduced by electrical stimulation of the amygdaloid nuclear region. This was true in five out of six of our patients. The one major feature of their illness that could not be reproduced was assaultive behavior. In no instance was any subjective or behavioral response evoked that remotely resembled aggressiveness. This finding was disconcerting as the major reason for selecting these patients for the electrical coagulation was intractable assaultiveness."

In other stimulation studies, the problem seems to be just the reverse. Drs. Kim and Umbach have observed that stimulation at a number of places in the amygdala may produce aggressive responses but only in violent patients, not in patients who have no aggressive tendencies (see page 90). The possibility that the response produced by the stimulation, therefore, may reflect the patient's personality rather than the specific function of the area stimulated may produce misleading conclusions concerning the brain area responsible for the behavior problem. Animal studies have also indicated that the temperament of the subject may contribute significantly to the response evoked by brain stimulation, and in some instances it may be a better predictor than the anatomical site of the electrode (see pages 87–90). This is not to imply that stimulation of any brain area elicits the same response, but it raises the possibility that stimulation at any one of a number of brain sites that commonly evoke such feelings as pain, fear, aversion, and anxiety may provoke aggression in some patients. If tissue is destroyed on the basis of the capacity of an electrode to elicit a particular response, the results are likely to be disappointing.

In addition to the fact that the effects of stimulation may be determined by the disposition of the subject rather than the discrete neural tissue surrounding the electrode tip, there are other problems as well. There is a practical limit to the number of sites one can explore with implanted electrodes. In the work of Mark and Ervin, for example, it was generally the practice to place two electrodes in the amygdala on a given side of the brain. Often only one side of the brain was explored. Although each electrode was made up of a strand of wires, which made it possible to explore a number of neural points along its depth, it is clear that the entire amygdala could not be adequately surveyed. It is very likely that many critical foci in the amygdala are missed because of the limited area surveyed. It may be recalled that Ajmone Marsan and Abraham (see page 206) observed that abnormal electrical discharge may not be evident in the recording from a depth electrode located only 1 centimeter away from a focus; these authors, as well as others, have pointed out that there often are multiple abnormal foci in the patient population usually studied with depth electrodes. There is also good reason for believing that similar stimulation and recording evidence could be obtained from very different parts of the brain. Brain tumors that produce aggressive outbursts, for example, can be associated with many other brain areas. There is a tendency to exaggerate the role of the amygdala in cases of brain tumors by stressing only the involvement of this structure, even though the tumor may have invaded other areas. It is very likely that in many ways preconceived ideas have served to selectively filter, and consequently distort, the clinical evidence. Finally, since the stimulating and recording amygdala electrodes (they are one and the same) are also used to ablate brain tissue, the site of destroyed tissue is predetermined by the arbitrarily positioned electrodes.

Furthermore, it is necessary to point out that we do not know what percentage of those individuals with a history of explosive aggression actually have specific brain sites that are triggering the violence. Mark and Ervin imply that there are patients, presumably those exhibiting the dyscontrol syndrome, in whom there is sufficient justification for implanting depth electrodes in the absence of either a history of epilepsy or any clear indication of abnormality obtained from the scalp electroencephalographic records. Almost all the cases they present, however, have had epileptic episodes, usually combined with evidence of an abnormal electroencephalographic record. It would seem essential, therefore, to know what proportion of patients who display the dyscontrol syndrome and a normal scalp electroencephalographic record actually have brain triggers of violence that could be treated.

A recent paper presented by Mark and Ervin (in collaboration with Dr. William Sweet) summarizes the clinical evidence on the effectiveness of their approach. To be noted from the outset is the fact that in spite of the claims of broad applicability, the 12 violent patients they describe all had intractable temporal lobe epilepsy. Brain electrodes were implanted to locate the focus of the disorders and in 10 of these patients permission was obtained to make amygdala lesions with a radiofrequency current. In regard to the three patients who received unilateral lesions, it was reported that for some months after the operation, episodic violence was absent, but in two of the patients it was clear that assaultiveness was returning—one of them having remarked that his "old feelings were coming back" after he fractured the jaw of a fellow worker. The third patient's seizures are returning, but under a condition where he formerly would have been provoked into violence he attempted suicide.

Better results are claimed for the seven patients

receiving bilateral amygdala lesions, but the fact that it is necessary to destroy tissue at several brain sites raises some serious questions in regard to the assertion by these investigators that they are destroying a specific trigger of the violence. Indeed, in another report Dr. Mark and his colleagues indicate that multiple foci are common in their patient population. Apparently there is considerable trial and error in the procedure; indeed, lesions are progressively enlarged until it appears that desirable results are obtained. There is a very disappointing amount of detail provided to back up the impression that is conveyed that the use of electrodes to stimulate and record provides a reliable basis for selecting the most effective brain sites to destroy. Moreover, a close scrutiny of the data does not reveal results that are nearly as impressive as the summary statements would imply.

Of the seven bilateral patients, one received no benefit at all, while another, in whom assaultiveness was absent for three years after the operation, became impotent and remained psychotic, continuing to have hallucinations. (This is not an uncommon result, as can be noted from Mark's comment at a symposium that "we found amygdaloidectomy in assaultive schizophrenic patients changes the assaultive character but not the schizophrenia.") A third patient developed a voracious appetite (hyperphagia) and gained 35 pounds in a little over three months. The patient still had seizures and rage attacks, but the latter were less frequent. A female patient who was suffering from uncontrollable fear (no evidence of violence is provided) was less incapacitated and able to hold a job, although the fears were not completely eliminated. In a fifth patient the assaultiveness disappeared for a year, but then "her intolerable assaultiveness recurred." A sixth patient had only been observed for a short period. The seventh patient is viewed as the most successful, but this is a very extreme case of a woman who received a head injury from a fall on ice. Afterward she had frequent seizures and physically assaulted almost everyone who came near her using her nails and teeth on delivery boys, a sick mother-in-law, her husband, and others. There was unquestionable evidence of brain damage. The bilateral amygdalectomy eliminated her rage attacks for seven years and reduced the seizure incidence from three to five a day to 20 a year.

Taking the evidence as a whole, there is hardly justification for the enthusiasm Mark and Ervin attempt to generate in the broad applicability of their procedure. Yet together with Dr. William Sweet they formed the Neuro Research Foundation, and according to Constance Holden (*Science,* March 16, 1973) who reviewed current trends in psychosurgery:

"In 1970, through various mysterious maneuvers that no one seems to be able to explain, they persuaded Congress to direct the National Institute of Mental Health (NIMH) to award them a $500,000 grant to carry on their work."

The Senate Labor, Health, Education and Welfare appropriations subcommittee headed by Warren Magnuson was so impressed by Sweet's testimony that they ordered $1 million for research in this area to be added to the budget of the National Institute for Neurological Diseases and Stroke. Moreover, the foundation obtained a grant from the Law Enforcement Assistance Administration of the Justice Department to test procedures for screening habitually violent prison inmates for brain damage.

Mark and Ervin speculate in their book that there are many more cases of assault resulting from brain pathology than previously suspected. They point out that the postmortem examination of Charles Whitman, who shot 44 people, killing 14, from the tower on the campus of The University of Texas, revealed brain cancer. Richard Speck, the murderer of eight nurses in Chicago, had symptoms of serious brain disease. Although Mark and Ervin usually qualify their remarks, the parallel statistics they cite throughout their book on the number of automobile accidents, murders, rapes, and assaults against infants and children that occur on the one hand and the incidence of epilepsy, cerebral palsy, head injuries, and other evidence of brain damage on the other hand are designed to create the impression a great amount of violence is triggered by abnormality in the brain. They suggest that "we need to develop an *early warning test* of limbic brain function to detect those humans who have a low threshold for impulsive violence, and we need better and more effective methods of treating them once we have found out who they are."

Citing instances of violence where there is some evidence of brain damage, as in the example of Charles Whitman, can be very misleading. In the first place, it is a highly selective process in that there is a tendency to mention only the cases where brain pathology was found. A greater shortcoming, however, is that there is no evidence that the brain damage was a cause of the violence or that an amygdalectomy would have been helpful. Sweet, in collaboration with Mark and Ervin, reported the results of a postmortem examination of Whitman's brain which revealed a highly malignant tumor (glioblastoma multiforme) in the region of the amygdala. It is possible that the tumor was a cause of the violence, since Whitman did complain of tremendous headaches. We will never know for certain, but it would be a mistake to assume that Charles Whitman's history conforms to the pattern of episodic violence described as part of the dyscontrol syndrome. In the case of Julia, which was described earlier, the violence was sudden and unplanned. Whitman's own diary, which he kept for four and one-half years before the killings, clearly indicates the pathological state of his thought processes and the fact that the events were planned rather than the product of a sudden, uncontrollable impulse. His diary contains great details of what he was going to wear when he climbed the tower, how he would defend his position, and many of his plans after his escape. The night before he climbed the tower,

Whitman stabbed and shot his mother and then returned home and stabbed his wife. He left a note confessing his love for his mother. It is abundantly clear that when Whitman positioned himself, armed with a high-powered hunting rifle, on the observation deck of the University Tower he was not in the throes of a sudden, episodic attack of violence. There are no strong reasons for believing that the removal of the brain tumor (even if this was the only tumorous site) would have cured the obviously pathological thought process expressed in the diary:

"It was after much thought that I decided to kill my wife, Kathy, tonight after I pick her up from work—I love her dearly, and she has been a fine wife to me as any man could ever hope to have. I cannot rationally pinpoint any specific reason for doing this. I don't know whether it is selfishness, or if I don't want her to have to face the embarrassment my actions would surely cause her. At this time though, the prominent reason in my mind is that I truly do not consider this world worth living in, and am prepared to die, and I do not want to leave her to suffer alone in it. I intend to kill her as painlessly as possible. . . ."

The extent to which Mark and Ervin attempt to convey the impression that brain pathology can explain a significant proportion of our present violence is mirrored in Michael Crichton's novel *The Terminal Man*. Although Crichton has exercised some literary license, the lines spoken by his character Ellis directly parallel the statistics and arguments presented in Mark and Ervin's book. Ellis is a neurosurgeon who is explaining on television why he implanted electrodes in a patient who had gone beserk and killed someone:[28]

"The reporters asked him about the operation and he explained it briefly but clearly. Then one asked, 'Why was this operation done?'

" 'The patient,' Ellis answered, 'suffers from intermittent attacks of violent behavior. He has organic brain disease—his brain is damaged. We are trying to fix that. We are trying to prevent violence.'

"No one could argue with that, he thought. . . .

" 'Is that common, brain damage associated with violence?'

" 'We don't know how common it is,' Ellis said. "We don't even know how common brain damage alone is. But our best estimates are that ten million Americans have obvious damage, and five million more have a subtle form of it.'

" 'Fifteen million?' one reporter said. 'That's one person in thirteen.'. . .

" 'Something like that,' he replied on the screen. 'There are three quarters of a million people with cerebral palsy. There are over four million with convulsive disorders, including epilepsy. There are six million with mental retardation. There may be as many as two and a half million with hyperkinetic behavior disorders.'

" 'And all of these people are violent?'

" 'No, certainly not. But an unusually high proportion of violent people, if you check them, have brain damage. Physical brain damage. Now, that shoots down a lot of theories about poverty and discrimination and social injustice and social disorganization. Those factors contribute to violence, of course. But physical brain damage is also a major factor. And you can't correct physical brain damage with social remedies.'. . .

" 'When you say violence——'

" 'I mean,' Ellis said, 'attacks of unprovoked violence initiated by single individuals. It's the biggest problem in the world today, violence. And it's a huge problem in this country. In 1969, more Americans were killed or attacked in this country than have been killed or wounded in all the years of the Vietnam war. Specifically——'·

"The reporters were in awe.

" '——We had 14,500 murders, 36,500 rapes and 306,-

500 cases of aggravated assault. All together, a third of a million cases of violence. That doesn't include automobile deaths, and a lot of violence is carried out with cars. We had 56,000 deaths in autos and three million injuries.'. . . .

"On the screen, a reporter was saying, 'And you think these figures reflect physical brain disease?'

"'In large part,' Ellis said. 'One of the clues pointing to physical brain disease in a single individual is a history of repeated violence. There are some famous examples. Charles Whitman, who killed seventeen people in Texas, had a malignant brain tumor and had told his psychiatrist for weeks before that he was having thoughts about climbing the tower and shooting people. Richard Speck engaged in several episodes of brutal violence before he killed eight nurses. Lee Harvey Oswald repeatedly attacked people, including his wife on many occasions. Those were famous cases. There are a third of a million cases every year that are not famous. We're trying to correct that violent behavior with surgery. I don't think that's a despicable thing. I think it's a noble and important goal.' "

My own view is that Mark and Ervin present a grossly inadequate amount of evidence to back up the impression their book gives that their clinical cases provide the insights that will enable us to control human violence. Their book contains many such sweeping statements as:

"Human violence is the most threatening problem in our world today. And although it is a problem that is both formidable and complex, we believe that it is potentially solvable." (Introduction)

"We have written this book to stimulate a new and biologically oriented approach to the problem of human violence." (Preface)

Sweet, Chief of the Neurological Service at the Massachusetts General Hospital, is a frequent collaborator of

Mark and Ervin. In the Foreward to *Violence and the Brain,* Sweet points out that most hospitals do not like to admit persons known to have poor control over dangerous impulses. The too frequent result, he maintains, is that such persons remain at large until some serious violence is committed, when they are incarcerated in jail or an institution for the criminally insane, at a great and usually permanent drain of the public purse. Sweet writes:

"Doctors Mark and Ervin present the evidence that there is now another option—that of providing a special institute or unit staffed not only by competent physicians but also by attendants specially trained to subdue a violent patient without significant injury to anyone involved. That tests may be developed to detect at an early stage the person with poor control of dangerous impulses is an especially appealing likelihood."

Sweet recognizes that "the ability to treat this special group of potentially violent persons represents only a small contribution to the solution of the total problem," but, he continues, "it holds out the hope that knowledge gained about emotional brain function in violent persons with brain disease can be applied to combat the violence-triggering mechanisms in the brains of the non-diseased."

I have every reason to believe that this group of clinicians is seriously concerned about violence and they have no desire to violate guaranteed freedoms, but it appears that they have not given sufficient thought to the ramifications of their proposed solutions. The possibility of developing a means to detect persons with poor control over dangerous impulses may be "appealing"when considered in a social vacuum, but there is a very dangerous precedent inherent in the suggestion of combatting "the violence-triggering mechanisms of the brains of the non-diseased." Implicit in the concept of early detection is the ability to predict violence and to take preventative measures before any serious crime has been committed. In an article entitled "Is There a Need to Evaluate the Individuals Producing Human Violence," Mark and Ervin conclude: "The aim of this research program would be to provide tools that could pinpoint and detect individuals with a low threshold for violence before they were placed in the environmental setting that triggers an episode of unrestrained assault." The only measures proposed, however, are incarceration in a "special institute" or brain surgery, thus it is not clear what course of action is suggested after detecting such individuals.

The suggestion by a neurosurgically oriented team that it would be desirable to screen people in order to prevent violence appears to be a poorly conceived plan as well as potentially dangerous precedent. The idea that brain surgery may be applicable to criminals who have repeatedly been involved in violent crimes has apparently found a sympathetic audience, including some people within state and federal government agencies. There have been several temporal lobe operations performed in a prison within the California penal system. The details of these cases are not available, and it is possible that there may have been convincing evidence that brain pathology was at the root of the behavior problems. Recently, however, the Law Enforcement Assistance Administration of the Department of Justice granted funds to investigate the appropriateness of more extensive use of brain surgery to control violence in prisons. Dr. M. Hunter Brown, a neurosurgeon at St. John's and Santa Monica Hospitals, California, has been quoted (*National Enquirer,* July 9, 1972) as saying:

"I've been invited to testify on this subject before the California legislature later this year. I have been talking to California authorities, and I really hope they will start a program. Once successful in one state it probably would expand across the country. The person convicted of a violent crime should have the chance for a corrective operation. A panel of doctors would give the pre-operation tests. After surgery, the patient would be kept in an institution for three months to see that the operation had worked. Then he would go before a parole board with powers to release him back to society. Obviously the usual checks would be kept to show the man had not reverted to a violent state. Each violent young criminal incarcerated from 20 years to life costs taxpayers perhaps $100,000. For roughly $6000, society can provide medical treatment which will transform him into a responsible well-adjusted citizen."

In 1970 Brown urged the delegates of the Second International Congress of Psychosurgery in Copenhagen "to initiate pilot programs for precise rehabilitation of the prisoner-patient who is often young and intelligent, yet incapable of controlling various forms of violence." Later, he referred to the "well intentioned but timid efforts with inadequate tools" presently being tried on hard-core violent prisoners at Vacaville, California. These "timid efforts" consist mainly of administering so-called minor tranquilizers such as Valium and "milieu conditioning." Brown is very skeptical about the possibilities of success of these treatments, for he writes:

"When this current effort fails, as it will, the state will turn to professionals for well-designed comprehensive programs including chromosome classification, activated electroencephalography, psychological testing, trials of newer medications that show promise, and finally neurosurgical intervention to specific targets as indicated. Until then, humanity must mark time."

There are some clear dangers inherent in Brown's suggestion. From the outset, it should be noted that in this quotation the only treatment listed is surgery and experimental drugs—the other procedures listed are diagnostic tools, not treatment. As is well recognized, there are good reasons for doubting that free consent can always be obtained within a prison or psychiatric institution. Furthermore, the medical and psychological screening Brown proposes would require a great number of skilled professionals and a large expenditure of funds if done properly. Regardless of the merits of Brown's comments about the huge expenses involved in maintaining a person in prison for life, it is not likely that the taxpayers or politicians would appropriate the additional money needed to do thorough testing of prisoners. There is every reason to suspect that practical considerations will reduce preoperative testing and exploration of nonsurgical alternatives to meaningless rituals so that surgery may be used prematurely. Another consideration that requires very close examination is that Brown is not restricting the potential application of neurosurgical procedures to prisoners who have unambiguous evidence of brain pathology. He is apparently sufficiently convinced that there are brain regions specifically devoted to regulating the expression of violence and has proposed surgery even in the absence of evidence of pathology.

A further danger that can result from an uncritical acceptance of the hypothesis that a considerable amount of violence is caused by biological factors is that it may lead to a neglect of social causes. In spite of all of their qualifying remarks, the "biological bias" of Mark and Ervin is quite evident. For example, they point out that although the cities of Boston and Montreal are both saturated with the same violent television shows, Boston leads Montreal in cases of aggravated assault by a ratio of 8 to 1. In the context within which these figures are presented they can create only one impression and that is that such social factors cannot explain the proliferation of violence. It is unquestionably true that one social factor, television violence, cannot completely explain the increase in incidence of assault. I do not seriously believe that Mark and Ervin would try to maintain that the crime ratio differences between the two cities can be explained by biological factors—but what other reason do they have for presenting the television statistics?

A letter to the *Journal of the American Medical Association* in 1967 by Mark, Sweet, and Ervin hit a very sensitive nerve. These investigators commented on the role of brain disease in riots and urban violence. While admitting that poverty is the underlying cause of most riots, they write:

"It is important to realize that only a small number of the millions of slum dwellers have taken part in the riots, and that only a sub-fraction of these rioters have indulged in arson, sniping and assault. Yet, if slum conditions alone determined and initiated riots, why are the vast majority of slum dwellers able to resist the temptations of unrestrained violence? Is there something peculiar about the violent slum dweller that differentiates him from his peaceful neighbor? . . . we need intensive research and clinical studies of the *individuals* committing the violence. The goal of such studies would be to pinpoint, diagnose, and treat those people with low violence thresholds before they contribute to further tragedies."

These same investigators also testified before those Congressional Committees which have been instrumental in appropriating over $900,000 of special funds since 1967 to study the causes of violence with special emphasis given to biological factors. As noted previously, a portion of these funds have been awarded directly for the support of studies of violent behavior related to brain function by Sweet, Mark, and Ervin. The financial support funneled through the Justice Department has particularly concerned a number of people in the United States because of its source and because it was awarded for the determination of the incidence of brain disorders in penal institutions and the development of means to detect such disorders in routine examinations. Although it clearly was not their intention, the fact that the letter by Mark, Sweet, and Ervin was written just after several race riots and that these investigators obtained funds from Congress and the Justice Department has created concern that black militants were the target of this program. It was not surprising, therefore, to learn that the now famous letter to the *Journal of the American Medical Association* was quoted in an article entitled *"New Threat to Blacks: Brain Surgery to Control Behavior,"* which appeared in *Ebony* magazine in February, 1973.

There are numerous studies that report a high incidence of abnormal electroencephalographic records among prisoners who have committed violent crimes. The fact that half of the murders, suicides, and fatal automobile accidents occur under the influence of alcohol has also been related to possible brain pathology, since alcohol is believed to facilitate temporal lobe epileptoid states. If one looks closely at much of the evidence, however, it often turns out to be considerably less than 100 percent convincing. Often the records are not read "blind"—that is, the person who interprets the EEG record knows the history of the subject. Also, in only a few studies are the criteria used for diagnosis completely objective. In neurological parlance, a distinction is made between "hard" and "soft" signs of organic involvement. The more objective "hard" signs consist of clearly identifiable EEG spikes and slow wave abnormalities, whereas the more subjective "soft" signs often are based on impressions from the clinical history and may include "blackouts," lapses of consciousness, and other suggestive, but not conclusive, types of evidence.

It is to Ervin's credit that he recently reported the result of a study at the Lewisburg Federal Penitentiary that is contradictory to the hypothesis presented in his and Mark's book. The results of this investigation of especially violent inmates was presented in March, 1972, at the Houston Neurological Symposium on the Neural Basis of Violence and Aggression. In spite of the fact that this population of inmates had received considerable "head abuse" during their violent lives, there was no more evidence of "hard" EEG signs of brain pathology than among a so-called normal population of equal size. The EEG screening was not intensive, however, and it is possible that it would have revealed more had the records been obtained during sleep or following various "activation procedures" (see footnote 27). Many "soft" signs of brain pathology were said to be present. Considering all the evidence available, it is probably true that the incidence of brain pathology is higher among a violent prison population than a control group, particularly if one selects a population in which the violence was unpredictable and impulsive rather than planned or committed in the course of carrying out a robbery. In any case the correlation is low and statistics usually cited probably exaggerate the contribution of brain pathology to violence. In many cases the brain pathology is caused by the frequent involvement with violence rather than the other way around. In other instances, the relation between violence and brain pathology may be an indirect result of the frustration and confusion caused by the inability of people with low intelligence to make an adequate adjustment.

Although it is possible that there are more cases of abnormal brain foci triggering violence than may have been suspected, there is little to support the view that this factor is a major contributor to the tremendous proliferation of violent crimes that we are now experiencing. The cases such as that of Julia (described earlier) have a very characteristic pattern, which is very different from that of the great majority of instances of violent assault. The number of people that are latent "Julias" would be extremely difficult to determine because there are undoubtedly many people with "abnormal" EEG patterns who never exhibit any unusual amount of violence. It is necessary to ask, therefore, what purpose would be served by the huge expenditure of money necessary to screen large segments of the population. Mark and Ervin have indicated that they operate on less than 1 percent of the patients referred to them as possible candidates for neurosurgery. In a paper on the self-referred patient, Drs. John Lion, George Bach y Rita, and Frank Ervin conclude that among patients who requested help because they were afraid they would kill someone, the largest group falls into the category of "borderline" or "schizoid" personality types. What would be the yield in a less selective population and how would the information be used? Few if any physicians would recommend the use of anticonvulsant drugs for people who have abnormal EEG records but no history of convulsive disorders. And all should agree that brain surgery would be out of the question.

The nature of the problem is clarified by contrasting two case histories. The first is described by Dr. Peter Gloor of the Montreal Neurological Institute of McGill University. The patient was operated on by Dr. Theodore Rasmussen of the same Institute and has been described as an exceptionally (not typical) clear instance of a relationship between the cure of the epileptic condition and the tendency toward unprovoked violence:

"The young man of 21 had suffered a head injury at age 15, with a lacerated wound in the right frontal region. Six months after the head injury, seizures began. . . . The referring physician stated that the patient had had seizures which were preceded or followed by temper outbursts and threats of violence. Frequent outbursts of rage, apparently unrelated to any seizure manifestations, began to present an increasingly serious problem until it became necessary to institutionalize the patient in a psychiatric hospital. The outbursts of rage were provoked by the most trifling stimuli. The intensity of anger provoked by these trifles was often extreme and certainly entirely out of proportion to the banality of the triggering event. During such episodes the patient was described as 'going beserk' and there were incidents of actual physical assault on people standing by. He once injured one of his co-workers with a razor blade, and openly voiced threats to kill the people around him. Between these outbursts of anger, the patient showed a hostile, threatening attitude.

"Upon his admission to the Montreal Neurological Institute, no positive neurological signs were found, but the patient showed a very clear-cut bilateral temporal epileptiform abnormality in the electroencephalogram, with a very strong predominance on the right side. It was apparent from sphenoidal [over temporal lobe] lead recordings that the firing was predominant in the uncinate region, an area just overlying the amygdaloid nucleus.

"The patient was operated on by Dr. Rasmussen, and the cortex of the temporal lobe showed gliosis [scarring] and yellowing in the vicinity of a deformity in the petrous bone, probably representing an old healed skull fracture. The surface and depth electroencephalogram showed during the operation, active discharge in the inferior temporal region.

"Since the operation and up to the present the patient has remained seizure-free. In a letter written by his mother soon after his surgery, she described him as 'happier, more interested, more relaxed, much more tolerant, considerate and understanding of others,' qualities he had not shown before the operation. The patient himself wrote in a letter. 'There is a happier feeling toward everything, especially people.' Only very early during the post-operative period were there three brief episodes of angry behavior, of which only one could be considered as irrational. None of these, however, involved attempted physical assault, and soon thereafter all abnormal manifestations of aggressive behavior ceased and have not reappeared. The underlying attitude of hostility also disappeared following surgery."

This patient is an excellent example of traumatic brain injury that has produced violent behavior. It should be emphasized that even though a certain percentage of head injuries may result in epileptic seizures, the relationship between seizures and violence is low. The belief that the relationship is higher than it actually is can be attributed to a few dramatic cases of violence committed during a psychomotor epileptic seizure and the fact that some criminal lawyers have attempted to use this argument as a defense for their clients. Sometimes rage may be expressed during a post-seizure confusional state when an epileptic is being forcibly restrained by a well-meaning person. Several accounts in our literature have also added to the false belief that a strong relationship between seizures and violence exists. Othello, for example, was subject to seizures and just before he killed Desdemona she uttered: "And yet I fear you; for you are fatal when your eyes roll so." There are statements in the older literature claiming that epileptics, particularly temporal lobe epileptics, exhibit a high tendency toward violence during the periods between seizures. More recently, most neurologists refute the earlier figures. Current estimates of the incidence of violence among epileptics is low. Estimates range from 4 to less than 1 percent and if one corrects for the fact that the onset of temporal lobe epilepsy (60 percent of epilepsy is diagnosed as temporal lobe) occurs at an older age than other epilepsies, the relationship is no higher among this particular subgroup.

The case described by Dr. Gloor should be contrasted with one presented by Drs. Jerome Kagen and Howard Moss in their book *Birth to Maturity:*

"Subject 1650 was examined at 3-1/2 years of age and had a spell of uncontrolled rage. When the doctor tried to get near him he screamed and held his breath. In his early years in school S was unusually destructive and violent. He gradually gave up holding his breath when he got irritated, but he was easily angered and provoked. When he was 8 he was observed to take some baby birds from a nest and torture them. In his preadolescent years his outbursts of temper continued and he was highly resistant to being interviewed by adults. At 12 he was a roughhouse when playing with other boys but was rebellious and openly resentful toward adults. In his twenties he remained easily angered and frustrated, and often verbally attacked his wife, child, and strangers. He felt that being tough and aggressive was the only way to get anywhere in the world and that hate and power strivings were basic qualities of human nature."

The probability of this subject being involved in violence may be greater than that of a subject with another personality, but in the absence of any crime or request for psychiatric help or evidence of organic pathology what preventative measures should be taken?

Psychosurgery

EARLY HISTORY

There is no doubt that many people today are horrified by any suggestion of destroying a portion of a person's brain for psychotherapeutic purposes. Some perspective can be gained, however, by appreciating that there was a strong conviction extending well into the present century that mental illness could be traced to abnormalities in the brain. The clinical literature reports numerous cases where the development of mental illness could be directly traced to a head injury; in some of these cases the symptoms could be dramatically eliminated by elevating the skull and removing pressure from the brain. It is not surprising that many believe that even in cases where there had been no injury to the brain, an underlying structural abnormality might be responsible for the mental illness.

The development of histological techniques that made it possible to study nerve cells in microscopic detail gave rise to the hope that the bases of psychiatric illness would be revealed. Because of our strong environmental bias we tend to forget that the majority of "informed people" formerly had no doubt that individual differences in psychiatric makeup as well as intelligence were organically based. The existence of a number of collections of the brains of scientific geniuses and outstanding public figures testifies to the prevailing conviction that individual differences could be traced to brain anatomy.[29] Many contributions to brain anatomy were made by investigators who were interested in psychiatry and motivated to search for the root of mental illness in the brain.

Although the logic underlying the belief was perfectly sound, the search for physical abnormalities (other than tumors and traumatic damage) in the brains of psychiatric patients has not been rewarding. Even in schizophrenia, where many psychiatrists believe there are underlying constitutional factors, there is no reliable anatomical evidence that explains the mental aberrations. Drs. Dionisio Nieto and Alfonso Escobar of the National Institute of Neurology in Mexico City have concluded that the morphological basis of schizophrenia remains controversial.[30] Neuropathologists quite understandably hope that the use of the electron microscope or new neurochemical techniques may reveal significant differences in the brains of schizophrenics, but at present there is no neuroanatomical information that helps to understand the process underlying schizophrenia, let alone the psychoneuroses. Most would agree with Dr. Fred Plum of the Cornell Medical Center in New York, who has concluded that "schizophrenia has been the graveyard of neuropathologists."

Many early neuropathologists spent a better part of their careers pursuing false leads that convinced them they had identified some structural change in the brains of schizophrenics. At the International Congress of Neuropathology in 1949, however, it became clear that there was no agreement on the nature of any brain change or its locus among the proponents of different structurally based theories of schizophrenia. Where there were adequately controlled studies, there was little evidence of structural changes in schizophrenic brains that were not also present in the brains of nonpsychotic individuals. Most of the earlier claims of brain differences were probably the effect of long periods of institutional confinement, malnutrition, and gradual deterioration prior to death, rather than the cause of schizophrenia. Clearly there never was any reliable evidence of brain pathology that provided a rationale for psychosurgery. Psychosurgical theory as it developed had to be based on presumed functional abnormalities in particular regions of the brain rather than demonstrable structural differences.[31]

PSYCHOSURGICAL THEORY

It is not surprising that the belief in the anatomical bases of mental illness encouraged people to explore the possibility that some surgical intervention might produce beneficial effects. It is true that there were not very many who subscribed to the idea that brain surgery might be therapeutic, since it did not necessarily follow that surgery would be helpful even if the problem could be related to brain structure. It was argued, however, that if the problem was produced by some functional excess in the activity of a portion of the brain, surgical intervention might be useful either in removing some of the source of the excess or in blocking its spread to other parts of the brain. This model seemed to apply especially to those hypermanic patients who were usually the greatest problem in mental institutions.

The first published account of psychosurgery was reported in 1891 by Dr. Gottlieb Burckhardt, who supervised the Insane Asylum in Préfargier, Switzerland. Burckhardt removed parts of the cerebral cortex to quiet patients who were responding to vivid hallucinations. He wrote: "If we could remove these exciting impulses from the brain mechanism, the patient might be transformed from a disturbed to a quiet dement." (My translation.) He was influenced by Frederich Goltz's report that dogs could be more easily provoked into a rage following complete removal of the neocortex, but if only the temporal cortex was destroyed, the dogs actually became calmer than normal.[32] Burckhardt was reflecting the dispute at the time over the question of localization of higher mental activity in the cortex when he argued:

"Who sees in psychoses only diffuse illness of the cortex . . . for him it will naturally be useless to remove small parts of the cortex in the hope to influence a psychosis beneficially by this means. One, therefore, has to be as I am, of a different opinion. That is, our psychological existence is composed of single elements, which are localized in separate areas of the brain. . . . Based on these and theories expressed earlier, I believe one has the right to excise such parts of the cortex, which one can consider as starting points and centers of psychological malfunctions and, furthermore, to interrupt connections whose existence is an important part of pathological processes."

Burckhardt commented on the poor prognosis of many of his patients and after acknowledging the insights gained from Goltz's experiments and the advances in brain surgery due to the contributions of Victor Horsley and others, he undertook surgery in six patients. He reasoned that:

". . . should excitement and impulsivity arise in our patients because stimuli in above normal quantity originating in the sensory areas enter the motor zone frequently and strongly, an improvement can only be brought about by inserting a resistance between both. . . . I was of the opinion that in the above instances it would be sufficient to remove a strip of cortical substance on both sides . . . so to say a ditch to be drawn, possibly up to the temporal lobe."

Burckhardt was vigorously opposed by the medical community (one patient died from the surgery), but he concluded that as modest as the improvement was (several patients, although still psychotic, were more peaceful on the wards), it represented progress compared to the otherwise hopeless condition of the patients. He concluded: "I would not allow myself to become discouraged, and hope that my colleagues will nonetheless, while utilizing my experience, themselves tread the path of cortical extirpation with ever better and more satisfactory results."

In 1910 in St. Petersburg, the pioneering Russian neurosurgeon Ludwig Puusepp cut the fibers between the parietal and frontal cortex on one side of the brain in three manic-depressive patients.[33] Puusepp was familiar with Burckhardt's investigations and his rationale for psychosurgery was essentially similar. He wrote:

"I introduced a slim knife with a double edge three centimeters into the brain (depth-wise) and precisely between the frontal and parietal lobes I cut the nerve fibers perpendicular to the longitudinal axis of the brain. . . . Unfortunately, the success of the operation was rather poor, so that I did not do any more operations of this kind," (My translation.)

Although Burckhardt and Puusepp had previously performed brain surgery on mental patients, it was Moniz' frontal lobe surgery that precipitated the large-scale adoption of psychosurgical techniques. The optimistic description of the results of Moniz' initial series of frontal lobe operations, the confirming reports from Freeman and Watts in the United States and many neurosurgeons in other countries, and the urgent need for a convenient treatment to cope with the many psychiatrically disturbed veterans during and after World War II [34] all combined to produce a wave of psychosurgery. The crest of the wave was reached at the end of the 1940s and the level remained high to the mid-1950s. Afterward, the tide receded in the face of a strong reaction against psychosurgery precipitated by reports of "dehumanized zombies," the overuse of the surgical approach, and the availability of psychoactive drugs as an alternative to surgery.[35]

The theoretical explanation of why partial destruction of the frontal lobes might be beneficial to psychiatric patients has been and remains at a very primitive level. In a sense it could not be otherwise, for in the absence of any clear understanding of the physiology underlying normal thought processes and emotions, it has not been possible to develop a sophisticated rationale for the surgical treatment of psychiatric disorders. At least initially, Moniz was concerned primarily with agitated patients, and the Jacobsen report on the lobectomized chimpanzees suggested that frontal lobe surgery might have a calming effect (see pages 50–54). The theory Moniz expressed later consisted of minor elements of Pavlovianism—Pavlov maintained that conditioned reflexes were established in the cerebral cortex—and the idea that fixed connections between nerve cells were developed during learning. He concluded that the psychiatric symptoms were the result of an abnormal stabilization of conditioned neural patterns in the brain and wrote:

"In accordance with the theory which we have just developed, one conclusion is derived: to cure these patients we must destroy the more or less fixed arrangements of cellular connections that exist in the brain, and particularly those which are related to the frontal lobes."

This theory (if it deserves to be called that) was about the only rationale that existed throughout the period of the

major application of psychosurgery. Different spokesmen
had their own way of expressing the same basic thought,
but the idea was essentially the same, only the words were
changed. One neurosurgeon found it helpful to refer to the
fixed connections and the ideas associated with them by
analogy to a cracked phonograph record and a stuck
needle. In reality, the theories underlying lobotomy had
no more explanatory power than the less pretentious statements of the youth of today who speak of "hangups,"
with the exception of the claim that the "hangups" were
somehow maintained by neural activity in the frontal
lobes.

Many of the physiological models used to explain why
prefrontal lobotomies should be psychiatrically helpful
were based on the now rejected theory that memories are
stored in "reverberating circuits" consisting of neurons,
whose branches form circular functional units capable of
perpetuating activity in feedback loops.[36] Walter Freeman
claimed that it was advantageous to perform transorbital
lobotomies, a technique to be described below, after electroconvulsive shock. He believed the shock would disorga-
nize the fixed cortical patterns and cutting the nerve fibers
would prevent them from reforming. A somewhat similar
idea was expressed by Norbert Wiener, the "father of
cybernetics":

"... the crowding of the brain is of importance, very
much as the traffic problem is of importance in every
large city. Combined with the absence of a complete
clearing process, we see that concomitant mental
processes in the same brain are likely to compete for
internuncial space and memory space and that this competition is likely to increase the traffic-jam still more. It
may be that, in the future, we can do something better
with situations where *circulating memories* have led to
bad traffic jams than to destroy a part of the connections
of the brain by a frontal lobotomy or to intervene brutally

in all synaptic connections by one or the other varieties of shock therapy." (Italics added)

The idea that *circulating memories* or preoccupying thoughts could lead to psychiatric problems was obviously not a new concept. Although Freud usually stressed the potentially disrupting influence of repressed thoughts, he as well as others also appreciated the fact that mental health may depend on a selective forgetting. Nietzsche also recognized the relevance of selective forgetting for maintaining the integrity of the personality thus: "My memory says that I did it, my pride says that I could not have done it, and in the end my memory yields." A recent Soviet film, *Solaris*, makes the point that only by forgetting some past events and blurring obsessions is it possible to achieve psychological health. The film depicts the story of space explorers who discover a new planet that emits a vapor causing everyone exposed to it to have total recall. Immediately, unpleasant and awful memories from the past become the totally absorbing substance of present thoughts. Everyone is completely corroded by guilt over past actions and the interpersonal relations on the space station all start to sour. In a sense, this was at the heart of the argument advanced by many of the advocates of psychosurgery. For example, Mary Robinson, who worked with Walter Freeman and James Watts, the leading American proponents of psychosurgery, commented in a paper delivered in 1949 at the American Psychological Association meeting:

"Lobotomy relieves the suffering with its attendant symptoms. But it does more. It frees the patient from the tyranny of his own past, from the anxious self-searching that has become too terrible to endure, and at the same time renders him largely indifferent to future problems and to the opinions of other people."

Freeman and Watts once remarked that without the frontal lobes there could be no functional psychoses, implying that it was this part of the brain that was responsible for the persistence of "fixed ideas" like those seen in phobias, obsessive thinking, and compulsions. Their theoretical statements differed very little from the initial, loosely formulated ideas of Moniz. In 1971, for example, Freeman wrote:

"The most tenable theory would seem to be that the fibers severed in transorbital lobotomy are collaterals of the thalamofrontal projections. It would further seem that these collaterals are highly unstable and thus unimportant in mental health, but that during the course of a functional mental disorder they become stabilized in their synaptic connections and thus serve to perpetuate the stereotyped thinking disorder and emotional reaction that underlie the pychosis. Thus *the original hypothesis of Egas Moniz appears more probable than ever.*"

Lobotomy does not erase the memory of fixed ideas. None of the standardized tests of memory have ever demonstrated any deficit following lobotomy. It is not the memory that is lost, but the degree of emotional involvement with the thoughts that is changed. Speaking of the mental state following the frontal operation, Freeman and Watts wrote: "The emotional nucleus of the psychosis is removed, the 'sting' of the disorder, is drawn. Even though the fixed ideas persist and the compulsions continued for a while, the fear that disabled the patient is banished." One patient remarked after the operation: "Doctor, you have removed my worry center." The thoughts that used to worry the patient were not erased, but they no longer seemed able to command the same emotional involvement.

The reports of deleterious effects that sometimes occurred after frontal lobe operations and the evidence that other parts of the brain, particularly the limbic system, are involved in emotional behavior combined to produce a change both in the type of surgery performed and the theoretical rationale for psychosurgery. Papez' theory that the limbic system of the brain plays the major role in modulating emotionality was not taken seriously at first, but a number of observations of dramatic emotional changes following destruction of limbic structures in experimental animals changed this attitude (see pages 47–50). Arguments that the main benefit resulting from the various frontal operations derived from a disruption of communicating pathways to and from the limbic system started to appear. These developments encouraged exploration of the advantages of either selective destruction of a portion of the fibers connecting the frontal lobes and the limbic system or the ablation of parts of the limbic system itself.

John Fulton, who was initially shocked by Moniz' suggestion that the Jacobsen chimpanzee experiment be applied to man (see pages 50–54), softened his attitude over the years and dedicated his 1951 book, *Frontal Lobotomy and Affective Behavior*, to "Egas Moniz and Almeida Lima *for their imagination, perseverance, and daring.*" However, as early as 1948, he wrote

"The results are of challenging interest to anyone who concerns himself with the functions of the brain, but the responsibility of those who undertake to interfere with the anatomical structure of the human brain is particularly grave, and I would close this preface with an earnest plea for caution on the part of the neurosurgeon lest in the absence of basic physiological data he unwittingly do irremediable harm to human beings who might be benefited by a far less radical operation than is now performed. I utter this word of caution not to discourage those who are performing leucotomies, but in the hope that they will not allow their zeal to outrun their knowledge of function."

This plea for more surgical precision and a more concerted effort to identify the function associated with different brain areas from a highly respected and influential brain scientist did not go unheeded. It fostered a search for more restricted psychosurgical procedures that might be better directed at those neural structures that were more specifically related to the different psychiatric problems.

Psychosurgical theory began to incorporate the newly developing emphasis placed on the limbic system's role in emotional expression. Two directions can be discerned as having developed out of this new emphasis. One was to attempt to make selective ablations of particular fiber tracts connecting the frontal lobes and specific limbic structures; the other approach involved selective ablation of limbic structures such as the cingulum, the midline thalamic areas, and the amygdala.[37] Reviewing this history in an article entitled "The Frontal Lobes Revisited. The Case for A Second Look," Dr. Kenneth Livingston of the University of Toronto writes:

"In retrospect, even as lobotomy fell from grace clinical evidence consistent with earlier physiological concepts was rapidly accumulating. It had been clinically established that a variety of anatomical lesions of the frontal lobes can produce beneficial change in the affect and behavior of patients suffering from severe psychotic and psychoneurotic disorders. It had been further demonstrated clinically that the areas most effective in producing such change are discrete regions of the medial and orbital frontal cortex, and demonstrated experimentally that stimulation of these "effective" frontal areas produced autonomic responses which presumably reached outflow pathways in the hypothalamus and brain stem through intermediate limbic circuits. On the basis of this evidence it could be postulated that the 'key' to understanding the effects of frontal lobotomy lay in the elucidation of functional frontolimbic relationships—the mechanisms by which frontal lesions may alter limbic system function."

In response to the emerging belief that the more medial fibers in the deeper parts of the frontal lobe constitute the most important connections with the limbic system, surgical procedures were developed to selectively interrupt these pathways. The evolution of the surgical procedures will be reviewed in the following section of this chapter, but it should be mentioned for the sake of continuity that in 1948, Dr. William Scoville developed his *orbital undercutting* approach to the medial and deep frontolimbic fibers while others began to adopt stereotaxic techniques for destroying fibers in the same general region. About the same time, Sir Hugh Cairns in Oxford and Dr. J. LeBeau of Paris began to report favorable results following destruction of the anterior regions of the cingulum, particularly in agitated and aggressive patients.

The theory that accompanied the development of these selective or "fractional" psychosurgical procedures has remained at a very speculative and tenuous level. The functions of the particular brain areas selected for ablation are still not understood, and for the most part theoretical statements simply paraphrase what is believed to be the more striking postoperative changes. For example, Dr. H. Crow of the Burden Neurological Institute in Bristol performs stereotaxic ablation of the deep (inferior) portion of the frontal lobes because of his conviction that:

". . . the cells of the inferior third of the frontal lobes are contained in a system, the function of which is to produce fear sensation. When the neuronal system is only slightly active, we may call the sensation 'apprehension,' and when it is very active we may call the sensation 'terror.' It can be plausibly argued that such a fear system is favorable, and possibly necessary, for survival among higher animals including man. I have also speculated that an essential component of what we call happiness is a suppression of the general level of activity of this hypothetical fear-system. In other words, happiness is the absence of fear at a time when we have in our consciousness a set of concepts which we have learned to consider attractive. I have come to consider that these particular patients were ill because they had inherited or through environmental influences in some way developed fear-systems which had become chronically overactive with intermittent paroxysms of severe overactivity; and because the intensity and duration of the fear sensations did not match the real threat of the world, they developed maladaptive concepts and behavior patterns which are labelled neurotic."

The attempts to provide a physiological rationale for destruction of any particular limbic structure inevitably are dependent on empirical results obtained initially from animal studies and later from reports of human cases following brain ablations. There is no theoretical way at present of predicting the consequences of destruction of a particular structure within the limbic system because almost all the structures are interconnected by many anatomical pathways. Knowledge of the details of how the limbic system regulates the emotions is very general at best and as a result essentially the same "theory" is presented as the rationale for different surgical interventions. Typical of these explanatory statements is that offered by Yakovlev:

"The cingulum is a bundle strategically situated to mediate activities of the limbic cortex to the entire forebrain. On general grounds one might speculate that these activities have something to do with the outward expression of the visceral, i.e., of the internal states or 'emotions.' Its interruption in cingulotomy modifies in some way the behavioral expression of the distraught internal states. The changes effected by cingulotomy apparently are not different in kind from those effected by the classical leucotomies. However, these effects appear to be more selective, less damaging to the intellectual facilities and obviously much less damaging to the brain."

This explanatory statement by Yakovlev was written in 1965; it is a sad but true commentary that no better explanation can be offered today.

THE EVOLUTION OF PSYCHOSURGICAL OPERATIONS

As noted previously, the evolution of psychosurgical operations has paralleled the prevailing theoretical view of brain function in psychiatric disorders. Moniz' original "core" operation was designed to cut the fiber tracts in the frontal lobes at several places (see Figure 38). This procedure was used very little by others because the anatomical reference points for the surgery could not be sufficiently standardized. This made it difficult to compare results and it also increased the potential danger of damaging the areas of the frontal lobe that controlled motor functions and speech. As described earlier, Watts and Freeman very quickly popularized their so-called *precision method*, a procedure involving the use of skull landmarks and an X-ray view of the lateral ventricles to guide the knife severing the fiber connections of the frontal lobes. They tried to find the best plane of section through the frontal lobes "that would give the patient relief from his emotional turmoil" and injected a contrast material into the incisions to show under X-ray where the cut was made. Depending on how much of the frontal lobes was separated from the rest of the brain, they called their operations *minimal, standard,* or *radical lobotomy.* If a minimal or standard operation did not achieve satis-

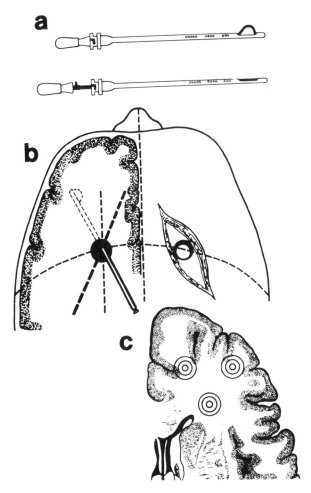

Figure 38. The "core" lobotomy procedure of Egas Moniz and Almeida Lima. *(a)* The leucotome, *(b)* The leucotome was inserted at different angles through a burr hole in the skull. When the leucotome was believed to be in place the cutting wire was extruded and the instrument rotated. *(c)* Sketch of a horizontal slice (parallel to the top of the head) through the brain illustrating three "cores" of destroyed nerve fibers in the frontal lobe.

278

factory results it was recommended that a radical operation be undertaken.

Although the Freeman-Watts operation was performed on a great number of people throughout the world, almost from the time of its introduction there was considerable concern over the fact that the small burr holes in the skull through which the knife was inserted did not provide the surgeon with an adequate view. Customarily, the wound was washed with a warm saline solution until bleeding stopped, but the surgeon was essentially working blind and consequently there was some danger of later hemorrhage from cut blood vessels. The dispute between the "open" and "closed" operations led to the development of

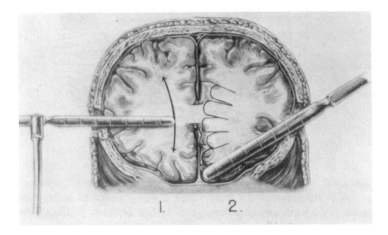

Figure 39. The Freeman-Watts lobotomy procedure. (1) The "precision" leucotome is inserted into the frontal lobes and a sweeping motion cut the fibers. (2) The more medial fibers could be cut with a blunt knife that was extended to the midline. The lobotomy was called "moderate," "standard," or "radical" depending on how posterior the incision was made. (From W. Freeman and J. W. Watts, *Psychosurgery in the Treatment of Mental Disorders and Intractable Pain*, 2nd Ed., 1950, Fig. 15. Courtesy of Charles C. Thomas, Publisher, Springfield, Ill.)

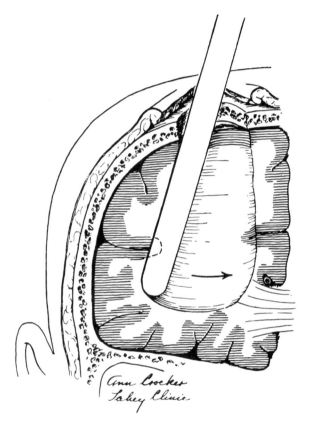

Figure 40. The technique of prefrontal lobotomy using a "superior" approach. By approaching from above it was possible to destroy the medial fibers while avoiding damage to the lateral fibers. Gradually the impression was formed that by limiting the destruction to the more medial fibers, particularly those in the depths of the frontal lobe, the emotional state could be modified without producing extensive intellectual deficits. (From James L. Poppen, "Technic of Prefrontal Lobotomy," *Journal of Neurosurgery*, 1948, Vol. 5, pp. 5l4-520, Fig. 3.)

a number of procedures involving the opening of a sufficient portion of the skull to provide the surgeon with a better view. In 1938, J. G. Lyerly of Jacksonville, Florida, described an "open" method which used the Freeman-Watts plane of sectioning, and in 1948 James Poppen of the Lahey Clinic in Boston described an approach to the frontal lobes from above (superior approach), which made it more convenient to destroy the medial or lateral fiber tracts separately (Figure 40). The latter procedure was significant because it contributed evidence to the growing conviction that destruction of the more medial fibers, particularly those deeper in the brain, produced the optimal results.

To evaluate the contribution of different regions of the frontal lobes, Dr. Lawrence Pool of Columbia University developed a technique called *topectomy*. This operation, which was used in the often cited Columbia-Greystone Study to be discussed later, involved the elimination of circular areas in the frontal lobes by cutting a circle with a pointed scalpel blade and attempting to remove a block of tissue as a whole after undercutting it with a curved dissecting tool. ("Gentle suction" was then applied "to smooth the edges of the cortical cavity.") Comparable "blocks" of brain were removed from each frontal lobe and these were weighed to allow quantification of the amount of tissue removed. Electrical stimulation was used to help locate functional areas within the frontal lobe and to avoid the critical regions controlling movement or speech.

In 1948 Freeman introduced the transorbital leucotomy procedure into the United States. This technique, which involves reaching the frontal lobes by penetration through the skull above the eye was originally developed by Fiamberti in Italy. The convenience of the procedure appealed to Freeman and after experimenting with an ice pick on cadavers he started to operate on patients. Essentially this

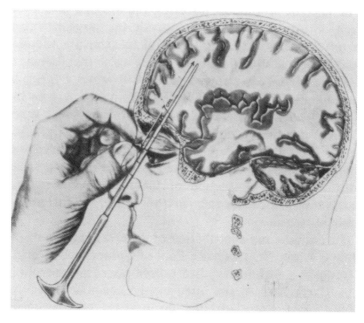

Figure 41. The transorbital lobotomy operation was first described by Fiamberti in Italy in 1937 and was popularized in the United States by Freeman in the late 1940s. A transorbital leucotome is inserted through the orbital roof into the brain and the handle is swung medially and laterally to sever fibers at the base of the frontal lobes. In addition to other objections, many surgeons believed that "closed operations" where severe hemorrhaging might not be detected were potentially dangerous. Watts, Freeman's collaborator up to this point, disagreed strongly with the extensive use of this procedure. Watts wrote: "It is Walter Freeman's opinion that transorbital lobotomy is a minor operation. This is clearly indicated by the fact that of the first ten cases he reported four were not disabled and six had been disabled less than six months. . . . It is my opinion that any procedure involving cutting of brain tissue is a major surgical operation, no matter how quickly or atraumatically one enters the intracranial cavity." (From W. Freeman, "Transorbital Leucotomy: The Deep Frontal Cut," *Proc. R. Soc. Med.*, 1949, Vol. 42, Suppl. pp. 8-12.)

technique consists of tapping the handle of the transorbital leucotome (surgical ice pick) with a mallet and driving it through the bony cavity above the eye into the base of the frontal lobes. The handle is then swung in an appropriate plane to cut the fibers in the lower depth of the frontal lobes. Due to the surgical simplicity of this procedure a great number of transorbital leucotomies were performed—some even in a physician's office rather than a hospital. There was continuous objection voiced over the fact that this operation, which many referred to as "ice pick psychosurgery," was done "blind" and Watts, who had been Freeman's collaborator up to the time, strongly disapproved of the wide-scale adoption of this procedure, especially by physicians who were inadequately trained in neurosurgery (see legend to Figure 41).

The transorbital leucotomy operation has been completely abandoned, partly in response to the reaction raised against it, partly as a function of the general decrease in psychosurgery, and partly because of the development of other procedures regarded as safer for gaining access to the base of the frontal lobes. As a matter of fact, none of the surgical techniques described up to this point is still being used. Frontal lobe psychosurgery has evolved from a point of swinging a knife relatively blindly within the frontal lobes to techniques that permit destruction of selective fiber tracts in the ventromedial portion of this lobe. Destruction is produced either under direct visual observation or with the guidance of stereotaxic instruments supplemented by X-ray visualization of landmarks within the brain.

In 1948 William Scoville introduced an "open" method for selective cutting of the fibers at the base of the frontal lobes. At first, the fibers under both the medial and lateral portions of the frontal lobes were cut, but with experience the impression was gained that cutting the medial fibers was most effective. Because the fibers are now cut only

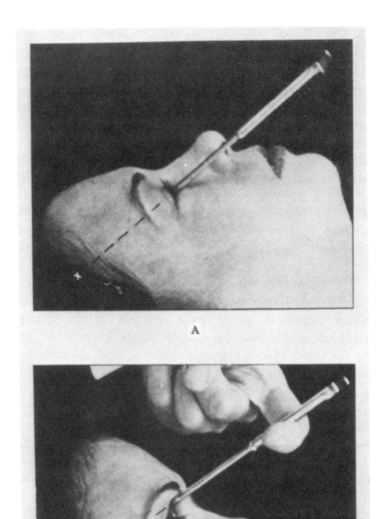

A

B

284

under the medial, so-called orbital region, of the frontal lobes, Scoville's procedure is referred to as *orbital undercutting*. To perform this operation, two trephine holes are drilled in the temple. A spatula is inserted into the holes and the frontal lobes are lifted so that the undersurface is exposed sufficiently to cut the medial fibers (see Figure 43). Scoville believes his procedure combines the precision and safety of an operation done under direct vision and is also sufficiently selective in the damage imposed to minimize blunting of the personality or intellect. In contrast to other contemporary psychosurgeons, Scoville does not believe that the type of mental illness should determine the location of the lesion. He recommends orbital undercutting as the operation of choice whenever psychosurgery is to be undertaken, but in the more intractable illnesses the area destroyed should be extended further posterior. Sadao Hirose introduced the Scoville technique in Japan in 1956 and soon modified the operation to limit the fibers cut to a more restricted area.

The realization that it was necessary to restrict the ablations to specific areas of the frontal lobes or limbic system to minimize intellectual deficits has led to the adoption of stereotaxic psychosurgery. First introduced by Spiegel and Wycis in 1949 as a technique for making rela-

---

Figure 42. Photograph illustrating transorbital lobotomy, (A) The initial cut, (B) The deep frontal cut. Freeman used electroconvulsive shock as the only "anesthesia." He wrote: "I believe the shock treatment disorganizes the cortical patterns that underlie the psychotic behavior, ánd the lobotomy, by severing the connections between the thalamus and the frontal pole prevents the pattern from reforming." The operation only took a few moments and in some later instances it was done as office surgery. The patient was often able to walk within an hour. Usually there was only a slight discoloration around the eyes. Freeman wrote: "Some of the 'black eyes' are beauties, however, and I usually ask the family to provide the patient with sun glasses rather than explanations. . . . Most patients deny having been operated on." (From W. Freeman "Transorbital Leucotomy: The Deep Frontal Cut," *Proc. R. Soc. Med.*, 1949, Vol. 42, Suppl. pp. 8-12.)

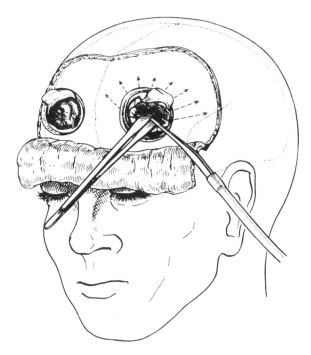

Figure 43. The "orbital undercutting" operation introduced by William Scoville. By lifting the frontal lobes with a spatula it is possible to selectively cut the fibers beneath the more medial (orbital) portion of the prefrontal area. (From A. Asenjo, *Neurosurgical Techniques,* 1963. Courtesy of Charles C. Thomas, Publisher, Springfield, Ill.)

tively circumscribed electrolytic lesions in the dorsomedial thalamus in psychotic patients (see pages 56–58), it is now used primarily to ablate other brain areas, even though there remain a few groups who continue to ablate portions of the medial thalamus in psychiatric patients. Dr. Orlando Andy of the University of Mississippi, for example, has performed such operations on "hyperresponsive" and aggressive patients, while Drs. R. Hassler and G. Dickmann of the Max-Planck Institute in Frankfurt use stereotaxic ablation of the medial thalamus for patients suffering from obsessional compulsive symptoms.

Dr. H. Crow and his colleagues at the Burden Neurological Institute in Bristol, England, have developed an elaborate system for restricted frontal lobe psychosurgery. Their technique, which is called a "controlled multifocal method," makes it possible to gradually increase the size and to vary the location of the neural destruction depending on the results achieved. The procedure involves the stereotaxic implantation of a number of gold electrodes in the frontal lobes. These can then be used to make electrolytic lesions over a period of three to six months during which time the patient's behavior can be monitored. The serial coagulations are usually made in intervals of one to four weeks and they can be progressively increased in size or the location can be changed by using another electrode. When the desired results are achieved the electrodes can be removed.

Crow has explored the possibility of using a polarizing electric current which disrupts but does not destroy nerve cells as a means of selecting the sites for coagulation. At active sites, the polarizing current may produce a decrease in fear or tension that might last from a few seconds to several hours after the termination of the current. This technique may be useful in selecting sites for destruction, but it has not yet been satisfactorily demonstrated that the effect achieved with polarizing current is a good predictor of the changes that would follow destruction of the area. Crow reports that his patients are progressively freed from morbid fear and obsessional thinking following each lesion and he argues that the method has the advantage of limiting the amount of tissue destroyed to the minimum necessary to achieve a therapeutically useful result. Moreover, to the extent that the polarizing current permits an accurate prediction of results that will be produced by coagulation, it may be possible to avoid errors that might be caused by individual differences in brain anatomy or localization of function.

The method of serial coagulations has also been used in cases of intractable pain. It has long been recognized that a major determinant of the intensity of pain sensation is the degree of concern or preoccupation with it. Therefore it is not surprising that psychosurgery would be tried with patients suffering from intractable and intense pain. Freeman and Watts had noted several instances of lobotomy appearing to relieve pain, but the initial impression was that this was hysterical pain that had a psychoneurotic rather than an organic origin—a distinction which may not be able to stand up to close scrutiny. By 1943 they became convinced that their observations were reliable and Watts performed the first lobotomy solely for pain and with Freeman published an article recommending this operation for the relief of pain in the absence of psychiatric symptoms.

A number of the *standard* Freeman-Watts operations have been done on patients suffering from intractable pain, but after reviewing the evidence Drs. James White and William Sweet of Massachusetts General Hospital concluded that an extensive bilateral lobotomy should be done only when the patient is unlikely to live more than several months because of the possibility of considerable intellectual deterioration. White has recommended a method of pain relief for patients suffering during a terminal malignancy which utilizes a type of implanted electrode that can be withdrawn in stages permitting serial coagulations. The coagulations are spaced about a week apart allowing time for an estimate of the pain relief achieved.

While frontal lobe psychosurgery was evolving other areas of the brain were being explored as potential targets for psychosurgery. In 1945 Wilbur Smith of the University of Rochester reported that electrical stimulation of the cingulum, a major limbic structure (see

Figures 25 and 26), produced bodily changes in animals that were characteristic of emotional states. Stimulation in this brain area elicited dilation of the pupils, hair standing on end (piloerection), heart rate changes, and other so-called autonomic reactions. Smith also noted that following destruction of a portion of the cingulum his monkeys became unusually tame and easy to handle. Shortly afterward in 1948, Arthur Ward of the University of Washington at Seattle introduced an experimental paper by relating an account in the year 1670 by Felix Plater, Professor of Medicine at Basel. Plater had described the case of "the good knight," Casper Bonecurtius, who gradually became mentally deranged over the course of two years. The knight suddenly died and an autopsy revealed a tumor over the anterior portion of the cingulum. In the main section of this paper, Ward presented data on the effects of destruction of the anterior cingulum of monkeys. Although he noted behavior which he believed was similar to what Smith had earlier called "tameness," Ward also pointed out that his operated monkeys seemed to have lost some "ability to accurately forecast the social repercussions of their own actions."

Although there was apparently much in the description of the changed behavior of the "cingulectomized monkeys" that might have cautioned neurosurgeons against its application to humans (see pages 327–328), the fact that the animals became tamed seemed to push all other observations into the background and encouraged several neurosurgical groups to risk performing cingulectomies on psychiatric patients. Groups headed by Sir Hugh Cairns (see Whitty, et al., 1952) in Oxford and Dr. J. LeBeau of the Neurosurgical Hospital in Paris destroyed portions of the cingulum in patients during the early 1950s. The former group reported that although the psychotics did not benefit, the majority of those suffering from severe obsessional and anxiety states were "definitely improved" and two patients were considered

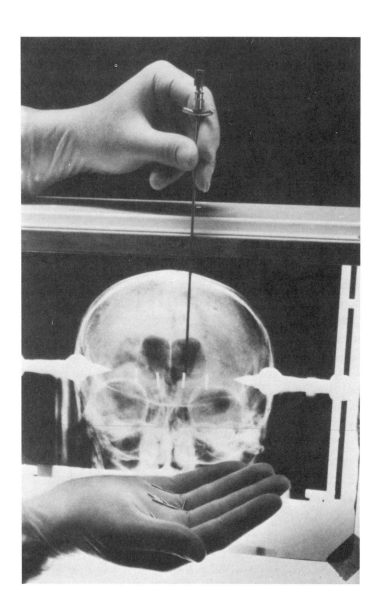

cured. It was also observed that "a striking feature of our results has been the very slight amount of unwanted personality change of the type seen after leucotomy." LeBeau came to similar conclusions and in addition remarked that "cingulectomy is especially indicated in intractable cases of anger, violence, aggressiveness and permanent agitation." Different psychosurgical procedures involving other limbic structures, or the midline thalamic nuclei, considered (on the basis of anatomical evidence) to be a part of the limbic system, have also been performed for psychiatric disorders.[38] The amygdalectomies and hypothalatomies performed for aggressive and violent behavior and the use of multitargeted limbic lesions for a variety of psychiatric symptoms have been discussed in the previous chapter.

To a great extent, neurosurgeons gain their reputations and the respect of their colleagues by developing new operations or new equipment or by being the first to apply a new technical advance. It has been said, for example, that there are as many different human stereotaxic instruments as there are neurosurgeons who use them. The value of technical achievements is obvious, but there are many instances where the progress that is claimed may be illusory. While there are new methods, for example, for destroying brain tissue that utilize ultrasonic waves or cobalt (lasers have also been suggested), unless they are paralleled by a more sophisticated understanding of brain mechanisms these developments are unlikely to achieve any great advances. Perhaps an example will make the point more effectively.

Figure 44. Implantation of radioactive yttrium seeds using an X-ray visualization of the ventricles to guide the positioning of the seeds. The radioactive half-life is 96 hours. It is estimated that up to 2 millimeters of tissue are destroyed around each yttrium seed. This psychosurgical technique is used by Geoffrey Knight. (Reprinted with permission of Time/Life Syndication Service, Bill Ray, *Life Magazine*, photographer, copyright 1972, Time Inc.)

Dr. Geoffrey Knight of the Brook General Hospital in London uses a novel technique to destroy the nerve fibers connecting the frontal lobes with the limbic system and hypothalamus. Knight, who is Vice President of the International Society of Psychosurgery, makes a lesion in a region called the substantia innominata (substance without a name), where the connecting fibers are dense.[39] What is most novel in Knight's psychosurgical method is the use of radioactive yttrium seeds to destroy the nerve fibers. (Yttrium is a metallic element that can be made radioactive.) Customarily, three to six yttrium seeds are implanted on each side of the brain of psychiatric patients. It is estimated that each seed, which has a radioactive half-life of 96 hours, destroys tissue up to 2 millimeters from its surface. The seeds are positioned with the aid of X-ray visualization and when in place they are extruded from the implanting tool into the brain (Figure 44). Knight reports that based on his experience with 450 cases the epileptic risk is less than 1 percent and although incontinence sometimes develops postoperatively it is only a temporary disability. He claims that there are no disabling personality changes and "in general the postoperative personality is bright, particularly in depressive syndromes with the release of normal emotions previously suppressed."

Although the yttrium seeds generally remain in place and the effectiveness is spent within 96 hours, the seeds have been known to travel to other parts of the brain. Drs. J. Corsellis and Alice Jack of the Runwell Hospital in Wickford, England, for example, have done autopsies on some of the brains and found seeds that migrated through the ventricles and destroyed tissue in the hypothalamus. In balance, the advantages of this technique are not apparent and the method is not very persuasively defended in the following quotation by Knight:

"There is, of course, no reason why similar lesions should not be produced by the formation of a series of small coagulating (electrolytic) lesions at multiple points, but for research purposes we have preferred to persevere with the use of yttrium which produces a well circumcised and accurate lesion."

It is a much easier task to describe the various psychosurgical procedures that have been used than to evaluate them, but it is necessary at this point to attempt the difficult task of evaluation. This is the subject of the next chapter.

Psychosurgery: An Evaluation

People don't ask for facts in making up their minds. They would rather have one good, soul-satisfying emotion than a dozen facts.

ROBERT KEITH LEAVITT, *VOYAGES AND DISCOVERIES,*
1939

It is difficult to find people who can remain objective on the topic of psychosurgery or psychosurgeons. Although it is an accepted medical practice under some circumstances to destroy a healthy organ, such as an endocrine gland, in order to arrest some serious disorder, the thought of destroying a part of the brain commonly provokes such a strong emotional reaction that the evidence cannot be evaluated objectively.[40] This is understandable in view of the readily acceptable conclusion that the brain, taken as a whole, is the basis of our capacity to learn, experience emotions, and express our individuality. Nevertheless, one would hope it would be possible to evaluate objectively the effect of destroying a specific part of the brain, but even opinions within the medical professions are not exempt from emotional reactions, as can be observed by contrasting the following two editorials:

"The Lobotomy Delusion

"Of recent years, a type of meddlesome surgery, originally instituted in Spain [actually Portugal], has been introduced into this country, frontal lobe lobectomy by name. Lobotomy for frontal lobe malignant tumor we can understand, but by this extended lobotomy, one is supposed to be able to 'pluck from the brain a hidden sorrow.' It is claimed it can ameliorate or cure people suffering from obsessional and compulsion neuroses, and even bring restitution to the more cyclical and obstinate disorder. . .we recommend these aspirants for neurosurgical honors to read and digest Karl Menninger's remarks on polysurgical castration devices, not those of strictly phallic significance but those that maim and destroy the creative functions of a non-mutilated body.

"In the name of Madame Roland who cried aloud concerning the many crimes committed in the cause of 'liberty' we would call the attention of these mutilating surgeons to the Hippocratic oath." (Unsigned editorial, *Medical Record*, 1940, **151**, 335)

"The 1949 Nobel Prize in Medicine

"The Nobel prize for 1949 in medicine has been awarded. . .Dr. Egas Moniz, a former professor of neurology in the University of Lisbon (who). . .devised the revolutionary brain operation of prefrontal leucotomy, later known as lobotomy, now widely used in the treatment of certain forms of mental disease. In the last thirteen years, since his report in 1936, thousands of such operations, now modified into various patterns, have been carried out in many parts of the world, greatly to the betterment of patients with the more serious and prolonged types of mental aberration. A new psychiatry may be said to have been born in 1935, when Moniz took his first bold step in the field of psychosurgery." (Editorial by Dr. Henry R. Viets, *New England Journal of Medicine*, 1949, **1241**, 1025-1026)

SOME PROBLEMS OF EVALUATION

Anyone who approaches the psychosurgical literature objectively cannot agree with either of the editorials quoted above, even though it would be no challenge for a zealot to select data that appear to provide strong support for one or the other position. The problem of evaluation is extremely difficult since the "evidence" often consists of the subjective impressions of those who cannot help but be concerned about the correctness of their decision to undertake psychosurgery as well as often being ego-involved in establishing the success of the particular surgical method employed. This is not to imply that the results have been consciously distorted, but in the absence of objective criteria and adequate experimental controls, it is very easy to find improvement when one looks for it and to attribute it to the particular psychosurgical procedure used. The amount of postoperative improvement that should be attributed to changes in the attitude and expectancy of the hospital staff, relatives, and the patient is usually impossible to determine.

It has long been recognized that the power of suggestion may influence behavior in dramatic ways.[41] Moreover, any serious operation or traumatic event may initiate a significant change in personality and behavior by interrupting some self-perpetuating behavior pattern. As early as 1937, the Russian neurosurgeon Ludwig Puusepp (see page 268) referred to a number of published cases of dramatic improvement in the mental status of psychotic patients following appendectomies, removal of stomach tumors, and operations on kidneys. People have been known to change their style of life and seemingly even their personality after a heart attack. In the case of psychosurgery, it is very difficult to know what the real relationship is between the excised brain tissue and any behavior change that might occur.

A striking example of the difficulty of determining the cause of any change observed after a brain operation was inadvertently provided by Rowland Krynauw of the Johannesburg Hospital in South Africa. In 1950 he removed one complete hemisphere of the brain—including the entire cerebral cortex, the putamen, and the globus pallidus—in 20 patients. The patients all had a paralysis on one side of their body from infancy (infantile hemiplegia) as a result of damage to one-half of the brain at birth or shortly thereafter. In addition to the paralysis, many of the patients exhibited marked personality disorders. Krynauw reported that after the operation there was not only an improvement in the paralysis, but there was also a "marked improvement in personality, behavior and mentality." In such instances it is extremely difficult to be certain of the cause of the improvement in behavior. Some of the improvement probably could be attributed to the elimination of the abnormal electrical activity emanating from the pathological side of the brain while some of the change may have been secondary to the reduction in spasticity—that is, as a result of the better psychological as well as physical adjustment possible after the severe disability was reduced. It is even possible that some of the improvement may have been the result of the "placebo effect" of the surgery.

Dr. Henry Beecher of Harvard's Massachusetts General Hospital has written about the placebo effect of surgery. Beecher demonstrated that a surgeon's enthusiasm for a technique can influence the patient's judgment of improvement following surgery. Using as an example an operation for the relief of angina pectoris that was later discredited, Beecher's statistics reveal a positive relationship between the surgeon's degree of enthusiasm for the procedure and the patient's report of relief from pain. Such studies show how factors unrelated to the specific surgery performed can influence results. In addition to the surgeon's attitude, it would be surprising if the patient's anxiety and stress before and after any major surgery and the changed attitude of the hospital staff did not exert a powerful placebo effect.

PSYCHOSURGERY AND THE PREFRONTAL SYNDROME

Even though the many deficiencies in the clinical literature make it very difficult to present a complete evaluation or to be certain of cause-effect relationships, some conclusions can be drawn with reasonable confidence. There seems to be little disagreement that the extensive transections of frontal lobe fibers can, but do not always produce an intellectual deficit characterized by a loss of ability to synthesize information and to maintain an energetic, goal-directed line of thought and behavior. The more distant the goal in time and space, the greater the possibility that the extensively lobotomized patient would become distracted by more immediate stimuli. Dr. Gösta Rylander of Stockholm described a patient whom he employed as a cook after she recovered from a prefrontal lobotomy. Originally she was very innovative in the kitchen, but after the operation she had difficulty in using new recipes and made ridiculous mistakes. She had no problem, however, with old recipes. When going out to buy food, she frequently disappeared for long periods, being distracted by one thing or another and often forgetting the food.

The Russian psychophysiologist Professor A. R. Luria studied a large population of patients who were suffering from damage to various parts of their brains as a result of injuries incurred during World War II. Professor Luria concluded that in cases of frontal lobe injury the patient is able to perform all the operations involved in different tasks, but there is a problem of motivation that is manifested by an inability to maintain directed activity:

". . .the patient begins to lose his stable system of interests and becomes indifferent, and his motives become narrow and primitive. He loses his intentions which he has formed; ideas coming into his head are transitory and put into operation with difficulty, or they easily disappear. This inability to concentrate on an internal intention, and the absence of persistent goal-directness are among the most characteristic features of behaviour in lesions of the frontal lobe."

Another Russian investigator, Dr. B. V. Zeigarnik, has taken advantage of the observation that most normal subjects tend to resume a task that has been interrupted. This tendency to complete tasks is viewed as a sign of the stability of motivation. Patients with large frontal lesions, however, usually do not return to a task after an interruption.

Dr. Walle Nauta of the Massachusetts Institute of Technology reached a similar conclusion after reviewing the clinical literature:

". . .the frontal lobe disorder is characterized foremost by a derangement of behavior programming. One of the essential functional deficits of the frontal-lobe patient appears to lie in an inability to maintain in his behavior a normal stability-in-time: his action programs, once started, are likely to fade out, to stagnate in reiteration or to become deflected away from the intended goal."

The evidence that damage to the frontal lobes might produce subtle changes in intellectual ability is not new and could have been noted in reports dating back to the last century. As early as 1876, David Ferrier described the deficits that follow frontal lobe destruction in monkeys:

"Removal or destruction by cautery of the antero-frontal lobes is not followed by any definite physiological results. The animals retain their appetites and instincts, and are capable of exhibiting emotional feeling. The sensory faculties, sight, hearing, touch, taste and smell remain unimpaired. The powers of voluntary motion are retained in their integrity, and there is little to indicate the presence of such extensive lesions, or removal of so large a part of the brain. I have removed the frontal lobes. . .almost completely in three monkeys, with the same negative results, and what is more remarkable, I found that the removal of these lobes in an animal which had recovered from ablation of the occipital lobes caused no symptoms indicative of affection or impairment of the special sensory or motor faculties.

"And yet notwithstanding this apparent absence of physiological symptoms, I could perceive a very decided alteration in the animals' character and behavior, though it is difficult to state in precise terms the nature of the change. The animals operated on were selected on account of their intelligent character. After operation though they might seem to one who had not compared their present with their past, fairly up to the average of monkey intelligence, they had undergone a considerable psychological alteration. Instead of, as before, being actively interested in their surroundings, and curiously prying into all things that came within the field of their observation, they remained apathetic or dull, or dozed off to sleep, responding only to the sensations or impressions of the moment, or varying their listlessness with restlessness and purposeless wanderings to and fro. While not actually deprived of intelligence, they had lost, to all appearance, the faculty of attentive and intelligent observation."

Leonardi Bianchi was a contemporary of Ferrier and as professor of nervous and mental disease at the University of Naples he concentrated his research efforts on frontal lobe function for about 40 years until his death in 1927. Although he did not use what would now be considered objective methods for studying behavior, his observational powers were said to have been remarkable. He noted that the removal of one frontal lobe had little effect on the monkey, but bilateral destruction had pronounced consequences:

"Removal of the frontal lobes does not so much interfere with the perceptions taken singly, as it does disaggregate the personality, and incapacitates for serializing and synthesizing groups of representations.

". . .What is more important is that in monkeys in which the operation was successful, there is complete lack of any initiative whatsoever. The movements performed by these animals lack any evident objective. . . . My experiments have demonstrated that although the fundamental and immediate emotions are preserved (some altered) after ablation of the frontal lobes, the higher sentiments or emotions, as these have been outlined in the monkey, are absent or profoundly disturbed, in correspondence to what is observed to follow severe lesions of the same lobes in man."

Some indication of the personality changes that might be produced by prefrontal lobotomy in man was available from the remarkable case of Phineas Gage, a 25-year-old construction foreman employed by the Rutland and Burlington Railroad in Vermont. In 1848, while he was preparing a hole for blasting powder, an accidental explosion drove an iron tamping rod (13-1/4 pounds, 3-1/2 feet long, and 1-1/4 inches in diameter) through Gage's left cheek and out the front side of his skull. Gage fell to the ground, but to the astonishment of his fellow workers who assumed he was near death, he sat up and asked for his tamping rod. He was taken to a local hotel in an ox cart and was attended by a physician, John M. Harlow, who later described the events immediately surrounding the accident and the long-term changes in Gage's behavior. The rod was smeared with pieces of brain and Dr. Harlow found that he could pass the entire length of his index finger through the 3-1/2-inch opening in the frontal bone "in the direction of the wound in the cheek, which received the other finger in like manner." To everyone's amazement, Gage recovered. Before the accident, Gage had been soft spoken, well liked by the workers, and one of the railroad's most reliable foremen. Harlow described his patient after he recovered from his physical disabilities:

". . . General appearance good; stands quite erect, with his head inclined slightly towards the right side; his gait in walking is steady; his movements rapid, and easily executed. . . . His physical health is good, and I am inclined to say that he has recovered. Has no pain in head, but says it has a queer feeling which he is not able to describe. Applied for his situation as foreman, but is undecided whether to work or travel. His contractors, who regarded him as the most efficient and capable foreman in their employ previous to his injury, considered the change in his mind so marked that they could not give him his place again. The equilibrium or balance, so to speak, between his intellectual faculties and animal propensities, seems to have been destroyed. He is fitful, irreverent, indulging at times in the grossest profanity (which was not previously his custom), manifesting but little deference for his fellows, impatient of restraint or advice when it conflicts with his desires, at times pertinaciously obstinate, yet capricious and vacillating, devising many plans of future operation, which are no sooner arranged than they are abandoned in turn for others appearing more feasible. A child in his intellectual capacity and manifestations, he has the animal passions of a strong man. Previous to his injury, though untrained in the schools, he possessed a well-balanced mind, and was looked upon by those who knew him as a shrewd, smart business man, very energetic and persistent in executing all his plans of operation. In this regard his mind was radically changed, so decidedly that his friends and aquaintances said he was 'no longer Gage'."

Gage flitted from one task to another and wandered to different places including Chile in South America for the purpose of establishing a line of coaches in the vicinity of Valparaíso and Santiago. He eventually returned to the United States and died in San Francisco in 1861 after a brief succession of what appeared to be epileptic seizures.

RESULTS OF OLDER PREFRONTAL PSYCHOSURGERY

Although the initial prefrontal psychosurgery did not produce as massive destruction of the frontal lobes as was involved in either the early animal research or the cases of traumatic injury in humans, similar deficits were often reported. However, even after admitting the deficits frequently produced by extensive frontal lobe destruction, it was still possible to conclude that in terms of the balance between gain and loss there often resulted a significant improvement in adjustment level. Drs. Milton Greenblatt and Harry Solomon of Harvard University and the Boston Psychopathic Hospital made an effort in 1953 to present a balanced picture of postlobotomy (Poppen "open" method) behavior:

"Reduction of cells and circuits theoretically may have the following consequences: (1) The individual loses drive,

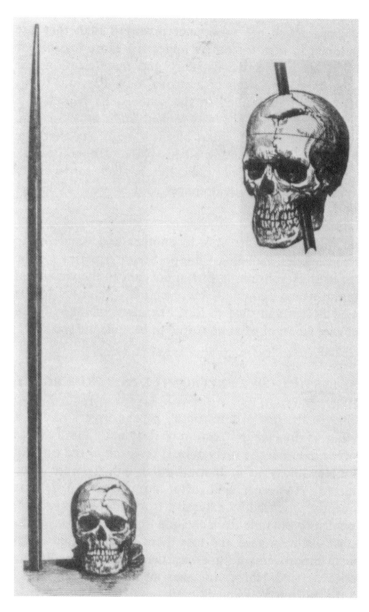

Figure 45. A sketch made by Harlow illustrating the relative size of the tamping bar that was driven by blasting powder through Phineas Gage's skull. The iron bar entered through the cheek and emerged at the top of the head.

force, energy. (2) He is less affected by past experience and more bound to immediate stimuli. (3) He is less able to elaborate experiences or to sustain experiences.

"At first glance the lobotomy operation appears as a serious and irreversible interference with brain activity. Some people are in principle opposed to all forms of destructive brain surgery on the grounds that nothing could possibly be gained by subtraction. Since pathologic studies have failed to demonstrate anatomic deviations in mentally ill patients, the removal of brain tissue is considered a reprehensible procedure which lowers the patient's powers of adaptation. Such convictions are often unshaken despite evidence purporting to show gain in level of adaptation; sometimes a neat theoretic explanation makes the objective findings more palatable.

"A loss of drive, force, energy, may theoretically be of benefit to a sick patient if troublesome motivation or maladaptive patterns of behavior are reduced in intensity. Impulses difficult to manage may then be kept within bounds. . . . If the patient is less affected by past experiences and more bound to immediate stimuli, he may be freed from past emotional entanglements and given an opportunity for a new line of development. . .abnormal emotional states might gradually evaporate, the distorted fantasy life becomes uncharged; tension, agitation, hostility, brooding and preoccupation would be less disorganizing, and although the individual might be more superficial and shallow, adaptation at a simpler level would be possible."

In essence, Greenblatt and Solomon were saying that given a choice it might be better to operate and sacrifice some intellectual potential that probably never was going to be fulfilled anyway than to leave someone uncommunicative, ridden with devastating and unbearable anxiety or obsessiveness, and totally unable to cope with everyday life. Many people have considered this argument to have merit. The difficult problem of course is at what point should it be decided that a patient's mental state cannot be improved by some as yet untried treatment that is less drastic than brain surgery.

It was even possible to maintain that intellectual loss did not necessarily follow one or another of the extensive lobotomy procedures. One can find examples of lobotomized persons functioning at a high professional and administrative level. Freeman, for example, has repeatedly described cases like the following:

"A physician who prior to the frontal operations had been discharged from two internships because of aggressive paranoid behavior. Following surgery he completed an internship, served as liaison officer among several military hospitals in Germany for three years, married and fathered two children. He established a ten man medical clinic and flies his own plane."

Although it is conceivable that even in such cases as this there may have been a significant decrement from a potentially much higher intellectual level, it is apparent that the surgery did not always have a devastating effect.

It cannot even be maintained that only psychosurgeons argue that extensive lobotomy need not produce serious intellectual loss. Donald Hebb, who is a distinguished psychologist at McGill University, studied the social and economic adjustment of a man with very extensive damage to the frontal lobes. The man had been severely injured by an overhead carrier in a saw mill; afterward, he had frequent epileptic convulsions and outbursts of violent rage. Between attacks he was a chronic behavior problem and was "irresponsible, childishly stubborn, restless and forgetful." Dr. Wilder Penfield of the Montreal Neurological Institute operated on the man, removing scar tissue and extending the incision into the region of the frontal lobe that appeared normal. In all, more than one-third of the total frontal lobes was removed. Hebb studied the man for over six years using many standardized intelligence tests as well as interviewing townspeople who had regular opportunities to observe the patient's daily behavior and general adjustment. The conclusion reached from studying this patient, as well as a careful review of the literature available up to 1945, was that "the frontal poles of the brain are not necessary to a good day by day adjustment in society or to a good performance on intelligence tests." Many of the deficits seen after frontal lobe damage were the result of scar tissue rather than being due to the absence of the frontal lobes. Although Hebb admitted that his study did not rule out the possibility that long-term planning, initiative, and creativity might be impaired by destruction of the frontal lobes, he concluded that "social and intellectual defects need not follow an uncomplicated excision of tissue from the anterior part of the frontal lobes."

Although it is certainly possible that some bias may have been introduced by the fact that most large-scale evaluations of the older lobotomy procedures were done by investigators associated with the surgery, it has to be recognized, nevertheless, that these reports were generally favorable. In 1948 the Connecticut Lobotomy Committee studied 200 lobotomy cases for periods ranging from three months to a year after the operation. About 90 percent of the patients were judged to have improved at least slightly, and approximately 25 percent were judged to have markedly improved. Five percent were considered to have been freed of symptoms. It was concluded that "the more troublesome symptoms to patient and society, such as anxiety, depression, etc., are eliminated in 75 percent or more of the cases." Study of the work adjustment of the lobotomized patients indicated that three months after the operation 42 percent of the 200 patients were able to hold a job, and 60 percent of the 49 patients who had been followed for a year were working at least part-time. A

British Board of Control study of 1000 lobotomized patients in mental hospitals in England and Wales was undertaken by Isable Wilson and her colleagues in 1947. Depending on the diagnosis, from 23 percent (the schizophrenics) to 50 percent (the manic-depressives) were discharged from the hospital. Of the 998 patients that could be found, the following evaluation was made of their general social behavior; 244 unchanged; 295 improved; 166 great improvement; 242 cured and living at home; 11 became worse.

In 1953, Jonathan Williams and Walter Freeman summarized the results obtained following 625 prefrontal lobotomies (Freeman-Watts series) and 500 transorbital lobotomies (Freeman series). The first series of patients had been followed from three to 15 years after the operation, while the second series had been observed for periods from one to five years. In both series, the statistics were approximately the same, indicating good results in 45 percent of the cases, 2 percent deaths attributable to the operation, and about 20 percent employed. All these statistics cited by psychosurgeons cannot be completely dismissed on the ground that they reflect biased reporting, since there are a number of instances of the same people admitting failures. Several examples of patients who showed no improvement, or even became worse after the lobotomy are described in considerable detail by Freeman and Watts in their book, *Psychosurgery*. Similarly, in Williams and Freeman's report on lobotomies performed on hyperkinetic and intensely destructive children it was readily admitted that the results were generally not encouraging.

Although all of the large-scale evaluations of prefrontal lobotomy appear to present favorable statistics, considerable skepticism toward these figures has to be maintained. In judging improvement, most of the studies gave exaggerated weighting to the elimination of behavior that was most troublesome to the hospital staff and society in general and attached considerably less importance to the qualitative aspects of the adjustment level. One of the more striking examples of this type of selective evaluation can be seen in a case described by Freeman and Watts. The patient was a young girl, age 6, who never made friends and was often destructive using toys as weapons and tearing her clothes. She may have had diffuse brain damage, for she frequently engaged in a characteristic rocking back and forth and at least one previous medical diagnosis was "unrecognized encephalitis." Prefrontal lobotomy was performed 22 days after she was admitted to the hospital. After a brief stay in the hospital, where it was observed that she could build "a tower of blocks to the height of 12," she was considered improved and discharged.

The patient reverted to the pattern of destructive behavior within two months and when she was returned to the hospital (eight months after the lobotomy) she was lobotomized again (15 millimeters behind the previous one and parallel to it) on the same day that she was admitted. Recovery was slower, but approximately two months later her mother wrote: "She has not had one temper tantrum since the operation. . .it is a pleasure to dress her now. . .she does not tear her clothes or show any signs of being destructive. . .she seems perfectly happy all the time and laughs a lot." Later she reverted to periods of destructiveness. Three years after the second operation she was described as "quite withdrawn, but less troublesome. She talked little and was making no progress in helping in the home." Freeman and Watts concluded that following the second operation "improvement has continued for nearly four years and the child is still making progress. In spite of her increased strength and speed, she can be more easily managed at home." It is impossible to determine now whether the child would have been better off without the lobotomy, but it is apparent that the evaluation of the postoperative change was influenced primarily by the fact that the patient was more manageable and less destructive.

During many of the debates over the value of lobotomy, Dr. Gösta Rylander of Sweden maintained that the major deficits seen after these operations were not revealed by tests or statistics. It was necessary to live with the patients (or at least observe them very thoroughly), he argued. Rylander conducted thorough follow-up studies and reported that all of the patients "have shown changes in behavior of the well-known type, namely, tactlessness, emotional lability with tendencies to outbursts, extrovertness and slight euphoric traits." The wife of a patient might say: "Doctor, you have given me a new husband. He isn't the same man" or "I have lost my husband. I'm alone. I must take over all responsibilities now."

A similar point related to the qualitative changes that may appear after a prefrontal lobotomy can be obtained from the literature on the use of brain surgery to relieve pain. It can be argued that the preoperative mental state of patients suffering from pain is a much better baseline to evaluate postoperative deficits than the mental state of psychotics. Drs. James C. White and William H. Sweet in their book, *Pain and the Neurosurgeon, a Forty-Year Experience*, make the important point that "there is no record of anyone on whom the bilateral *radical operation* (see pages 288–289) was carried out for the relief of pain and suffering ever returning to productive work. Some, after too radical sacrifice of frontal lobe tissue, required institutional care. . . . The majority became serious burdens to their families." A wife of a patient who received such an operation for relief of a chronic backache wrote:

"That operation was performed on my husband in Sept. 1949 and it has also been a very sad affair, and if the doctor had of spoke of it as you do we would never of have it done, but he said it would slow him up but he would be able to do the things he always did and even be able to get at his place of business, but he can not do anything and do it right, he can't even take care of himself in the bathroom, and does not take any interest in anything. When he went into it mentally he was fine, kept in contact with his business, even done some of the book work, but he had suffered pain for years from back trouble. . . . I some days think I will lose my mind going through this with him."

Another point that has to be considered when evaluating the lobotomy statistics is that an insufficient allowance was normally made for the percentage of patients who might have improved without surgery. For example, in the British Board of Control study the greatest improvement was observed among manic-depressive disorders, but this is a category that would be expected to exhibit improvement even without treatment.

Very few studies have contrasted the results that followed psychosurgery with the changes that occurred over a comparable period of time in a matched, un-operated control group. One study that attempted to do this was published by Tan, Marks, and Marset, who studied a group of 24 obsessive-compulsive patients that had received a standard lobotomy (called leucotomy in England) performed at the Maudsley Hospital between 1951 and 1965. An assessor, who did not know what treatment the patients had, read the case records and matched patients in pairs based on symptom type, du-ration and severity of illness, age, and sex. Thirteen pairs that were adequately matched could be established and their behavior change over a five-year period was com-pared by assessors who also did not know which patients had. been lobotomized. The lobotomized patients had a significantly greater reduction in anxiety and obsessive tendencies over their matched controls immediately after the operation. This trend continued for several years, but by five years after the operation, the differences were very slight and probably not reliable. The work adjustment of the two groups was more variable, with the lobotomized patients having only a very slightly better record by the end of the five-year postsurgery period.

The Columbia-Greystone study is probably referred to more than any other evaluation of psychosurgery, but in actuality it is not very decisive one way or the other (see Mettler, 1949 and 1952). The strength of this study lies in the extensive series of physiological and psychological tests that were given to the patients before and after psychosurgery and in the distinguished group of scientists who participated in this testing program. The latter reason probably explains why it is always cited. From a list of over 100 psychological tests, 35 were selected for the test battery to be used on all patients. However, several of these were the type of standard intelligence tests that most previous reports had shown to be insensitive to frontal lobe damage, and a number of the other tests were new and had not been adequately standardized for a brain-damaged population. Moreover, the patient population was quite small, originally consisting of 24 surgical patients and 24 unoperated control patients. Actually, because some of the patients were either inaccessible or uncooperative, only 19 surgical and 13 unoperated control patients were studied extensively. The psychosurgical operation primarily used was a topectomy, a procedure involving removal of portions of the prefrontal area (see page 281). (At a later point, some additional patients received one of several different psychosurgical procedures. Among the procedures explored were the Freeman-Watts lobotomy, thermocoagulation, dorsomedial thalotomy, venous ligation which restricted the blood supply to the frontal areas, and with the help of Walter Freeman 9 transorbital lobotomies were performed.) Emphasis was given to the topectomy operation, because it seemed most useful for correlating postoperative behavioral changes with specific prefrontal areas, but it was not the most commonly used psychosurgical procedure, and for this as well as other reasons it may not have been the best to generalize from. The small group of 19 surgical patients had to be further subdivided into groups depending on which part of the prefrontal area was destroyed.

In spite of the reputation of the more than 50 participating investigators (representing 12 medical and scientific specialties) working on the Columbia-Greystone report, there was much that could be criticized in the selection and assignment of patients into the different surgical subgroups. Dr. Robert Heath, who wrote the psychiatric report, concluded: "The present series of topectomy patients is so small and contains so many variables that it would be a mistake to develop statistics relating to improvement. Significant, however, is the finding that many patients with poor prognostic expectations did improve." The battery of psychological tests revealed very little. For a short period following surgery, some defects were detected, but after a few months there were very few differences to point to between the surgical and nonsurgical groups. There was no evidence that the psychosurgery produced any permanent loss in learning ability, memory, creativity, imagination, intellectual achievement, social or ethical attitudes, or even sense of humor (see Landis, Zubin, and Mettler, 1950).

The surgical group achieved improved scores on the Complaint and Anxiety Inventories and the neurosurgeon Dr. Lawrence Pool reported that 40 percent of a total of 106 topectomized patients (only a small proportion of these were included in the Columbia-Greystone study) were significantly improved and 34 percent were "socially rehabilitated." However, Dr. Carney Landis, who wrote the psychological report for the project, did not believe this was a specific effect of the operation and he concluded:

"There is no clear-cut evidence of a consistent or uniform personality change which resulted from any particular variety of topectomy in which the operation could clearly be said to be solely responsible for the change. The amelioration from psychosis and social improvement which occurred in many of the operatees is easiest understood as an indirect effect of the operation."

Landis argued that one often sees improvement in the mental status of psychiatric patients after any type of physical injury or unrelated operations—even after an appendectomy. However, Landis did raise the rhetorical question: "But why does an appendectomy patient show a relapse when healing is complete while certain topectomy patients were still lucid at the end of a year?" Drs. Landis, Zubin, and Mettler wrote: ". . .the result of psychosurgery in approximately one-third of operated psychotic patients is an improvement from psychosis which is marked by a variable decrease in vigilence, anguish and zeal." They also wrote: "Within a few days after the operation a few patients will remark, quite spontaneously, 'I'm well. The torment is gone. The voices are quiet.' As time passes still others will remark that the distress or anguish is lessening." Taken as a whole, the Columbia-Greystone report provided no *substantial* evidence that psychosurgery produced either significant deficits or improvement. It is often claimed that the reports, which were published in 1949 and 1952 was responsible for decreasing the number of psychosurgical operations performed. There is little justification for that conclusion as some psychiatric improvement was claimed and no permanent deficits could be detected by the tests used. Probably the most damaging aspect of the study was the inability to find any convincing evidence that destruction of any one part of the frontal area produced distinctive and predictable results. At any rate, psychosurgery continued at a high level until the mid 1950s. It was the introduction of psychopharmacologic agents and public awareness of many abuses in the practice that were mainly responsible for the rapid decline in psychosurgery.

In general, there seems to be strong suggestive evidence (if not absolutely convincing) that some patients may have been significantly helped by psychosurgery. There is certainly no grounds for either the position that all psychosurgery necessarily reduces people to a "vegetable status" or that it has a high probability of producing miraculous cures. The truth, even if somewhat wishy-washy, lies in between these extreme positions. There is little doubt, however, that many abuses existed especially during the 1945–1955 decade when these operations were performed in the greatest numbers. Quite aside from any evaluation of the effectiveness of the surgery, it should not be forgotten that there were always some risks. Patients did occasionally die from the operation, epilepsy was not an uncommon aftermath, prolonged urinary incontinence was sometimes produced, and various symptoms from infections and neurological damage could be attributed directly to the surgery. Judgment of psychosurgical practices, however, should be tempered by recognition of the few alternatives available at the time. Psychoactive drugs were not available and most mental institutions were pitifully understaffed by psychiatrists, who were generally ineffective in treating the more severely disturbed patients. Overall, the evidence does not support the position taken by those extremists who, while refusing to examine the record, charge that lobotomy was generally used by sadistic, self-seeking, or indifferent doctors. This is not to deny that there existed much that could be criticized, not the least of which involved a decision to perform surgery without sufficient exploration of psychiatric alternatives. The statements customarily made in the literature saying that the patient had not been helped by previous psychiatric treatment over a period of years often have little meaning, since the psychiatric treatment was frequently of a perfunctory nature. During their greatest popularity, so many lobotomies were performed that it is unlikely that a thorough examination could possibly have been made in all cases. Walter Freeman once remarked that an enterprising neurologist could perform 10 to 15 supraorbital lobotomies (see Figures 41 and 42) in a morning.

There is little doubt that there were instances of psychosurgery performed without an adequate exploration of alternatives. There is also little doubt that in some cases surgeons were attempting to establish the success of a particular procedure, so that the patient's interest did not completely govern the selection of treatment. Often a second operation was performed before sufficient time had elapsed to adequately judge the results of the first operation. Without meaning to single out Freeman for special criticism, as one of the active lobotomists during the early period of psychosurgery and a prolific spokesman he is often most convenient to cite as an example of trends that were common. For example, Freeman commented at the conclusion of a presentation of the Connecticut Lobotomy Committee:

"While we can often tell at the end of three months whether a patient is going to be benefited, we are required in certain instances to make the judgment within three days, because a patient may come from a distance, and if relief is not considered sufficient, we may have to reoperate."

THE NEWER PSYCHOSURGICAL PROCEDURES

In a sense the evaluation of the extensive lobotomy procedures is academic since these operations are almost never performed any more. As already discussed, the number of psychosurgical operations was drastically reduced during the second half of the 1950s. The psychosurgery that is now performed are the so-called fractional or restricted operations on the deep and medial fibers of the frontal lobes or operations on limbic system structures, particularly the cingulate and amygdala. Dr. William Scoville, the current president of the 150-member International Society of Psychosurgery, has written that approximately 600 brain operations are performed each year in the United States for purely psychiatric disease. This figure excludes operations done to alleviate pain, epilepsy, movement disorders, and aggression. Scoville calculates that this figure represents only one case for every four neurosurgeons in this country or one case per month for the approximately 50 surgeons performing these operations. Many of the procedures now use stereotaxic techniques combined with electrolytic lesions, or they use an operative approach that permits the tissue to be destroyed under direct vision.

The problem of evaluation of the newer psychosurgical techniques remains difficult, since many of the shortcomings of the earlier lobotomy studies are still evident. It is also necessary to recognize that there has been a clear shift in the type of patients selected for psychosurgery. Originally, only chronic psychotic patients who were considered otherwise hopeless were picked for surgery. Gradually it became clear that the prognosis was very poor for such patients. Today the patients considered to be the best candidates are those with tensions, anxieties, phobias, depressions, obsessions, compulsions, and severe hypochondriacal symptoms. As a group the patients are not nearly as deteriorated as the earlier lobotomy patients, but this does not mean that their symptoms are mild. The patients may be constantly anxious or depressed and suicide attempts are not uncommon. In some, the phobias, obsessions, or physical complaints may completely block any kind of normal existence.

The general impression is that the best results are obtained in patients who have a great amount of tension. Those who have been emotionally spent for a long time are poor candidates for psychosurgery. As a result the comment has been made on several occasions that psychosurgery should not be considered a last effort to help a patient. In contrast it has been suggested by Freeman that it may be dangerous to wait too long:

"It would seem that lobotomy rather than being a final heroic remedy, marks the turning point in effective therapy. . .frontal lobotomy is more successful in early cases of schizophrenia. In the chronic case it has limited value. In a dangerous disease such as schizophrenia it may prove safer to operate than to wait."

The evaluative studies of the newer psychosurgical procedures tend to have smaller numbers of subjects who have been followed for shorter periods of time. In general, insufficient details are provided, but the results reported are favorable in terms of psychiatric improvement, work adjustment, and low incidence of serious intellectual and personality changes or physical complications. It may be important to bear in mind, however, that these reports have customarily been presented by those doing the surgery—there has not been sufficient interest generated to sponsor a more impartial, as well as more thorough, evaluation.

One earlier study deserves special mention because it may be the only instance of an evaluation of a psychosurgical procedure that utilized the type of experimental controls demanded of acceptable animal studies. Between 1949 and 1953, Dr. Kenneth Livingston performed approximately 100 anterior cingulate lesions on psychiatric patients at the Veterans Administration Hospital at Roseburg, Oregon. The average duration of hospitalization was over four years and all the patients were considered to have very low prospects of rehabilitation and discharge. Many of the patients were very aggressive and dangerous to others. Operations were performed under local anesthetic and, because some patients refused to cooperate during the surgery, some of the operations were terminated after a skull "button" was removed and only a superficial incision was made in the cerebral cortex. Some of the "sham" operations were also planned in advance. All of the patients were sent back to the ward with the same bandages and instructions, and the surgical notes were kept secret so that none of the attendants, nurses, or staff knew what had been done in surgery.

Dr. Livingston reported that none of the sham-operated patients "showed even slight improvement during their period of control study and all were subjected to cingulate isolation one to three months later." In contrast, it was reported that of those who received the anterior cingulotomy, "the majority show a striking mood change characterized by pleasantness and evidence of contentment, absence of hostility and fear, and exhibit an emotional coloring and reactivity which often is strikingly normal in quality." Although there were several instances of patients who showed improvement suddenly reverting to their preoperative status, many patients continued to progress toward normalcy and were discharged about one year following surgery.

Livingston's study provides some important evidence that many of the improvements observed after cingulotomy are probably due to the surgery and not to any change in attitude of the hospital staff or any placebo effect on the patient. It also raises some interesting ethical issues concerning the use of experimental controls in medicine. On the one hand, it certainly could be argued that surgery always involves some risks and that the control population was subjected to this risk even though it was unlikely that they would be helped by the sham operation. On the other hand, it can be argued that the scientific information was important to obtain and could affect many other people, the risks to the control group were slight, and these patients were given the treatment considered most beneficial, cingulotomy, after the relatively short time required to compare results. Moreover, it was not absolutely clear at the time that patients in the control group might not benefit from the placebo effect of the sham operation. Had there been a serious challenge, it might have been difficult to defend the use of this procedure against cross-examination by a clever attorney, who would exaggerate the risks and stress the fact that this was experimentation with little realistic hope of benefiting the control patients. The difficulty in defending a position, however, does not necessarily make it wrong, It is not always easy to decide where to draw the line that will allow sufficient opportunity to do research that may eventually help many people while protecting the rights of individual patients.

In a relatively recent (1967) publication, Dr. H. Thomas Ballantine of Harvard and his associates at the Wiswall Hospital in Wellesley, Massachusetts, described favorable results following anterior cingulotomy in 40 psychiatric patients. The 40 patients had been considered intractably ill, but following surgery 30 were judged to have been at least "usefully improved." In a note appended to the report, Ballantine and his associates indicated that up to December, 1966, they had performed 117 operations on 84 patients (some had to be reoperated) without any deaths occurring. Since "neither the patients, their relatives, nor their doctors have observed serious physical or psychological complications of the operations," it was concluded "that the risk of cingulotomy is negligible." The immediate stimulus for this study was an earlier report by Dr. E. Foltz and L. White that of the 16 patients who underwent cingulotomy for the relief of pain those who had anxiety or depression had the best results.[42] In contradistinction, Dr. William Scoville, who indicated that he introduced the operation and subsequently communicated his results to Sir Hugh Cairns at Oxford and LeBeau in Paris, repeatedly reports that he has not observed any psychiatric improvement following cingulotomy. Scoville claims good results only with his technique for undercutting the fibers beneath the orbital surface of the frontal lobes and he challenges proponents of the cingulotomy technique to compare the two operations.

As already noted, the results following various types of fractional prefrontal procedures are generally reported to be favorable, but most of the data are uncontrolled and presented in terms of improvement on vaguely defined scales. There have been few attempts to explore ways to provide objective evidence for the statements that no intellectual loss has occurred. This is not an easy task, however, because there are no generally accepted tests to measure the more subtle capacities that may be lost. It will be recalled that intelligence tests scores did not detect any loss, even following extensive prefrontal damage. One of the problems in evaluating changes in intellect is caused by difficulty in obtaining meaningful estimates of preoperative potential. At the time of surgery, the patients are often functioning much below their potential, and therefore test performance immediately before surgery can be a very inadequate base line to use for comparison with postoperative performance.[43] Generally, what has been demonstrated is that the average intelligence test scores after psychosurgery do not differ significantly from those of the population at large. Sometimes the data consist mainly of examples of patients who, after surgery, seem capable of holding a position that normally requires more than average intellectual capacity.

Dr. Sadao Hirose of Tokyo modified the Scoville orbital undercutting operation (see Figure 43) so that an even more restricted area of fibers can be destroyed. He has had considerable experience with this procedure, but during the last few years he has performed only five to ten operations per year. Hirose commented that "the preju-

dice that all psychosurgical operations are followed by undesirable deficit of personality and damage to human
dignity ought to be dispelled." To support this point,
Hirose cites a case of a former patient, a 40-year-old
statistical officer who is presently employed in the
Japanese Prime Minister's Office. Before surgery he was
hospitalized five times during 13 years. Electroconvulsive
therapy, insulin coma treatment, and antidepressant drugs
helped for short periods, but each time he relapsed into his
former state characterized by incapacitating depression,
delusions of reference and persecution, fear, anxiety, and
general emotional turmoil. Three years have elapsed since
the operation and during this time no personality deficits
have been detected. The man married, made an official
trip to Okinawa, represented Japan at a meeting in
Bangkok, and in general seems to be functioning satisfactorily. In spite of such favorable reports, a careful reading
of all the published data on the behavior of patients after
the fractional psychosurgical procedures does reveal
instances of increased hostility, lowered personal standards and initiative, and some memory loss. Although
there is not much information available, there does not
appear to be any evidence of the *severe* deficits that were
often observed during the first few months following extensive prefrontal lobotomy.

The shift toward more restrictive psychosurgical operations has emphasized the need to delineate the function of
different areas. There is a generally accepted belief that
destruction of the more lateral prefrontal areas is likely to
produce intellectual deficits whereas destruction of the
medial areas causes emotional changes. This belief is not
founded on any solid evidence from the psychosurgical
studies, but animal experiments seem to support this impression. A recent conference on frontal lobe function in
Jablonna, Poland, made it apparent that even though
there is still considerable mystery surrounding frontal lobe
function, there is general agreement that in monkeys,
destruction of the more lateral portions of the prefrontal

area produces intellectual deficits whereas destruction of the more medial region along the inferior (bottom) surface of this part of the brain is likely to result in emotional changes and to modify social behavior. (See Teuber, 1972, for a summary of the Jablonna Conference.) It is, however, much easier to indicate an agreement on the general differences that appear following medial and lateral frontal lobe damage than it is to provide specific descriptions of the basic deficits.

In spite of all the animal studies, the fundamental deficit following removal of the prefrontal cortex remains elusive. Jacobsen's initial impression that the lobectomized animal's inability to do delayed response tasks was due to a recent memory loss did not stand up. Later, in a resumé of the long-term loss of problem-solving ability suffered by the lobotomized chimpanzees Becky and Lucy, Jacobsen and his colleagues (see Crawford et al, 1948) concluded:

"The deficit appears to be primarily an inability to maintain a behavioral set and organization against the competition of newly impinging internal and external stimulation for dominance of the action system."

As already noted, many investigators have reached essentially the same conclusions (see pages 298–303), but it is still difficult to specify the precise deficit that makes it difficult to maintain goal-directed behavior. Some investigators have stressed either the distractibility or impulsivity of the operated animals. It was noted, for example, that lobotomized monkeys were often easily distracted from the task at hand or responded so rapidly they tended not to be able to utilize previously acquired information. Dr. Robert Malmo demonstrated that the performance of "frontal monkeys" was improved if distractions were minimized by testing them in the dark, and Dr. Karl Pribram improved the performance of frontal lobotomized baboons by partially sedating them with small doses of barbiturates. Although much remains to be explained, it seems to be well established now that at least in monkeys the lateral aspects of the prefrontal area are essential to the ability to perform on a delayed response task. There is even reasonably good evidence that it is a specific part (sulcus principalis) of the lateral area that is critical for delayed response performance in monkeys.[44]

What these results mean for man is not clear, for these deficits, which can be reliably demonstrated in monkeys, are not seen in man. The ability of man to encode information in words ("It's on the left") makes it possible to bridge the time gap and compensate for deficits that might otherwise appear. Dr. Brenda Milner of the Montreal Neurological Institute reported that epileptic patients who underwent surgical destruction of frontal areas analogous to the lateral area in monkey have a deficit in tests requiring sorting of objects into different categories such as shape or color—a task which demonstrates a capacity for abstraction. It is possible that this decreased capacity to abstract may underlie the lobectomized humans' difficulty in maintaining long-term goals and the increased tendency to respond to the more concrete aspects of the immediate environment. Following destruction of the ventromedial (orbital) portion of the frontal lobes the same deficits do not appear, according to Milner.

The emotional changes that are produced by damage to the more medial (orbital) region at the base of the prefrontal area are equally hard to specify. Several investigators have electrically stimulated this region in animals and man and observed changes in such autonomic activity as respiration, heart rate, and blood pressure.[45] It is possible that the reduction in blood pressure observed by Freeman and Watts to occur in hypertensive lobotomized patients might have been due to destruction of the orbital prefrontal area. In regard to behavior, monkeys with damage to this region tend to have difficulty inhibiting learned response habits, even though a change in the test situation makes the responses incorrect. This perseverative tendency of the "orbital animal" is not observed in animals with only lateral prefrontal damage. To date, the known anatomical connections do not help us understand these differences in function between the two prefrontal areas. There is enough overlap in the anatomical connections so that even if we knew what the connections implied—which we do not—we would not have been able to predict the differences. Nor is it clear why orbital destruction may produce an alleviation of certain psychiatric problems. Perhaps the best guess is that an increased perseverative tendency, which at first glance seems like a deficit that should not help anyone, may reflect a general disinhibition (or increased impulsiveness) that may counteract the immobility of thought and action that is characteristic of obsessive and anxiety-ridden personalities. However, if there is a tendency toward hostile behavior, the heightened impulsiveness may increase the amount of hostility expressed.

There are several formidable obstacles that make it very difficult to reach any firm conclusions regarding frontal lobe function in humans. The inability to readily transfer experimental results from one species to another—even between different primates—makes it clear that animal brain research can provide only tentative suggestions about human brain function. The intellectual capacities of man are obviously different from those of any animal, comparable anatomical areas often do not have the same connections to other brain regions, and only in man have functional differences between the right and left half of the cerebral cortex been demonstrated. Moreover, even the observations restricted to humans seem to indicate that the same damage in two individuals often produces very different results. Dr. Hans-Lukas Teuber has observed that behavior of patients with similar shell-fragment wounds to the prefrontal area may range from apathy and seemingly slothful attitude to overactivity and impulsiveness. As a result of such differences, the predictions of postoperative changes will always fall short of what would be desirable. Most psychosurgeons agree that the changes produced by an operation are determined partly by the personality of the patient. In reality, such a view implicitly accepts the idea that the brain functions as a whole. Although we may speak of its parts in terms of relative importance for a particular function, we can never completely separate one part from the whole.

ANIMAL RESEARCH AND PSYCHOSURGERY

The point has been made several times in this book that the results of animal research cannot be applied to humans (or for that matter to other animal species) without a great amount of careful consideration. This note of caution should certainly not lead anyone to conclude that we cannot learn anything about human brains and behavior from animal studies or that animal experimentation has not had a great influence on developments in psychosurgery. In regard to the latter point, the influence of animal research has often been so immediate that it becomes frightening to contemplate.

Almost every new development in psychosurgery has been directly inspired by animal experimentation. From the very first psychosurgical experiment by Burckhardt—who was influenced by Goltz's experiments on the cerebral cortex of dogs (see page 266)—to the most recent developments in psychosurgery, animal research has had a very direct influence. It will be recalled that it was Jacobsen's observations of the prefrontal lobectomized chimpanzee that encouraged Moniz to begin the exploration that subsequently led to a wave of psychosurgery (see pages 50–54). The taming of monkeys, which was described as part of the Klüver-Bucy syndrome (see page 131), contributed to the adoption of temporal lobe psychosurgery for aggressive patients. In every instance where animal experimentation led to the adoption of a psychosurgical procedure, there is evidence that attention was paid to a selective part of the total animal data. We have seen several examples of this trend to focus on postoperative changes that seemed as though they might be beneficial to some patients while ignoring the evidence of significant deficits. It may be helpful to provide two further examples.

Shortly after Smith, and later Ward, reported that cingulectomized monkeys became tamer, there was considerable interest in investigating the usefulness of this operation on humans. John Fulton, for example, received a grant from the Veterans Administration to secure basic information on whether the benefit of frontal operations could be obtained with fewer undesirable side effects by either more restrictive frontal operations or destruction of portions of the limbic system, particularly the cingulum. In 1948 at the William Withering Lectures at the University of Birmingham in England. Fulton asked whether a partial destruction of the anterior cingulate area might not be chiefly responsible for the behavioral changes that occur in man after a radical frontal lobotomy. He indicated that "the suggestion was based largely on behavioral changes reported in monkeys by Wilbur Smith and Arthur Ward." It is generally believed that Fulton's speech encouraged Dr. LeBeau in Paris and Sir Hugh Cairns in Oxford to try cingulotomies in agitated patients (see page 289). A closer examination of Ward's description of the postoperative behavior of the monkeys reveals the inadequacy of the term "tameness" to summarize all the changes that occurred. Ward wrote:

". . .there is an obvious change in personality. The monkey loses its preoperative shyness and is less fearful of man. It appears more inquisitive than the normal monkey of the same age. In a large cage with other monkeys of the same size, such an animal shows no grooming behavior or acts of affection towards its companions. In fact, it treats them as it treats inanimate objects and will walk on them, bump into them if they happen to be in the way, and will even sit on them. It will openly eat food in the hand of a companion without being prepared to do battle and appears surprised when it is rebuffed. Such an animal never shows actual hostility to its fellows. It neither fights nor tries to escape when removed from a cage. It acts under all circumstances as though it had lost its 'social conscience.' This is probably what Smith saw and called 'tameness.' It is thus evident that following removal of the anterior limbic area, such monkeys lose some of the social fear and anxiety which normally governs their activity and thus lose the ability to accurately forecast the social repercussions of their own actions."

An even more striking example of the selective perception of the results of animal experimentation is reflected in a new psychosurgical procedure used by Drs. F. Roeder, Hans Orthner, and Dieter Müller of the University of Göttingen in Germany. For a number of years these investigators have treated "sexual deviants," particularly a group diagnosed as *pedophilic homosexuals*—men who seek out sexual opportunities with young or teenage boys. At the International Neurological Congress in Brussels, they had an opportunity to see Schreiner and Kling's film picturing the hypersexuality of amygdalectomized male cats and monkeys. The operated animals shown in the film exhibited highly exaggerated sexual activity directed toward males as well as females and even toward animals of other species (see Figure 27). A later study by Kling indicated that the hypersexuality could be eliminated by a second brain operation that destroyed the ventromedial nucleus of the hypothalamus. Roeder, Orthner, and Müller considered the animal studies "a mine of information for human sexual pathology" and wrote ". . .the behavior of male cats with lesions of the amygdalar region in some respects closely approached that of human perversion. The films convinced us that there was a basis for a therapeutic, stereotaxic approach to this problem in man."

Roeder, Orthner, and Müller's psychosurgical procedure involves destruction of the ventromedial hypothalamic nucleus by using an electrode to make an electrolytic lesion in this structure. As its name implies, the ventromedial nucleus is close to the base of the brain at the midline, situated just above the pituitary gland, which is suspended from a "stalk" (infundibulum) just below the hypothalamus (see Figure 25). To avoid damaging the critical structures in the midline of the brain, a cannula is inserted approximately 10 millimeters lateral to the ventromedial nucleus, and the electrode is then pushed to its target through a side hole as illustrated in Figure 46. In general, about three-quarters of the ventromedial nucleus is destroyed on one side, but in one patient the operation was performed bilaterally. The unilateral lesion is made on what is called the nondominant side of the brain (right side for right-handed persons), although there is little evidence that there is any assymetry in the function of the hypothalamus. Their typical patient is a 27- to 55-year-old man with a compulsive desire for homosexual relations with younger men or boys. Some of the patients have been referred by the courts, while others have sought out help voluntarily. Over the past 10 years, stereotaxic electrolytic lesions have been made in the hypothalamus of 20 male patients.

In addition to the studies of amygdalectomized cats that subsequently were given ventromedial lesions, Roeder and his colleagues found experimental support for their surgical approach to pedophilic homosexuality in the reports of "sex centers" in the brains of rats by G. Dorner and his associates at Humboldt University in Berlin. Dorner's group believes they identified a separate male and female sex center in rat brains. These centers respond to the appropriate hormonal stimulation and regulate sexual behavior. Normally one of these centers is dominant over the other, depending on the sex of the animal; furthermore, it is maintained that if the dominant sex center is destroyed, the other will take over. Ac-

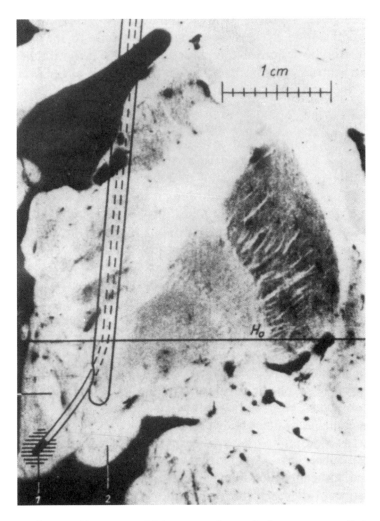

cording to Dorner and his co-workers, if the ventromedial hypothalamic "female sex center" is destroyed, male sexual behavior would become more dominant providing male hormone is present.

Most investigators studying the physiology of sex behavior believe that there is a great abundance of evidence refuting Dorner's view that there is only one "center" regulating the behavior of each sex and that these centers are completely separate. Moreover, it is generally agreed that in animals where learning plays an important role in establishing sexual roles, as is especially the case in humans, it is very unlikely that brain operations and hormonal treatment could radically alter an established sexual orientation. Nevertheless, the rat experiments by Dorner and his associates and Kling's report that ventromedial hypothalamic ablations reduce the hypersexuality of amygdalectomized cats provided sufficient justification for Roeder and his colleagues to use psychosurgery on patients with sexual pathology.

The ventromedial portion of the hypothalamus is generally believed to regulate many functions, including critical endocrine and visceral activity, appetite and body weight, and other important physiological regulations as well.[46] There are also a number of reports in the animal literature that destruction of the ventromedial nucleus may produce irritability and aggressiveness, and there exist several clinical reports that tumors in this area have produced episodes of rage in humans. The idea of destroying a large percentage of this sensitive region in humans would be a frightening thought to most scientists knowledgeable in this field. One can only wonder how Roeder and his colleagues were able to muster the

Figure 46. Technique used to destroy the ventromedial hypothalamic nucleus in sexual deviants. (Only the right side of the brain is shown. The black area at the left is the third ventricle in the midline of the brain.) The cannula is positioned with a stereotaxic instrument; the coagulating electrode is pushed through a side hole and guided into the ventromedial nucleus (1). The position of the ventromedial nucleus is estimated from the X-ray view of the third ventricle and the ability to produce the sensation of light flashes by stimulating the optic tract (2). (From F. Roeder, H. Orthner, and D. Müller. The Stereotaxic Treatment of Pedophilic Homosexuality and Other Sexual Deviation, in E. Hitchcock, L. Laitinen, and K. Vaernet (Eds.), *Psychosurgery*, 1972, Fig. 8-2. Charles C. Thomas, Publisher, Springfield, Ill.

"courage" to perform their first ventromedial hypothalamic operation on a human.

Although it is said that metabolic side effects or obesity
do not develop postoperatively and in a number of cases
the "homosexual libido, fantasies and impulses have
permanently vanished," the physiological and the psychiatric descriptions of the patients are insufficiently
documented to adequately support the conclusion
presented. After one of the operations judged to be most
successful it was stated: "Pedophilic drive has disappeared. Can watch small boys playing without getting
erection as before the operation." It is also claimed that a
desire for heterosexual contacts develops after the
operation, but the evidence presented makes it clear that
the major effect of the surgery is to produce a general
lowering of sexual drive. The patients generally report a
decreased capacity for erection and ejaculation. Nocturnal
emissions and masturbatory activity also decreased. One
patient reported he masturbated only once during the year
following the operation and that was motivated by
curiosity rather than sex drive. Description of the postoperative behavior of another patient included such statements as: "No more exhibitionistic drives, also no
onanism. No erections after awakening as before
operation. . . . The operative effect absolutely came up to
that of castration."

There is little in the description of the cases operated on
by Roeder and his colleagues, or the underlying animal research, that can even begin to justify the extreme confidence they express in their psychosurgical procedure. For
example:

"In conclusion there is no doubt that experimental behavioral research has afforded us a basic method to
eliminate or to control pedophilic homosexuality by
means of an effective psychosurgical operation in the area
of the sex-behavior center. *Virtually no forensic and juri-
dical problems exist, since neither surgical nor chemical*

castration is involved by this stereotaxic procedure."
(Italics in original)

Roeder and his associates believe that the reduction in
homosexuality that they report occurs postoperatively "is
due to the restoration of a previously disturbed equilibrium in brain function." They apparently conceive of their
operation as establishing a more normal balance between
the "male and female sex-behavior centers." Without
analyzing the many assumptions underlying the belief that
pedophilic homosexuality reflects an overactive "female
sex-behavior center," it is only necessary to point out that
there is no convincing evidence that the operation has only
affected the homosexual behavior. Describing the sexual
adjustment of one patient after surgery, Roeder and his
colleagues write: "The sexual drive is significantly
reduced. This concerns the normal and also the homosexual components." When allowance is made for the
fact that the patients generally want to change their behavior, there is no reason to believe that the surgery
produced a change in sexual orientation. The major effect
of the surgery seems to be a general reduction of sexual
drive to the point where it is possible for the patient to
control his deviant behavior. Moreover, considering the
many functions in which the ventromedial nucleus has
been implicated, very little information is provided about
other behavioral and physiological changes that might
have occurred. Clearly, this is an example of a group
adopting a psychosurgical procedure based on an arbitrary selection from the total animal data available and
then reporting their clinical results in a completely inadequate form. No indication has been presented that these
investigators have or intend to employ the type of behavior testing necessary for an objective evaluation of
postoperative changes.

Other examples could be provided to illustrate what
amounts to tunnel vision perception of the relationship of
animal brain research to clinical applications. There is

often a very limited appreciation displayed of the complexity of the results of the animal research that initially triggered the exploration of a particular surgical approach. A wider perspective would not only influence the adoption of particular procedures, but it would also have a marked influence on the testing programs used to evaluate postoperative changes. There is clearly a need for closer cooperation and a more critical exchange of ideas between clinicians and investigators doing basic research in the field of brain and behavior. In the past the relationship has often been superficial. Most neurosurgeons do not have the time or appropriate training to undertake the kind of investigations that must be done if any meaningful conclusions are to be drawn. The comment made by the neurosurgeon James Poppen in 1948 is still relevant:

"I feel strongly that it is the neurosurgeon's duty to perform the operation as safely and accurately as possible, but that the burden of deciding whether a mental patient should be subjected to the procedures falls on the shoulders of competent neuropsychiatrists who had had an opportunity to study many patients before and after operation.

"No neurosurgeon wishes to be a technician only. In most instances, however, the neurosurgeon has not had the proper training nor has he the time to devote the many weeks and perhaps months of intimate contact with the patient and his relatives to reach a just decision. Therefore, he is not in a position to weigh justly the merits for or against operative interference."

Although some neurosurgeons may have a little more sophistication about psychiatry and the behavioral sciences today than they did in 1948, the argument raised by Poppen is essentially true. The decision to undertake psychosurgery should not be allowed to rest in the hands of any one person. The appropriate way of preventing the abuses that occurred in the past is not by outlawing psychosurgery and thereby establishing a precedent that could stultify progress in medicine. What is needed are procedures for maximizing the critical exchange of views between experimentalists (not only psychiatrists) and clinicians and for assuring a meaningful review of experimental therapeutic practices. Problems related to review committees and other ethical and social considerations are discussed in the last chapter.

Comments On Ethical and Social Considerations

As a stream cannot rise above its source, so a code cannot change a low-grade man into a high-grade doctor, but it can help a good man to be a better man and a more enlightened doctor. It can quicken and inform a conscience, but not create one.

International code of Medical Ethics, Adopted by the General
Assembly of the World Medical Association, London, 1949.

One of the main purposes in writing this book was to provide the historical perspective and experimental evidence necessary for an informed discussion of the ethical and social issues raised by the possibility of applying various brain interventions to clinical and social problems. The difficult task of setting up specific codes of conduct in this area will be left to others, who will be able to draw in part on established guidelines such as the American Psychological Association's definition of informed consent and the Federal government's regulation of the use of new drugs. The difficulty always is in finding the proper balance that assures maximum protection of individuals without eliminating all leeway for testing new therapeutic techniques. It is much easier to dwell on mistakes of the past than to face the complex problem of obtaining the proper balance. Throughout this book, examples were presented to illustrate some of the subtleties of the ethical decisions that have to be faced when considering the various attempts to modify behavior by altering the brain. Often the distinction between "past abuses" and medically useful "discoveries" could only be made by hindsight. My own view is that we should resist those individuals who relate past abuses only for the purpose of gaining support for their position that broad categories of experimental medicine should be outlawed. Such a solution would stultify research and close the door to future progress that might be based on new findings or principles that are unknown at present. Nevertheless, restraints are necessary and it is to be hoped that this book can stimulate some badly needed constructive dialogue on this subject.

Although it has been argued, only partly in jest, that the possibility of a malpractice lawsuit is one of the major deterrents that protect patients, an independent review of experimental therapeutic procedures might potentially provide more meaningful protection. An independent review of questionable brain interventions can prevent a research-oriented physician's scientific goals or personal ambition from gaining priority over the interest of the patient. It has become increasingly common for hospitals to require some review process before permission is granted to undertake any procedures that go beyond the limits of general acceptability. When federal research funds are used, a review is now mandatory. To protect patients, many hospitals have set up "review committees" made up of psychiatrists, neurosurgeons, lawyers, ministers, scientists, and lay persons. No formal review process or set of regulations, however, can substitute for good judgment and moral integrity. Several studies have shown that review committees often do not provide adequate protection for patients. Too frequently, these "peer" committees have served only to "rubber stamp" the research projects of professional colleagues. This has happened not only in small private hospitals and state hospitals for the indigent, but in many of the largest, most prestigious institutions in the country. It is clear that approval has been granted in a number of cases where there have been few legitimate arguments in favor of the proposed procedures. This is not to deny that there are a number of instances where equally well-trained and well-intentioned physicians will disagree on the best treatment for a given patient. Two review committees can also reach different conclusions, and both may be based on reasonable arguments. There have been, however, too many cases where the legitimacy of a review committee's approval would never stand up to the light of day. Several such cases have been described in the press, but there are many more that might have been exposed. One of the ways of strengthening the review process is to challenge committees that approve procedures that seem to involve a violation of patients' rights.

It would serve no purpose to try to present an exhaustive list of all the factors that have to be considered by a review committee. Most of these are obvious and routine, but it might help to focus a dialogue if the areas where there have been abuses in the past are listed.

1. Review committee members must be as independent as possible from those recommending an equivocal procedure. It is not uncommon for such a committee to have to pass judgment on the recommendation of a very prestigious and influential member of the hospital staff. Those serving on a committee should be selected not only on the basis of their knowledge and the special interest they represent, but also on their professional, economic, and psychological independence from the physician whose case is being reviewed. There is little doubt that this has not always been the situation in the past and as a result it

has been a major source of violation of the rights of patients.

2. There is clear need to include in the review process the specific details concerning the alternative treatment methods that have been said to have been exhausted. This would include details about the drugs that have been used and the amount of meaningful contact with psychiatrists and psychologists. Too often in the past there has been an uncritical acceptance of the statement that drugs and psychiatric treatments have been adequately tried and found unsuccessful. The burden of proof that alternative treatments have been adequately explored should always be on those recommending psychosurgery. Often in the past when it was claimed that drugs were ineffective, there has been no indication of what drugs were used, in what doses, and for how long. Similarly, there is ample reason to suspect that in a number of instances, years of only custodial care in a psychiatric institution has been accepted as evidence of the failure of psychiatric treatment. It is likely that in the future new treatment methods such as the various forms of behavior therapies (counterconditioning, behavior modification) will also have to be considered. Particularly in the case of children, there should be a thorough exploration of familial and environmental factors that may have caused or exaggerated the behavioral symptoms. Traditionally, medical practice has focused on the doctor-patient relation to the neglect of therapeutic possibilities that may involve factors outside this relationship. All members of the review committee should hold the patient's interest as the foremost consideration, but it would be a good practice to have one member serve as the patient's ombudsman. It would be the ombudsman's specific responsibility to protect the patient by questioning in detail whether alternative therapies were sufficiently explored and also to determine if consent was given under conditions that assured the patient or guardian was maximally informed. The

ombudsman would have to be sensitive to the fact that there may be a need to protect children from the consent of their own parents, who in some instances act in their own, rather than their child's interest.

3. There should be a clear rationale for the proposed procedure. Several instances have been cited throughout the book where it has not been evident at all how the patient might be helped by the brain intervention undertaken. It would be unreasonable to require that a completely adequate scientific explanation always be provided since so much of medicine is an art based on empirical evidence that a procedure has worked in the past, rather than on any clear understanding of the underlying physiology. A list of the arguments as they relate specifically to the patient being discussed, however, would tend to make transparent those instances where the justification is very weak. Admittedly, this is a difficult area in which to achieve the proper balance. When a controversial method works, we are likely to judge its originator as bold and imaginative; when it does not work, we may consider such a person callous, naive, and unethical. Although it is difficult to do otherwise, the ethicality of behavior should not be judged by its outcome. Judgments after the fact are so much easier. It is interesting, for example, to consider the implications of the fact that a substantial number, if not a majority, of psychiatrists believe that electroconvulsive shock is a useful treatment in cases of depression. However, if the method was not known and Dr. Cerletti (see pages 156–162) came along today and requested permission to pass a crude electric current through the brain of a patient, it is unlikely that he could offer any rationale that could justify this experimentation.

4. One source of violation of the rights of patients stems from the tendency to deny what is obviously true, that patients are used in experimentation. By ignoring this reality and pretending, sometimes with a fair amount of deceit, that everything that is done to a patient has a

therapeutic purpose, many procedures have escaped adequate review. Dr. Henry Beecher of the Harvard Medical School described a number of such cases in his article on the ethics of clinical research. Beecher maintains that the fact that promotions at most medical schools are contingent on doing research and that the editors of scientific journals are usually willing to publish investigations involving questionable ethical practices created a climate where potentially dangerous procedures that had no therapeutic value for the patient might be employed. A 1964 search through 100 consecutive articles in a major medical journal revealed 12 investigations that seemed unethical. A number of patients were exposed to such dangerous procedures as receiving transplants of cancer cells, having abnormal heart beats induced, arteries cannulated, and blood supply to the brain modified—none of which could possibly benefit them.

There is little doubt that electrodes have been inserted in diverse regions of the brain where the probability of obtaining information of direct benefit to the patient has to be regarded as extremely remote. It is often claimed that the extra electrodes serve some diagnostic purpose, but the supporting evidence has frequently been easily disputed. On a number of occasions the questionable brain electrodes have been used to evoke strong emotional states capable of precipitating psychological reactions whose consequences could not be anticipated. Electrodes have also been left in the brain for periods exceeding any need for therapeutic or diagnostic purpose in order to fulfill research requirements. Sometimes the nontherapeutic aspects are quite innocuous and may involve only a slight prolongation of a procedure, at no risk or discomfort to the patient, in order to obtain some potentially useful scientific information. The range of experimental possibilities is great—some are minor and some serious procedures. (It is not uncommon, for example, for extra blood to be drawn in a hospital to accommodate a member of the hospital staff who is conducting an experiment sometimes unrelated to the patient's therapy.) In every case, however, the experimental aspects should be explicitly stated and made contingent upon the patient's informed consent and subject to examination by a review committee.

PSYCHOSURGERY IN PRISONS

Not too long ago I attended a public discussion in Detroit on the topic of psychosurgery on prison inmates. The meeting was called mainly in response to the publicity given to a case of a person who had apparently volunteered for experimental psychosurgery in the hope that he might be released from the psychiatric institute to which he was committed. Eighteen years earlier the man had been committed to a psychiatric institute and while there he had strangled a nurse and sexually assaulted her dead body. He was then classified as a criminal sexual psychopath, but he was now being offered an opportunity to volunteer for psychosurgery and thereby increase the possibility that he might be released. The proposed psychosurgery was part of an experimental program to be conducted at the Lafayette Clinic in Detroit and was to be supported by $228,000 grant from the Michigan legislature. (In response to the public reaction, the grant has since been rescinded.) The purpose of the experimentation was to compare the relative effectiveness of psychosurgery (amygdalectomy) and hormonal treatment (using antiandrogens) as a means of combating the criminal impulses of a sexual psychopath. The physicians involved in the study had asked the courts to make a "declarative judgment" on the legality of the experiment, and the newspaper accounts of the pending judicial hearing had aroused strong public reactions which served as a catalyst for public meetings such as the one I attended.

There are good reasons, as will be explained subsequently, for us to be concerned about psychosurgical experiments, but the mood at most public meetings is more conducive to hurling accusations of Nazi tactics rather than seriously discussing the ethical and legal principles that might guide our decisions about such matters. In spite of the heated discussion, however, the major issues were raised, although generally in a much too emotional a manner to permit constructive discussion. One of the main issues that comes up in any discussion of medical experimentation concerns the matter of consent, which all agree should be given only after the subject is informed and under conditions that are free of coercion. It is often argued, with insufficient thought, that free consent is not possible by those subjected to involuntary confinement. I am not certain that this is necessarily true, although I clearly recognize that it is a problem that bears close monitoring. Anyone who thinks that it is impossible to freely volunteer as an experimental subject while confined in a prison would be advised to read Nathan Leopold's book, *Life Plus 99 Years.* Leopold describes the conditions under which he and a number of other prison inmates volunteered for testing antimalarial drugs. The men were thoroughly informed of the risks and the discomforts as well as given absolutely no explicit or even implicit promises of shortened prison terms. On the contrary, attempts were made to talk some of the men out of volunteering when they seemed to be responding impulsively, and they were given time to reflect and change their minds. Leopold writes:

"The young docs and Dr. Alving leaned over backward in handling the matter of volunteering in a scrupulously ethical manner. The large-scale use of human volunteers in medical experiments was still something rather new and not too clearly defined from an ethical point of view, and the fact that all of us here were prisoners made it even more a moot point. Indeed, at the famous Nuremberg trials of German war criminals, some of the defendants who were scientists introduced testimony about the Stateville experiments to show that our side was doing the very same thing of which they were accused. That was absolutely false. The docs explained in great detail to each and every volunteer before he was used just what it was planned to do. We were told that there was danger, that we might be sick, that we might die. No man was coerced or even persuaded. If anything, the Army officers threw their weight the other way. Every man who went on the project at Stateville did so because he wanted to, almost because he insisted on it. The problem was never that of finding volunteers, rather it was the difficult one of selecting among the large number who wanted to become subjects."

It is probably true that some of the men had hopes that the fact of their volunteering would influence the parole board. Volunteering, however, is never completely made in a social and psychological vacuum. The important point is whether they volunteered without coercion or the promise of irresistible rewards, and on the basis of the best information at hand. It cannot be assumed that the conditions of volunteering necessarily are completely different inside and outside a prison. There can be great pressures to volunteer, even at considerable personal risk, outside of a prison. In his book, *The Patient as Person,* Paul Ramsey discusses the tremendous psychological pressure placed on a twin to volunteer a kidney for transplantation into a twin who would otherwise die. Indeed, the pressure may be recognized as so great that in the Masden case, it was necessary for a psychiatrist to testify that Leonard, a 19-year-old, would suffer "grave emotional impact" if he was not allowed to give a kidney to his brother, Leon. Judge Edward A. Counihan, Jr., ruled:

"I am satisfied from the testimony of the psychiatrist that grave emotional impact may be visited upon Leonard if the defendants refuse to perform this operation and Leon should die, as apparently he will. . . . Such emotional disturbance could well affect the health and physical well-being of Leonard for the remainder of his life. I therefore find that this operation is necessary for the continued good health and future well-being of Leonard and that in performing the operation the defendants are conferring a benefit upon Leonard as well as upon Leon."

As school children we all learned that the construction of the Panama Canal was made possible by Walter Reed solving the problem of how yellow fever was transmitted. Perhaps less remembered is the fact that Army volunteers were needed to expose themselves to infected mosquitoes and injections of virulent substances. It might be argued today that it is not possible for someone in the Army to truly volunteer. Such arguments, however, can be dangerous and irresponsible, as Dr. Robert Marston, the former Director of the National Institutes of Health, argued in a speech at the University of Virginia. Marston pointed out there is a dual responsibility with respect to research on human subjects. One is to assure that the subjects are as fully protected as possible, the other involves a recognition "that there is immorality in *not* carrying out necessary research involving human subjects". Not to have tested the polio vaccine on children, for example, might also be considered irresponsible and possibly even unethical. The struggle for the proper balance between the welfare of the individual and that of society will always be with us and cannot be permanently resolved by decrees that prohibit experimentation in one situation or another.

Nevertheless, there is an essential distinction that has to be made between a prisoner volunteering under closely supervised conditions for an experiment that may help others and a person volunteering for some experimental procedure that is claimed may directly affect the psychiatric condition responsible for his confinement.

Nicholas Kittrie has discussed the very special conditions that apply to the "quarantining" of those people who are considered criminally inclined psychopaths. There is no agreement among psychiatrists on the definition of a criminal psychopath, and yet a number of states have laws governing their confinement that in effect deprive them of those constitutional protections that are provided ordinary criminals. A psychopath is not considered mentally ill by most psychiatrists. Instead, they are said to have some "personality disorder" which is responsible for their committing crimes without the ordinary restraints of a social conscience. The laws vary in different states, but basically a person may be committed to an institution on the testimony of one or several psychiatrists. The period of confinement is usually unspecified, but to obtain release he must prove he is cured. Usually it is necessary for a person so committed to convince the psychiatrists of the confining institute that he is cured, since outside psychiatrists are not permitted to visit on the grounds that such visits might be disruptive. According to Kittrie, it is practically impossible for a patient to be released from a psychopathic institute without staff approval, but the criteria that have to be met can be very vague.

D. L. Rosenhan, a Professor of Psychology and Law at Stanford University, performed an experiment demonstrating the lack of objective criteria in psychiatric diagnosis. Eight pseudopatients gained admission into 12 psychiatric hospitals (located in five different states) by claiming during their initial interview that they had been hearing voices. On questioning, they said the voices were unclear, but seemed to be saying "empty," "hollow," and "thud." No other symptoms were reported and immediately after admission to the hospital the pseudopatients behaved as they did normally. All but one of the pseudopatients received the diagnostic label of "schizophrenia" and in no case was it detected that they were not psychotic. Rather than the normal behavior exhibited on the ward influencing the diagnostic label, the converse was true. The perception of the pseudopatients' behavior and past history tended to be distorted by the staff to conform to a theory of the dynamics of schizophrenia.

The difficulties in establishing objective criteria for diagnosis and cure are compounded in a psychopathic institution. The whole process has a nightmarish quality, or as Kittrie remarks in *The Right to be Different*:

" Like a Kafka-esque characater, the psychopath is a man to whom no clear-cut social standards are applicable. He suffers from a disputed mental disorder. . . . To secure release, he must be cured of a condition that is not clearly definable and that some say is not treatable. Finally his return to society depends upon ambiguous conditions."

Quite aside from the matter of the vague definition of a psychopathic personality and the illusory criteria for a cure is the great pressure on those who might recommend release to err on the cautious side. Since there have been several tragic cases of persons released from these institutions committing terrible crimes, it is understandable that those who have to make such decisions are likely to be conservative. To consider psychosurgical experiments on the violent or sexual psychopath in the context of such a legal and definitional morass and under conditions where the inmate's chances of release are so completely dependent on the satisfaction of the psychiatric staff is very dangerous. The severe pressure placed on people who are confined for indefinite periods under completely unstructured circumstances makes a sham of any pretense that meaningful volunteering is possible. In his book, *Prisoners of Psychiatry*, Bruce Ennis vivdly describes the helplessness of people committed to some mental institutions where they may receive virtually no treatment for 15 years or more and in spite of the fact that they may never have meaningful contact with a psychiatrist, they are routinely declared unfit for release. Many of these "patients" have never even committed a crime, but have been declared mentally incompetent under conditions in some regions where physicians (often not psychiatrists) and a sheriff can provide the legally required testimony. There may be a place for experimental psychosurgery under carefully controlled conditions, but there should be serious doubts whether the group of people already committed as criminal psychopaths is the right population for such experimentation.

I have made a point of seeking out opportunities to learn the opinion of lawyers and judges on the legal aspects of psychosurgery. In general, what I heard is quite disappointing. There seem to be few existing legal precedents that either provide clarification of issues or offer protection against unjustified experimentation. Legal clarification and more specific guidelines are badly needed in this area. In general, lawyers who have voiced strong opposition to experimental psychosurgery have based their arguments on medical and scientific evidence that the procedures do not work or have undesirable side effects rather than on legal considerations. These lawyers may find themselves on weak ground if they have to argue against neurosurgeons such as Dr. M. Hunter Brown of Santa Monica Hospital who claim that their specifically targeted stereotaxic surgery has had no adverse effect on memory, intellect, or judgment (see page 239). Dr. Brown claims that based on his experience on over 260 patients over a 24-year period the operation has "converted violent patients to useful citizens." He also strongly argued during an extensive radio interview (Station CJOR, Vancouver, Canada) as well as in his publications that his surgical technique should be applied to prison inmates as a humane and tax-saving alternative to a life of confinement.[47] The great majority of neuroscientists are very skeptical of Dr. Brown's claims that he has the scientific evidence to support his statements, and many would testify to this effect. It seems inescapable, but nevertheless ironic, that a judge who is unlikely to have any technical knowledge or experience in this field will have to evaluate conflicting testimony and make a judgment. In the Lafayette Clinic case in Detroit described earlier, for example, the three presiding judges ruled that the proposed psychosurgery could not be performed on persons confined against their will—even if consent is formerly obtained—because the procedure "is clearly experimental, poses substantial danger to research subjects, and carries substantial unknown risks." In their decision, however, the judges also wrote that when psychosurgery "becomes an accepted neurosurgical procedure and is no longer experimental" the decision could be reviewed and changed.

One additional comment should be made with respect to experimental therapeutics. It can surely be argued that any experiment on humans is immoral if people are subjected to risks and discomfort under conditions where little scientific information can be gained. Many proposals of experimental psychosurgery within the confines of a prison or psychopathic institute can be criticized on this ground. There has been almost no discussion of the problem of evaluating the effectiveness of the psychosurgery within the limits of the confining institution. If a prisoner were to be subjected to brain surgery, how should he be tested before it is decided that the operation has been successful and it is safe to release the person into society? Should a series of *Clockwork Orange* type tests be given to determine if the person could be provoked into violence or sex crimes? There is no evidence that those who have proposed the experimental psychosurgery have adequately considered this problem.

SOCIAL IMPLICATIONS

There is at present both a serious concern over the rapidly increasing number of violent crimes and a strong feeling of frustration over the inability to develop means to effectively combat this trend. Such a situation will assuredly increase the pressure to come up with new types of solutions. It is not surprising, therefore, that solutions involving biological approaches to the problem have been proposed. Although these proposals often receive a great amount of publicity, the ideas expressed generally reflect desperation over the problem rather than familiarity with the physiological mechanisms that are incorporated into the suggested solutions. An excellent example of this trend can be seen in the following recent proposal by the social psychologist Dr. Kenneth B. Clark:

"Given the urgency of the immediate survival problem, the psychological and social sciences must enable us to control the animalistic, barbaric and primitive propensities in man and subordinate these negatives to the uniquely human moral and ethical characteristics of love, kindness and empathy. . . . We can no longer afford to rely solely on the traditional prescientific attempts to contain human cruelty and destructiveness.

". . . Given these contemporary facts, it would seem that a requirement imposed on all power-controlling leaders—and those who aspire to such leadership—would be that they accept and use the earliest perfected form of psychotechnological, biochemical intervention which would assure their positive use of power and reduce or block the possibility of using power destructively. It would assure that there would be no absurd or barbaric use of power. It would provide the masses of human beings with the security that their leaders would not sacrifice them on the altars of their personal ego. . . ." (Dr. K. B. Clark, Presidential Address, American Psychological Association, 1971)

Undoubtedly Dr. Clark is seriously concerned about the problem, but stripped to its essentials his proposal is revealed as a modern phrenology based on the belief that the brain is organized into neat functional compartments that conform to our social needs. We need only exorcise those regions of the brain that regulate undesirable behavior—or suppress them biochemically—and we will permit goodness to dominate. Even if the unlikely possibility that future leaders would submit to brain manipulations or biochemical interventions is unchallenged, there is no known way to eliminate aggression without reducing and distorting a number of desirable capacities that we would hope our leaders would possess. If our leaders were "stoned" on drugs, it is unlikely that anyone would be sacrificed on the altars of their personal ambition, but in what sense could they remain our leaders? Drugs may have the potential for accomplishing many useful ends such as facilitating learning and memory and counteracting manic states, depression, and anxiety. That is quite different, however, from drugs determining *what* we learn and remember, assuring moral integrity, and eliminating socially maladaptive behavior.

It is indeed surprising to find a social psychologist accepting the questionable hypotheses that wars are caused by man's animal-like, aggressive tendencies and that biological interventions may prevent them. Wars are often planned over a number of years and they involve geopolitical, economic, and social considerations that have little to do with any presumed, innate propensities of man that are thought to be revealed by brain stimulation studies of animals. Stimulation techniques have helped to identify regions of animal brains that seem to possess the capacity to coordinate a number of the muscular and visceral responses involved in aggressive and predatory behavior. Animals stimulated in critical regions may bare their fangs, arch their backs, and strike out with their paws at a suitable target. The killing responses of some animals may be stereotyped and unlearned—rats, for example, almost always kill mice by biting through the spinal cord in the region of the back of the neck and opposums kill by holding their prey in their mouths and rapidly moving their heads in a figure-eight pattern until the prey's neck is broken. The relationship of these stereotyped predatory and defensive responses to warfare is very remote.

Some of the responses displayed by humans engaged in an unarmed conflict undoubtedly reflect circuits built into the nervous system, but this factor probably contributes very little to our understanding of the dynamics of warfare where modern weaponry has virtually eliminated hand-to-hand combat. Furthermore, these responses are relevant only to the form of fighting rather than the causes. It should be pointed out that these biologically important predatory and aggressive responses have multiple representations in the nervous system and, as explained earlier (see pages 122–124), they cannot be eliminated by drugs or even by destroying the brain tissue surrounding the eliciting electrode. It is almost impossible to eliminate these response patterns by any brain interventions short of those involving such extensive destruction of the brain that the subject is reduced to a "vegetable status."

The surgical procedures that may at times eliminate aggression and rage in humans are not affecting innate, stereotyped response patterns. Their mode of action is much more global; they seem to be reducing responsiveness to many significant aspects of the environment. It is very unlikely that any of the ablation or stimulation techniques, or for that matter drugs, presently being investigated are capable of reducing undesirable aggression in a normal population without also reducing such qualities as sensitivity, ambition, and intellectual alertness. Unfortunately, the nervous system is not organized in a way that makes it possible to separate functions in terms of their social implications. The amount of violence prevalent at different times and among different people has varied greatly. Few people, if any, would seriously maintain that the rapidly increasing crime rate in urban centers can be attributed to brain pathology. There is a real possibility, however, that the frustration produced by our inability to effectively reverse this trend may create a mood that makes it possible for some policy makers to be seduced into believing that surgical or biochemical interventions can make a significant contribution to the problem.

If drug-related crimes are excluded, most of the present upsurge in violence can be related to a rejection of previously accepted values and social roles and to the existence of large groups of people who feel that they have no vested interest in the stability of the society in which they live. It may not be easy to find or to implement the changes that are necessary, but there is a great danger in accepting the delusion that biological solutions are available for these social problems. It is likely that there are some biological factors that contribute to a propensity toward violence, but we would be in serious trouble if a number of influential people became convinced that violence is mainly a product of a diseased brain rather than a diseased society.

Bibliography

Adams, D., & Flynn, J. P. Transfer of an escape response from tail shock to brain stimulated attack behavior. *J. Exp. Anal. Behav.*, 1966, **8**, 401–408.

Adams, J. E., & Rutkin, B. B. Visual responses to subcortical stimulation in the visual and limbic systems. *Confin. Neurol.*, 1970, **32**, 158–164.

Agranoff, B. W. Effects of antibiotics on long-term memory formation in the goldfish. In W. K. Honig & P. H. James (Eds.), *Animal Memory*, New York: Academic Press, 1971, pp. 243–258.

Ajmone Marsan, C., & Abraham, K. Considerations on the use of chronically implanted electrodes in seizure disorders. *Confin. Neurol.*, 1966, **27**, 95–110.

Akert, K., Gruesen, R. A., Woolsey, C. N., & Meyer, D. R. Klüver-Bucy syndrome in monkeys with neocortical ablations of temporal lobes. *Brain*, 1961, **84**, 480–498.

Allen, W. F. Effects of ablating the pyriform, amygdaloid areas, and hippocampi on positive and negative olfactory conditioned reflexes and on conditioned olfactory differentiation. *Am. J. Physiol.*, 1941, **132**, 81–92.

Alonso-de Florida, F., & Delgado, J. M. R. Lasting behavioral and EEG changes in cats induced by prolonged stimulation of amygdala. *Am. J. Physiol.*, 1958, **193**, 223–229.

Anand, B. K., & Brobeck, J. R. Hypothalamic control of food intake. *Yale J. Biol. Med.*, 1951, **24**, 123–140.

Anand, B. K., Dua, S., & Singh, B. Electrical activity of the hypothalamic "feeding centers" under the effect of changes in blood chemistry. *EEG Clin. Neurophysiol.*, 1961, **13**, 54–59.

Andersen, R. Differences in the course of learning as measured by various memory tasks after amygdalectomy in man. In E. Hitchcock, L. Laitinen, & K. Vaernet (Eds.), *Psychosurgery*, Springfield, Ill.: Charles C Thomas, 1972, pp. 177–183.

Andersson, B., & McCann, S. M. Further study of polydipsia evoked by hypothalamic stimulation in the goat. *Acta Physiol. Scand.*, 1955, **33**,333–346.

Andersson, B., & Wyrwicka, Wanda. The elicitation of a drinking motor conditioned reaction by electrical stimulation of the hypothalamic "drinking area" in the goat. *Acta Physiol. Scand.*, 1957, **41**, 194–198.

Andrew, R. J. Intracranial self-stimulation in the chick. *Nature*, 1967,- **213**, 847–848.

Andy, O. J. Neurosurgical treatment of abnormal behavior. *Am. J. Med. Sci.*, 1966, **252**, 232–238.

Andy, O. J. Thalamotomy in hyperactive and aggressive behavior. *Confin. Neurol.*, 1970, **32**, 322–325.

Andy, O. J., & Jurko, M. F. Thalatomy for hyperresponsive syndrome. In E. Hitchcock, L. Laitinen, & K. Vaernet (Eds.), *Psychosurgery*, Springfield, Ill.: Charles C Thomas, 1972, pp. 127–135.

Antelman, S. M., Lippa, A. S., & Fisher, A. E. 6-Hydroxydopamine, noradrenergic reward, and schizophrenia. *Science*, 1972, **175**, 919–920.

Baker, E. F. W., Young, M. P., Gauld, D. M., & Fleming, J. F. R. A new look at bimedial prefrontal leukotomy. *Can. Med. Assoc. J.*, 1970, **102**, 37–41.

Balasubramaniam, V., Kanaka, T. S., & Ramamurthi, B. Surgical treatment of hyperkinetic and behavior disorders. *Int. Surg.*, 1970, **54**, 18–23.

Balasubramaniam, V., Kanaka, T. S., Ramanujam, P. V., & Ramamurthi, B. Sedative neurosurgery. *J. Indian Med. Assoc.*, 1969, **53**, (8), 377–381.

Balasubramaniam, V., & Ramamurthi, B. Stereotaxic amygdalotomy in behavior disorders. *Confin. Neurol.*, 1970, **32**, 367–373.

Baldwin, M. Sensory responses from the human temporal lobe. In M. Baldwin & P. Bailey (Eds.), *Temporal Lobe Epilepsy*, Springfield, Ill.: Charles C Thomas, 1958, pp. 69–77.

Baldwin, M. Electrical stimulation of the mesial temporal region. In E. R. Ramey & D. S. O'Doherty (Eds.), *Electrical Studies on the Unanesthetized Brain*, New York: Paul B. Hoeber, 1960, pp. 159–176.

Ballantine, T. H., Cassidy, W. L., Flanagan, N. B., & Marino, R. Stereotaxic anterior cingulotomy for neuropsychiatric illness and intractable pain. *J. Neurosurg.*, 1967, **26**, 488–495.

Bandler, R. J., Chi, C. C., & Flynn, J. P. Biting attack elicited by stimulation of the ventral midbrain tegmentum of cats. *Science*, 1972, **177**, 364–366.

Barbeau, A., Doshay, L. J., & Spiegel, E. A. (Eds.). *Parkinson's Disease: Trends in Research and Treatment*. New York: Grune & Stratton, 1965.

Barfield, R. J., & Sachs, B. D. Sexual behavior: Stimulation by painful electric shock to the skin of male rats. *Science*, 1968, **161**, 392–394.

Bartholow, R. Experimental investigations into the functions of the human brain. *Am. J. Med. Sci.*, 1874, **67**, 305–313.

Bartholow, R. *Medical Electricity. A Practical Treatise.* Philadelphia: Lea Bros., 1881.

Bechterewa, N. P. (Ed.) *Physiologic und Pathophysiologic der tiefen Hirnstrukturen des Menschen.* Berlin: Veb Verlag Volk und Gesundheit, 1969. (Translated into German from the Russian publication of the Academy of Medical Sciences of the USSR, 1967.)

Beecher, H. K. Surgery as placebo. A quantitative study of bias. *J. Am. Med. Assoc.*, 1961, **176**, 1102–1107.

Beecher, H. K. Ethics and clinical research. *New Eng. J. Med.*, 1966, **274**, 1354–1360.

Bianchi, L. *The Mechanism of the Brain and the Function of the Frontal Lobes*, J. H. Macdonald, Trans. New York: Wm. Wood, 1922.

Bickford, R. G., Dodge, H. W., Jr., & Uihlein, A. Electrographic and behavioral effects related to depth stimulation in human patients. In E. R. Ramey & D. S. O'Doherty (Eds.), *Electrical Studies on the Unanesthetized Brain*. New York: Paul B. Hoeber, 1960, pp. 248–261.

Bickford, R. G., Mulder, D. W., Dodge, H. W., Jr., Svien, H. J., & Rome, H. P. Changes in memory function produced by electrical stimulation of the temporal lobe in man. In H. C. Solomon, S. Cobb, & W. Penfield (Eds.), *The Brain and Human Behavior*.

Res. Pub. Assoc. Res. Nerv. Mental Dis., Vol. 36. Baltimore: Williams & Wilkins, 1958, pp. 227–243.

Bishop, M. P., Elder, S. T., & Heath, R. G. Intracranial self-stimulation in man. *Science*, 1963, **140**, 394–396.

Bishop, M. P., Elder, S. T., & Heath, R. G. Attempted control of operant behavior in man with intracranial self-stimulation. In R. G. Heath (Ed.), *The Role of Pleasure in Behavior*. New York: Harper & Row (Hoeber Med. Div.), 1964, pp. 55–81.

Blanchard, D. C., & Blanchard, R. J. Innate and conditioned reactions to threat in rats with amygdaloid lesions. *J. comp. physiol. Psychol.*, 1972, **81**, 281–290.

Bower, G. H., & Miller, N. E. Rewarding and punishing effects from stimulating the same place in the rat's brain. *J. comp. physiol. Psychol.*, 1958, **51**, 669–674.

Boyd, E., & Gardner, L. Positive and negative reinforcement from intracranial self-stimulation in teleosts. *Science*, 1962, **136**, 648.

Boyle, R. *Experimenta et observationes physicae*. London: John Taylor, 1691 (26), 158, 32 pp.

Brady, J. V., & Nauta, W. J. H. Subcortical mechanisms in emotional behavior: Affective changes following septal forebrain lesions in the albino rat. *J. comp. physiol. Psychol.*, 1953, **46**, 339–346.

Brazier, M. A. B. Stimulation of the hippocampus in man using implanted electrodes. In M. Brazier (Ed.), *Brain Function, Vol. II*. Los Angeles: University of California Press, 1964, pp. 299–308.

Breggin, P. R. The return of lobotomy and psychosurgery. *Congressional Record*, **118**(26), Feb. 24, 1972.

Brickner, R. M. *The Intellectual Functions of the Frontal Lobe. A Study Based Upon Observations of a Man After Partial Frontal Lobectomy*. New York: Macmillan, 1936.

Brindley, G. S., & Lewin, W. S. The sensations produced by electrical stimulation of the visual cortex. *J. Physiol.*, 1968, **196**, 479–493.

Brindley, G. S. & Lewin, W. S. The sensations produced by electrical stimulation of the visual cortex. In. T. D. Sterling, E. A. Bering, S. V. Pollack & H. G. Vaughn (Eds.), *Visual Prosthesis, The Interdisciplinary Dialogue*. New York: Academic Press, 1971, pp. 23–40.

Brown, M. H. The changing role of cingulate surgery. In *Symposium on Cingulotomy, 1972, Hahnemann Medical College*. Springfield, Ill.: Charles C Thomas. In press.

Brown, M. H. Further experience with multiple limbic lesions for schizophrenia and sociopathic aggression. Presented at the Third

World Congress of Psychosurgery (Cambridge, England, August 14–19, 1972).

Brügger, M. von. Fresstrieb als hypothamisches Symptom. *Helv. Physiol. Acta*, 1943, **1**, 183–198.

Bruner, A. Self-stimulation in the rabbit: An anatomical map of stimulation effects. *J. comp. Neurol.*, 1967, **131**, 615–629.

Burckhardt, G. Ueber Rindenexcisionen, als Bertrag zur operativen Therapie der Psychosen. *Allg. Z. Psychiat.*, 1891, **47**, 463–548.

Bursten, B., & Delgado, J. M. R. Positive reinforcement induced by intracranial stimulation in the monkey. *J. comp. physiol. Psychol.*, 1958, **51**, 6–10.

Caggiula, A. R. Analysis of the copulation-reward properties of posterior hypothalamic stimulation in male rats. *J. comp. physiol. Psychol.*, 1970, **70**, 399–412.

Caggiula, A. R., & Eibergen, R. Copulation of virgin male rats evoked by painful peripheral stimulation. *J. comp. physiol. Psychol.*, 1969, **69**, 414–419

Caggiula, A. R., & Hoebel, B. G. "Copulation-reward site" in the posterior hypothalamus. *Science*, 1966, **153**, 1284–1285.

Cannon, W. B. *The Wisdom of the Body.* New York: Norton, 1932.

Cerletti, U. Electroshock therapy. In F. Marti-Ibanez, A. M. Sackler, M. D. Sackler, & R. R. Sackler (Eds.), *The Great Psychodynamic Therapies in Psychiatry.* New York: Hoeber-Harper, 1956, pp. 91–120.

Chapman, W. P. Studies of the periamygdaloid area in relation to human behavior. In H. C. Solomon, S. Cobb, & W. Penfield (Eds.), *The Brain and Human Behavior.* Res. Pub. Assoc. Nerv. Ment. Dis. Vol. 36. Baltimore: Williams & Wilkins, 1958, pp. 258–270.

Chapman, W. P. Depth electrode studies in patients with temporal lobe epilepsy. In E. R. Ramey & D. S. O'Doherty (Eds.), *Electrical Studies on the Unanesthetized Brain.* New York: Paul B. Hoeber, 1960, pp. 334–350.

Chatrian, G. E., & Chapman, W. P. Electrographic study of the amygdaloid region with implanted electrodes in patients with temporal lobe epilepsy. In E. R. Ramey & D. S. O'Doherty (Eds.), *Electrical Studies on the Unanesthetized Brain.* New York: Paul B. Hoeber, 1960, pp. 351–373.

Chitanondh, H. Stereotaxic amygdalotomy in the treatment of olfactory seizures and psychiatric disorders with olfactory hallucination. *Confin. Neurol.*, 1966, **27**, 181–196.

Chow, K. L. Effects of partial extirpation of posterior association cortex on visually mediated behavior in monkeys. *Comp. Psychol. Monogr.*, 1951, **20**, 187–217.

Chow, K. L., Lindsley, D. F., & Gollender, M. Modification of response patterns of lateral geniculate neurons after paired stimulation of contralateral and ipsilateral eyes. *J. Neurophysiol.*, 1968, **31**, 729–739.

Clark, E., & O'Malley, C. D. *The Human Brain and Spinal Cord.* Berkeley: University of California Press, 1968.

Clark, K. Cited in *Am. Psychol. Assoc. Monit.*, 1971, **2**, (October)

Clarke, A. C. *Profiles of the Future*, New York, Bantam, 1964.

Clarke, R. H. Investigation of the central nervous system. Part I, Methods and instruments. *Johns Hopkins Hospital Report*, Baltimore, 1920.

Connecticut Lobotomy Committee (B. Moore, S. Friedman, B. Simon, & J. Farmer) A co-operative clinical study of lobotomy. *Res. Publ. Assoc. Nerv. Ment. Dis.*, 1948, **27**, 769–794.

Cooper, I. S. *Parkinsonism: Its Medical and Surgical Therapy.* Springfield, Ill.: Charles C Thomas, 1961.

Cooper, I. S. A cryogenic method for the physiologic inhibition and production of lesions in the brain. *J. Neurosurg.*, 1962, **19**, 853–858.

Cooper, I. S. *Involuntary Movement Disorders.* New York: Harper & Row Hoeber Med. Div., 1969.

Cooper, I. S. Motor functions of the thalamus with recent observations concerning the role of pulvinar. *Int. J. Neurol.*, 1971, **8**, 238–259.

Cooper, I. S. *The Victim is Always the Same.* New York: Harper & Row, 1973.

Cooper, I. S., Riklan, M., Stellar, S., Waltz, J. M., Levita, E., Ribera, V. A. and Zimmerman, J. A multidisciplinary investigation of neurosurgical rehabilitation in bilateral Parkinsonism. *Amer. Geriat. Soc.*, 1968, **16**, 1177–1306.

Cooper, I. S., Waltz, J. M. and Amin, I. A multi-disciplinary study of the effects of cryopulvinectomy (Ablation of the pulvinar). *Int. J. Neurol.* (in press).

Cooper, R. Physiological data from electrodes implanted for investigation and treatment of psychiatric and other disorders. In N. S. Kline & E. Laska (Eds.), *Computers and Electronic Devices in Psychiatry.* New York: Grune & Stratton, 1968, pp. 169–178.

Cox, V. C., and Valenstein, E. S. Attenuation of aversive properties of peripheral shock by hypothalamic stimulation. *Science*, 1965, **149**, 323–325.

Cox, V. C. & Valenstein, E. S. The effect of extensive mesencephalic central gray lesions on responses to reinforcing brain stimulation. *Psychon. Sci.*, 1966, **4**, 1–2.

Cox, V. C., & Valenstein, E. S. Distribution of hypothalamic sites yielding stimulus-bound behavior. *Brain Behav. Evol.*, 1969, **2**, 359–376.

Crawford, M. P., Fulton, M. D., Jacobson, C. F., and Wolfe, J. B. Frontal lobe ablation in chimpanzee: a resume of "Becky" and "Lucy". *Ass. Res. Nerv. & Ment. Dis.*, 1948, **27**, 3–57.

Crichton, M. *The Terminal Man.* New York: Alfred Knopf, 1972.

Crow, H. J. Electronic devices in psychiatry. In N. S. Kline & E. Laska (Eds.), *Computers and Electronic Devices in Psychiatry.* New York: Grune & Stratton, 1968, pp. 158–168.

Crow, H. J., Cooper, R., & Phillips, D. G. Controlled multifocal frontal leucotomy for psychiatric illness. *J. Neurol. Neurosurg. Psychiat.*, 1961, **24**, 353–360.

Crow, H. J., Cooper, R. & Phillips, D. G. Progressive leucotomy. *Curr. Psychiat. Ther.*, 1963, **3**, 98–113.

Crowley, W. R., Poplow, H. B., & Ward, O. B., Jr. From dud to stud: Copulatory behavior elicited through conditioned arousal in sexually inactive male rats. *Physiol. Behav.*, 1973, **10**, 391–394.

Delgado, J. M. R. Permanent implantation of multilead electrodes in the brain. *Yale J. Biol. Med.*, 1952, **24**, 351–358.

Delgado, J. M. R. Evaluation of permanent implantation of electrodes within the brain. *EEG Clin. Neurophysiol.*, 1955, **7**, 637–644.

Delgado, J. M. R. Prolonged stimulation of brain in awake monkeys. *J. Neurophysiol.*, 1959, **22**, 458–475.

Delgado, J. M. R. Cerebral heterostimulation in monkey colony. *Science*, 1963a, **141**, 161–163.

Delgado, J. M. R. Telemetry and telestimulation of the brain. In L. Slater (Ed.), *Biotelemetry.* New York: Pergamon Press, 1963b, pp. 231–249.

Delgado, J. M. R. Free behavior and brain stimulation. In C. C. Pfeiffer & J. R. Smythies (Eds.), *Int. Rev. Neurobiol.*, 1964, **6**, 349–449.

Delgado, J. M. R. *Physical Control of the Mind.* New York: Harper & Row, 1969.

Delgado, J. M. R., & Anand, B. K. Increase of food intake induced by electrical stimulation of the lateral hypothalamus. *Am. J. Physiol.*, 1953, **172**, 162–168.

Delgado, J. M. R., DeFeudis, F. V., Roth, R. H., Ryugo, D. K., & Mitruka, B. M. Dialytrode for long term intracerebral perfusion in awake monkeys. *Arch. int. Pharmacodyn. Thér.*, 1972, **198**, 9–21.

Delgado, J. M. R., & Hamlin, H. Spontaneous and evoked electrical seizure in animals and in humans. In E. R. Ramey & D. S. O'Doherty (Eds.), *Electrical Studies on the Unanesthetized Brain.* New York: Paul B. Hoeber, 1960, pp. 133–158.

Delgado, J. M. R., Hamlin, H., & Chapman, W. P. Techniques of intracranial electrode implacement and stimulation and its possible therapeutic value in psychotic patients. *Confin. Neurol.*, 1952, **12**, 315–319.

Delgado, J. M. R., Mark, V. H., Sweet, W. H., Ervin, F. R., Gerhardt, W., Bach y Rita, G., & Hagiwara, R. Intracerebral radio stimulation and recording in completely free patients. *J. Nerv. Ment. Dis.*, 1968, **147**, 329–340.

Delgado, J. M. R., Roberts, W. W., & Miller, N. E. Learning motivated by electrical stimulation of the brain. *Am. J. Physiol.*, 1954, **179**,587–593.

Delgado, J. M. R., Rosvold, H. E., & Looney, E. Evoking conditioned fear by electrical stimulation of subcortical structures in the monkey brain. *J. comp. physiol. Psychol.*, 1956, **49**, 373–380.

Denny-Brown, D., & Chambers, R. A. The parietal lobe and behavior. *Res. Publ. Assoc. Res. Nerv. Ment. Dis.*, 1958, **36**, 35–117.

Detre, T. P., & Jarecki, H. G. *Modern Psychiatric Treatment.* Philadelphia: Lippincott, 1971.

Dörner, G., Döcke, F., & Hinz, G. Homo- and hypersexuality in rats with hypothalamic lesions. *Neuroendocrinology*, 1969, **4**, 20–24.

Downer, J. L. de C. Changes in visual gnostic functions and emotional behaviour following unilateral temporal pole damage in the "split-brain" monkey. *Nature*, 1961, **191**, 50–51.

Downer, J. L. de C. Interhemispheric integration in the visual system. In V. B. Mountcastle (Ed.), *Interhemispheric Relations and Cerebral Dominance.* Baltimore: Johns Hopkins Press, 1962, pp. 87–100.

Dubos, R. The despairing optimist. *Am. Scholar*, 1971, **40**, 565–572.

Egger, M. D. & Flynn, J. P. Effects of electrical stimulation of the amygdala on hypothalamically elicited attack behavior in cats. *J. Neurophysiol.*, 1963, **26**, 705–720.

Ellison, G. D., & Flynn, J. P. Organized aggressive behavior in cats after surgical isolation of the hypothalamus. *Arch. Ital. Biol.*, 1968, **106**, 1–20.

Endroczi, E., & Lissak, K. Behavioral reactions evoked by electrical stimulation in the medial forebrain bundle region. *Physiol. Behav.*, 1966, **1**, 223–227.

Ennis, B. *Prisoners of Psychiatry: Mental Patients, Psychiatrists and the Law.* New York: Harcourt Brace Jovanovich, 1972.

Epstein, A. N. Reciprocal changes in feeding behavior produced by intrahypothalamic chemical injections. *Am. J. Physiol.*, 1960, **199**, 969–974.

Erofeyeva, M. Contribution a l'étude des reflexes conditionnels destructifs. *Compt. Rendu. Soc. Biol. (Paris)*, 1916, **79**, 239–240.

Ewald, J. R. Über künstlich erzeugte Epilepsie. *Berliner Klin. Wochenschr.*, 1898, **35**, 689.

Fedio, P., & Ommaya, A. K. Bilateral cingulum lesions and stimulation in man with lateralized impairment in short-term verbal memory. *Exp. Neurol.*, 1970, **28**, 84–91.

Fedio, P., & Van Buren, J. Cerebral mechanisms for perception and immediate memory under electrical stimulation in conscious man. Presented at Symposium, "Human Memory: Cortical and Subcortical Mechanisms," Annual Meeting of the American Psychological Association, Washington, D. C., September 1971.

Ferrier, D. Experimental researches in cerebral physiology and pathology. *West Riding Lunatic Asylum Medical Report*, 1873, **3**, 30–96.

Ferrier, D. *The Functions of the Brain.* London: Smith Elder & Co., 1876.

Fiamberti, A. M. Proposta di una technica operatoria modificata e semplificata per gli interventi alla Moniz sui lobi prefrontali in malati di mente. *Rassegna di studi psichiat.*, 1937, **26**, 797.

Fisher, A. E. Maternal and sexual behavior induced by intracranial chemical stimulation. *Science*, 1956, **124**, 228–229.

Fisher, A. E., & Coury, J. N. Cholinergic tracing of a central neural circuit underlying the thirst drive. *Science*, 1962, **138**, 691–693.

Fisher, A. E., & Coury, J. N. Chemical tracing of the neural pathways mediating the thirst drive. In M. J. Wagner (Ed.), *Thirst.* First Internation Symposium on Thirst in the Regulation of Body Water. New York: Macmillan, 1964, pp. 515–529.

Flam, E. S., & Van Buren, J. M. The reliability of reconstructed ventricular landmarks for localization of depth electrodes in man. *J. Neurosurg.*, 1966, **25**, 67–72.

Flynn, J. The neural basis of aggression in cats. In D. C. Glass (Ed.),

Neurophysiology and Emotion. New York: Rockefeller University Press, 1967, pp. 40–60.

Flynn, J. P., Edwards, S. B., & Bandler, R. J. Changes in sensory and motor system during centrally elicited attack. *Behav. Sci.*, 1971, **16,** 1–19.

Flynn, J. P., Vanegas, H., Foote, W., & Edwards, S. Neural mechanisms involved in a cat's attack on a rat. In R. E. Whalen, R. F. Thompson, M. Verzeano, & N. M. Weinberger (Eds.), *The Neural Control of Behavior.* New York: Academic Press, 1970, pp. 135–173.

Foltz, E., & White, L. E. Experimental cingulumotomy and modification of morphine withdrawal. *J. Neurosurg.*, 1957, **14,** 655–673.

Foltz, E. L., & White, L. E. Pain "relief" by frontal cingulumotomy. *J. Neurosurg.*, 1962, **19,** 89–100.

Fonberg, E. The motivational role of the hypothalamus in animal behavior. *Acta Biol. Exp. (Warsaw)*, 1967, **27,** 303–318.

Fonberg, E. The normalizing effect of lateral amygdalar lesions upon the dorsomedial amygdalar syndrome in dogs. *Acta Neurobiol. Exp. (Poland)*, 1973, **33,** 449–466.

Freeman, W. J. Transorbital leucotomy: The deep frontal cut. *Proc. Roy. Soc. Med.*, 1949, **42,** Suppl. 8–12.

Freeman, W. J. Comparison of thresholds for behavioral and electrical responses to cortical electrical stimulation in cats. *Exp. Neurol.*, 1962, **6,** 315–331.

Freeman, W. J. Frontal lobotomy in early schizophrenia: Long followup in 415 cases. *Br. J. Psychiat.*, 1971, **119,** 621–624.

Freeman, W. J., & Watts, J. W. *Psychosurgery in the Treatment of Mental Disorders and Intractable Pain,* 2nd ed. Springfield, Ill: Charles C Thomas, 1950.

Fritsch, G., & Hitzig, E. Ueber die elektrische Erregbarkeit des Grosshirns. *Arch. Anat. Physiol., Leipzig,* 1870, **37,** 300–332.

Fry, W. J., & Meyers, R. Ultrasonic method of modifying brain structures. 1st Int. Symp. Stereoencephalotomy, Philadelphia 1961. *Confin. Neurol.*, 1962, **22,** 315–327.

Fry, W. J., Mosberg, W. H., Barnard, J. W., & Fry, F. J. Production of focal destructive lesions in the central nervous system with ultrasound. *J. Neurosurg.*, 1954, **11,** 471–478.

Fulton, J. F. *Functional Localization in Relation to Frontal Lobotomy. The William Withering Memorial Lectures.* New York: Oxford University Press, 1949.

364 Bibliography

Fulton, J. F. *Frontal Lobotomy and Affective Behavior. A Neurophysiological Analysis.* New York: W. W. Norton, 1951.

Galef, B. G., Jr. Aggression and timidity: Responses to novelty in feral Norway rats. *J. comp. physiol. Psychol.*, 1970, **70**, 370–381.

Gallistel, C. R. Self-stimulation: The neurophysiology of reward and motivation. In J. A. Deutsch (Ed.), *The Physiological Basis of Memory*, New York, Academic Press, 1973, pp. 176–267.

Gardner, D., & Kandel, E. R. Diphasic postsynaptic potential: A chemical synapse capable of mediating conjoint excitation and inhibition. *Science*, 1972, **176**, 675–678.

Gellhorn, E. The physiological basis of shock therapy. *Roy. Soc. Med. Proc. (Suppl.)*, 1949, **42**, 55–70.

Gellhorn, E. *Autonomic Imbalance and the Hypothalamus.* Minneapolis: University of Minnesota Press, 1957.

Gerard, R. W. What is memory? *Scientific American*, 1953 (September), San Francisco: W. H. Freeman.

Gibbs, E. L., & Gibbs, F. A. A purring center in the cat's brain. *J. Comp. Neuro.*, 1936, **64**, 209–211.

Gibbs, F. A. Abnormal electrical activity in the temporal regions and its relationship to abnormalities of behavior. In H. C. Solomon, S. Cobb & W. Penfield (Eds.), *The Brain and Human Behavior*, Res. Publ. Assoc. Res. Nerv. Ment. Dis., Vol. 36, Baltimore: Williams & Wilkins, 1958, pp. 278–294.

Gibson, W. E., Reid, L. D., Sakai, M., & Porter, P. B. Intracranial reinforcement compared with sugar-water reinforcement. *Science*, 1965, **148**, 1357–1359.

Glickman, S. E., & Schiff, B. B. A biological theory of reinforcement. *Psychol. Rev.*, 1967, **74**, 81–109.

Gloor, P. Discussion. In C. D. Clemente & D. B. Lindsley (Eds.), *Aggression and Defense, Neural Mechanisms and Social Patterns*, Los Angeles: University of California Press, 1967, pp. 116–124.

Goddard, G. V. Functions of the amygdala. *Psychol. Bull.*, 1964, **62**, 89–109.

Goddard, G. V., McIntyre, D. C., & Leech, C. K. A permanent change in brain function resulting from daily electrical stimulation. *Exp. Neurol.*, 1969, **25**, 295–330.

Gol, A. Relief of pain by electrical stimulation of the septal area. *J. Neurol. Sci.*, 1967, **5**, 115–120.

Goltz, F. Der Hund ohne Grosshirn. *Pflüger's Arch. ges. Physiol.*, 1892, **51**, 570–614.

Goodall, J. *In the Shadow of Man.* New York: Dell Publishing Co., 1972.

Grastyán, E., Lissack, K., & Kekesi, F. Facilitation and inhibition of conditioned alimentary and defensive reflexes by stimulation of the hypothalamus and reticular formation. *Acta Physiol. Acad. Sci. Hung.*, 1956, **9**, 133–151.

Gray, J. *The Psychology of Fear and Stress.* New York: World University Library (McGraw-Hill), 1971.

Green, J. D., Clemente, C. D., & de Groot, J. Rhinencephalic lesions and behavior in cats. *J. Comp. Neurol.*, 1957, **108**, 505–545.

Greenblatt, M., & Solomon, H. C. *Frontal Lobes and Schizophrenia.* New York: Springer, 1953.

Greenblatt, M., & Solomon, H. C. Studies of lobotomy. In H. C. Solomon, S. Cobb, & W. Penfield (Eds.), *The Brain and Human Behavior*, Res. Publ. Assoc. Res. Nerv. Ment. Dis., Vol. 36, Baltimore: Williams & Wilkins, 1958, pp. 19–34.

Greer, M. A. Suggestive evidence of a primary "drinking center" in the hypothalamus of the rat. *Proc. Soc. Exp. Biol. Med.*, 1955, **89**, 59–62.

Grimm, R. J. Feeding behavior and electrical stimulation of the brain of *Carassius auratus. Science*, 1960, **131**, 162–163.

Gross, M. D. Violence associated with organic brain disease. In J. Fawcett (Ed.), *Dynamics of Violence.* Chicago: American Medical Association, 1971, pp. 85–91.

Grossman, S. P. Eating or drinking elicited by direct adrenergic or cholingergic stimulation of hypothalamus. *Science*, 1960, **132**, 301–302.

Grossman, S. P. Chemically induced epileptiform seizures in the cat. *Science*, 1963, **142**, 409–411.

Halstead, W. C. *Brain and Intelligence; a quantitative study of the frontal lobes.* Chicago: University of Chicago Press, 1947.

Harlow, J. M. Passage of an iron through the head. *Boston Med. Surg. J.* (now *New Eng. J. Med.)*, 1848, **39**, 389–393.

Harlow, J. M. Recovery from the passage of an iron bar through the head. *Mass. Med. Soc. Publication*, 1866–1868, **2**, 329–347.

Harwood, D., & Vowles, D. M. Defensive behavior and the after effects of brain stimulation in the ring dove *(Streptopelia risoria). Neuropsychologia*, 1967, **5**, 345–366.

Hassler, R., & Dieckmann, G. Stereotaxic treatment of compulsive and obsessive symptoms. *Confin. Neurol.*, 1967, **29**, 153–158.

Heath, R. G. *Studies in Schizophrenia. A Multidisciplinary Approach to Mind-Brain Relationships.* Cambridge: Harvard University Press, 1954.

Heath, R. G. Electrical self-stimulation of the brain in man. *Am. J. Psychiat.*, 1963, **120**, 571–577.

Heath, R. G. Pleasure response of human subjects to direct stimulation of the brain: Physiologic and psychodynamic consideration. In R. G. Heath (Ed.), *The Role of Pleasure in Behavior.* New York: Hoeber Medical Div., Harper & Row, 1964, pp. 219–243.

Heath, R. G. (Ed.), *The Role of Pleasure in Behavior.* New York: Hoeber Medical Div., Harper & Row, 1964.

Heath, R. G. Perspectives for biological psychiatry. *Biol. Psychiat.*, 1970, **2**, 81–88.

Heath, R. G. Depth recording and stimulation studies in patients. In A. Winter (Ed.), *The Surgical Control of Behavior.* Springfield, Ill.: Charles C Thomas, 1971, pp. 21–37.

Heath, R. G. Marihuana. Effects on deep and surface electroencephalograms of man. *Arch. Gen. Psychiat.*, 1972, **26**, 577–584.

Heath, R. G. Pleasure and brain activity in man. *J. Nerv. Ment. Dis.*, 1972, **154**, 3–18.

Heath, R. G., John, S. B., & Fontana, C. J. The pleasure response: Studies by stereotaxic technics in patients. In N. Kline & E. Laska (Eds.), *Computers and Electronic Devices in Psychiatry*, New York: Grune & Stratton, 1968, pp. 178–189.

Heath, R. G., & Mickle, W. A. Evaluation of seven years' experience with depth electrode studies in human patients. In E. R. Ramey & D. S. O'Doherty (Eds.), *Electrical Studies on the Unanesthetized Brain.* New York: Paul B. Hoeber, 1960, pp. 214–248.

Heath, R. G., Monroe, R. R., & Mickle, W. A. Stimulation of the amygdaloid nucleus in a schizophrenic patient. *Am. J. Psychiat.*, 1955, **111**, 862–863.

Hebb, D. O. Man's frontal lobes: A critical review. *Arch. Neurol. Psychiat.*, 1945, **54**, 10–24.

Hebb, D. O., & Penfield, W. Human behavior after extensive bilateral removal from the frontal lobes. *Arch. Neurol. Psychiat.,* 1940, **44**, 421–438.

Heimburger, R. F., Whitlock, C. C., & Kalsbeck, J. E. Stereotaxic amygdalectomy for epilepsy with aggressive behavior. *J. Am. Med. Assoc.*, 1966, **198**, 741–745.

Herberg, L. J. & Blundell, J. E. Lateral hypothalamus: Hoarding behavior elicited by electrical stimulation. *Science*, 1967, **155**, 349–350.

Herrick, C. J. The functions of the olfactory parts of the cerebral cortex. *Proc. Nat. Acad. Sci. (U.S.A.)*, 1933, **18**, 7–14.

Herrick, C. J. *The Brain of the Tiger Salamander.* Chicago: University of Chicago Press, 1948.

Herrick, C. J. Analytic and integrative nervous functions. *Dialectica,* 1957, **11,** 179–186.

Hess, W. R. *Diencephalon: Autonomic and extrapyramidal functions.* New York: Grune & Stratton, 1954. (Original publication in German: *Die funktionelle Organisation des vegetativen Nervensystems.* Basel: Benno Schwabe, 1948.)

Hess, W. R. *Das Zwishchenhirn: Syndrome, Lokalisationen, Funktionen,* 2nd ed. Basel: Schwabe, 1954.

Hess, W. R. *The Functional Organization of the Diencephalon.* New York: Grune & Stratton, 1957.

Hess, W. R. The Central Control of the Activity of Internal Organs. Nobel Lecture, December 12, 1949. In *Nobel Lectures, Physiology or Medicine* 1942–1962. New York: Elsevier, 1964.

Hetherington, A. W., & Ransom, S. W. Hypothalamic lesions and adiposity in the rat. *Anat. Rec.,* 1940, **78,** 149–172.

Higgins, J. W., Mahl, G. F., Delgado, J. M. R., & Hamlin, H. Behavioral changes during intracerebral electrical stimulation. *Arch. Neurol. Psychiat.,* 1956, **76,** 399–419.

Hirose, S. Orbito-ventromedial undercutting 1957–1963: Follow-up study of 77 cases. *Am. J. Psychiat.,* 1965, **121,** 1194–1202.

Hirose, S. Present trends in psychosurgery. Excerpts Med. Int. Cong. Series No. 150. Proc. of the IV World Congress of Psychiatry, Madrid, Sept. 5–11, 1966, pp. 1156–1165.

Hirose, S. The case selection of mental disorder for orbitoventral undercutting. In E. Hitchcock, L. Laitinen, & K. Vaernet (Eds.), *Psychosurgery.* Springfield, Ill.: Charles C Thomas, 1972, pp. 291–203.

Hitchcock, E., Laitinen, L., & Vaernet, K. (Eds.), *Psychosurgery.* (Proceedings of the Second International Conference of Psychosurgery, Copenhagen, Denmark.) Springfield, Ill: Charles C Thomas, 1972.

Hitzig, E. Physiologisches und therapeutisches über einige elektrische Reizmethoden. *Berlin klin. Swchr.,* 1870, **7,** 137–138.

Hitzig, E., & Fritsch, G. T. Über die elektrische Erregbarkeit des Grosshirns. *Arch. Anat. Physiol.,* **1870,** 300–332. (English translation in G. von Bonin, *Some Papers on the Cerebral Cortex.* Springfield, Ill.: Charles C Thomas, 1960, pp. 73–96.)

Hoch, P. H. Clinical and biological interrelations between schizophrenia and epilepsy. *Am. J. Psychiat.,* 1943, **99,** 507–512.

Hoch, P. H. Introduction: The achievements of biological psychiatry. In J. Wortis (Ed.), *Recent Advances in Biological Psychiatry*, Vol. III. New York: Grune & Stratton, 1961, pp. 1–10.

Hodos. W. Evolutionary interpretation of neural and behavioral studies of living vertebrates. In F. O. Schmitt (Ed.), *The Neurosciences. Second Study Program*. New York: Rockefeller University Press, 1970, pp. 26–39.

Hodos, W., & Campbell, C. B. G. *Scala natural:* Why there is no theory in comparative psychology. *Psychol. Rev.*, 1969, **76,** 337–350.

Hoebel, B. G., & Teitelbaum, P. Hypothalamic control of feeding and self-stimulation. *Science*, 1962, **135,** 375– 377.

Hofstatter, L., & Girgis, M. Depth electrode investigations of the limbic system of the brain by radiostimulation, electrolytic lesion and histochemical studies. Presented at the Third International Congress of Psychosurgery, Cambridge, England (August 15–18, 1972).

Holden, J. M. C., & Hofstatter, L. Prefrontal lobotomy: Stepping-stone or pitfall? *Am. J. Psychiat.*, 1970, **127,** 51–58.

Holst, E. von, & Saint Paul, U. Electrically controlled behavior. *Sci. Amer.*, 1962, **206,** 50–59.

Holst, E. von, & St. Paul, U. Von wirkungsgefuge der Triebe. *Naturwissenschaften*, 1960, **18,** 409–422. (Translated in *Anim. Behav.*, 1963, **11,** 1–20.)

Horel, J. A., & Keating, E. G. Recovery from a partial Klüver-Bucy syndrome in the monkey produced by disconnection. *J. comp. physiol. Psychol.*, 1972, **79,** 105–114.

Horsley, V., & Clarke, R. H. The structure and functions of the cerebellum examined by a new method. *Brain*, 1908, **31,** 45–124.

Hosobuchi, Y., Adams, J. E., & Weinstein, P. R. Preliminary percutaneous dorsal column stimulation prior to permanent implantation. Technical note. *J. Neurosurg.,* 1972, **37,** 242–245.

Hutchinson, R. R., & Renfrew, J. W. Stalking attack and eating behaviors elicited from the same sites in the hypothalamus. *J. comp. physiol. Psychol.*, 1966, **61,** 360-367.

Ito, M. Hippocampal electrical correlates of self-stimulation in the rat. *Electroenceph. clin. Neurophysiol.*, 1966, **21,** 261–268.

Jacobsen, C. F. Functions of frontal association areas in primates. *Arch. Neurol. Psychiat. (Chicago)*, 1935, **33,** 558–569.

Jacobsen, C. F. Studies of cerebral function in primates. *Compar. Psychol. Monogr.*, 1936, **13,** 1–60.

Jacobsen, C. F., Wolfe, J. B., & Jackson, T. A. An experimental analysis of the functions of the frontal association areas in primates. *J. Nerv. Ment. Dis.*, 1935, **82,** 1–14.

Jasper, H. H., & Rasmussen, T. Studies of clinical and electrical responses to deep temporal stimulation in man with some considerations of functional anatomy. In H. C. Solomon, S. Cobb, & W. Penfield (Eds.), *The Brain and Human Behavior*, Res. Publ. Assoc. Res. Nerv. Ment. Dis., Vol. 36, Baltimore: Williams & Wilkins, 1958, pp. 316–334.

Jessner, L., & Ryan, G. V. *Shock Treatment in Psychiatry: A Manual.* New York: Grune & Stratton, 1941.

John, E. R. *Mechanisms of Memory.* New York: Academic Press, 1967.

Jurgens, U., Maurus, M., Ploog, D., & Winter, P. Vocalization in the squirrel monkey *(Saimiri sciureus)* elicited by brain stimulation. *Exp. Brain Res.*, 1967, **4,** 114–117.

Kaada, B. R. Brain mechanisms related to aggressive behavior. In C. D. Clemente & D. B. Lindsley (Eds.), *Aggression and Defense, Neural Mechanisms and Social Patterns.* Los Angeles: University of California Press, 1967, pp. 95–116.

Kagan, J., & Moss, H. A. *Birth to Maturity: A Study in Psychological Development.* New York: John Wiley & Sons, 1962.

Kalinowski, L. B., & Hippius, H. *Pharmacological, Convulsive and Other Somatic Treatments in Psychiatry.* New York: Grune & Stratton, 1969.

Karplus, J. P., & Kreidl, A. Gehirn und Sympathicus. VIII. *Mitt. Arch. ges Physiol.*, 1928, **219,** 613–618.

Katzenelbogen, S. (Ed. & Trans.). The Treatment of Schizophrenia, Insulin Shock, Cardiazol, Sleep Treatment. Proc. 89th Meeting of the Swiss Psychiatric Assoc., Munsingen, Berne, May 29–31, 1937. *Am. J. Psychiat.*, 1938, **94** (suppl.), 1–354.

Kaufman, H. *Aggression and Altruism.* New York: Holt, Rinehart and Winston, 1970.

Kellaway, P. The part played by electric fish in the early history of bioelectricity and electrotherapy. The William Osler Medical Essay. *Bull. Hist. Med.*, 1946, **20,** 112–137.

Kesey, K. *One Flew Over the Cockoo's Nest.* New York: Viking Press, 1962.

Kety, S. S. The biogenic amines in the central nervous system: Their possible roles in arousal, emotion, and learning. In F. O. Schmitt (Ed.), *The Neurosciences, Second Study Program.* New York: Rockefeller University Press, 1970, pp. 324–336.

Kim, Y. K. Effects of basolateral amygdalectomy. In W. Umbach (Ed.), *Special Topics in Stereotaxis.* Stuttgart: Hippokrates-Verlag, 1971, pp. 69–81.

Kim, Y. K., & Umbach, W. Combined stereotaxic lesions for treatment of behavior disorders and severe pain. Paper presented at the Third World Congress of Psychosurgery, Cambridge, England (August 14–18, 1972).

King, H. E. Psychological effects of excitation in the limbic system. In D. E. Sheer (Ed.), *Electrical Stimulation of the Brain.* Austin: University of Texas Press, 1961, pp. 477–486.

Kittrie, N. N. *The Right to be Different. Defiance and Enforced Therapy.* Baltimore: Johns Hopkins Press. 1971.

Kline, N. S., & Laska, E. (Eds.), *Computers and Electronic Devices in Psychiatry.* New York: Grune & Stratton, 1968.

Kling, A. Effects of amygdalectomy on social-affective behavior in nonhuman primates. In B. E. Eleftheriou (Ed.), *The Neurobiology of the Amygdala.* New York: Plenum Press, 1972, pp. 511–536.

Kling, A., Lancaster, J., & Benitone, J. Amygdalectomy in the free-ranging vervet (Cercopithecus althiops). *J. Psychiat. Res.,* 1970, **7,** 191–199.

Kling, J. W., & Matsumiya, Y. Relative reinforcing values of food and intracranial stimulation. *Science,* 1962, **135,** 668–670.

Klüver, H., & Bucy, P. C. "Psychic blindness" and other symptoms following bilateral temporal lobectomy in rhesus monkeys. *Am. J. Physiol.,* 1937, **119,** 352–353.

Klüver, H., & Bucy, P. C. An analysis of certain effects of bilateral temporal lobectomy in the rhesus monkey with special reference to "psychic blindness." *J. Psychol.,* 1938, **5,** 33–54.

Klüver, H., & Bucy, P. C. Preliminary analysis of functions of the temporal lobe in monkeys. *Arch. Neurol. Psychiat. Chicago,* 1939, **42,** 979–1000.

Knight, G. G. Bi-frontal stereotactic tractotomy: An atraumatic operation of value in the treatment of intractable psychoneurosis. *Br. J. Psychiat.,* 1969, **115,** 257–266.

Knight, G. G. Bifrontal stereotaxic tractotomy in the substantia inominata. An experience of 450 cases. In E. Hitchcok, L. Laitinen, & K. Vaernet (Eds.), *Psychosurgery.* Springifeld, Ill., Charles C Thomas, 1972, pp. 267–277.

Kopa, J., Szabo, I., & Grastyan, E. A dual behavioral effect from stimulating the same thalamic point with identical stimulus parameters in different conditional reflex situations. *Acta Physiol. Acad. Sci. Hung.,* 1962, **21,** 207–214.

Koikegami, H., Fuse, S., Yokoyama, T., Watanabe, T., & Watanabe, H. Contributions to the comparative anatomy of the amygdaloid nuclei of mammals with some experiments of their destruction or stimulation. *Folia Psychiat. Neurol. Jap.*, 1955, **8**, 336–370.

Kornblith, C., & Olds, J. T-maze learning with one trial per day using brain stimulation reinforcement. *J. comp. physiol. Psychol.*, 1968, **66**, 488–491.

Krynauw, R. A. Infantile hemiplegia treated by removing one cerebral hemisphere. *J. Neurol. Neurosurg. Psychiat.*, 1950, **13**, 243–267.

Kubie, L. S. Some implications for psychoanalysis of modern concepts of the organization of the brain. *Psychoanalyt. Q.*, 1953, **22**, 21–52.

Landis, C., Zubin, J., & Mettler, F. The functions of the human frontal lobe. *J. Psychol.*, 1950, **30**, 123–138.

Larsson, K. Non-specific stimulation and sexual behavior in the male rat. *Behaviour*, 1963, **20**, 110–114.

Larsson, S. Hyperphagia from stimulation of the hypothalamus and medulla in sheep and goats. *Acta Physiol. Scand.*, 1954, **32**, Suppl. 115, 8–40.

LeBeau, J. The cingular and precingular areas in psychosurgery (agitated behavior, obsessive compulsive states, epilepsy). *Acta Psychiat. Neurol. Scand.*, 1952, **27**, 305–316.

Leksell, L. A stereotaxic apparatus for intracerebral surgery. *Acta Chir. Scand.*, 1949, **99**, 229–233.

Leksell, L. *Stereotaxis and Radiosurgery: An Operative System.* Springfield, Ill.: Charles C Thomas, 1971.

Leopold, N. *Life Plus 99 Years.* Garden City, N. Y.: Doubleday, 1958.

Levison, P. K., & Flynn, J. P. The objects attacked by cats during stimulation of the hypothalamus. *Animal Behav.*, 1965, **13**, 217–220.

Liberson, W. T., Holmquest, H. J., Scott, D., & Dow, M. Functional electrotherapy: Stimulation of the peroneal nerve synchronized with the swing phase of the gait of hemiplegic patients. *Arch. Phys. Med.*, 1961, **42**, 101–105.

Lilly, J. C., & Miller, A. M. Operant conditioning of the bottlenose dolphin with electrical stimulation of the brain. *J. comp. physiol. Psychol.*, 1962, **55**, 73–79.

Lindstrom, P. A. Prefrontal sonic treatment—Sixteen year's experience. In E. Hitchcock, L. Laitenen, & K. Vaernet (Eds.), *Psychosurgery*, Springfield, Ill.: Charles C Thomas, 1972, pp. 357–376.

Lion, J. R. Bach y Rita, G., & Ervin, F. R. The self-referred violent patient. In J. Fawcett (Ed.), *Dynamics of Violence*. Chicago: American Medical Association, 1971, pp. 79–83.

Lippold, O. C. J., & Redfearn, J. W. T. Mental changes resulting from the passage of small direct currents through the human brain. *Br. J. Psychiat.*, 1964, **110**, 768–772.

Livingston, K. E. Angulate cortex isolation for the treatment of psychoses and psychoneuroses. *Assoc. Res. Nerv. Ment. Dis.*, 1953, **31**, 374–378.

Livingston, K. E. The frontal lobes revisited. The case for a second look. *Arch. Neurol.*, 1969, **20**, 90–95.

Livingston, K. E., & Escobar, A. Anatomical bias of the limbic system concept. A proposed reorientation. *Arch. Neurol.*, 1971, **24**, 17–21.

Lloyd, C. W., & Weisz, J. Hormones and aggression. In W. S. Fields & W. H. Sweet (Eds.), *Neural Bases of Violence and Aggression*. St. Louis: Warren H. Green, In press.

London, P. *Behavior Control*. New York: Harper & Row, 1969.

Lorenz, K. *On Aggression*. New York: Harcourt, Brace, and World, 1966.

Luria, A. R. *Restoration of Function after Brain Injury*. New York: Macmillan, 1963.

Lyerly, J. G. Transection of the deep association fibers of the prefrontal lobes in certain mental disorders. *South. Surgeon*, 1939, **8**, 426–434.

MacDonnell, M. F., & Flynn, J. P. Control of sensory fields by stimulation of hypothalamus. *Science*, 1966, **152**, 1406–1408.

MacLean, P. D. Psychosomatic disease and the "visceral brain." Recent developments bearing on the Papez theory of emotion. *Psychosom. Med.*, 1949, **11**, 338–353.

MacLean, P. D. Chemical and electrical stimulation of hippocampus in unrestrained animals. II. Behavioral findings. *A.M.A. Arch. Neurol. Psychiat.*, 1957, **78**, 128–142.

MacLean, P. D., & Delgado, J. M. R. Electrical and chemical stimulation of frontotemporal portion of limbic system in the waking animal. *Electroenceph. clin. Neurophysiol.*, 1953, **5**, 91–100.

MacLean, P. P., & Ploog, D. W. Cerebral representation of penile erection. *J. Neurophysiol.*, 1962, **25**, 29–55.

McCleary, R. A. Response-modulating functions of the limbic system: Initiation and suppression. In E. Stellar & J. M. Sprague (Eds.),

Progress in Physiological Psychology, Vol. I. New York: Academic Press, 1966, pp. 209-272.

MacLeish, K. The Tasadays, stone age cavemen of Mindanao. *National Geographic,* 1972, **142**(2), 219-249.

Mahl, G. F., Rothenberg, A., Delgado, J. M. R., & Hamlin, H. Psychological responses in the human to intracerebral electric stimulation. *Psychosom.Med.,* 1964, **26**, 337-368.

Maire, F. W. Eating and drinking responses elicited by diencephalic stimulation in unanesthetized rats. *Fed. Proc.,* 1956, **15**, 124.

Malmo, R. B. Interference factors in delayed response in monkeys after removal of the frontal lobes. *J. Neurophysiol.,* 1942, **5**, 295-308.

Manen, J. van *Stereotactic Methods and Their Applications in Disorders of the Motor System.* Essen: Van Gorcum & Company N. V., 1967.

Mark V. H., & Ervin, F. R. Is there a need to evaluate the individuals producing human violence? *Psychiat. Opinion,* 1968, **5**, 32-34.

Mark, V. H., & Ervin, E. P. *Violence and the Brain.* New York: Harper & Row, 1970.

Mark, V. H., Sweet, W. H., & Ervin, F. R. Role of brain disease in riots and urban violence (letter to the journal). *Am. Med. Assoc.,* 1967, **201**, 895.

Mark, V. H., Sweet, W. H., & Ervin, F. R. The effect of amygdalectomy on violent behavior in patients with temporal lobe epilepsy. In E. Hitchcock, L. Laitinen, & K. Vaernet (Eds.), *Psychosurgery*, Springfield, Ill.: Charles C Thomas, 1972, pp. 139-155.

Marti-Ibañez, F., Sackler, A. M., Sackler, M. D., & Sackler, R. R. (Eds.), *The Great Physiodynamic Therapies in Psychiatry. An Historical Reappraisal.* New York: Hoeber-Harper, 1956.

Masserman, J. H. Is the hypothalamus a center of emotion? *Psychosom. Med.,* 1941, **3**, 1-25.

Masterton, B., & Skeen, L. C. Origins of anthropoid intelligence: Prefrontal system and delayed alternation in hedgehog, tree shrew, and bush baby. *J. Comp. Physiol. Psychol.,* 1972, **81**, 423-433.

Matteucci, C. *Essai sur les phénomènes électrique des animaux. Carillian.* Paris: Goeury & Dalmont, 1840.

Matteucci, C. *Traité des phénomènes électro-physiologiques des animaux.* Paris: Fortin, Masson, 1844.

Matteucci, C. *Lectures on the physical phenomena of living beings.* Translated by J. Pereira.) London: Longman, Brown, Green & Longman, 1847.

Mayer, D. J., Wolfle, T. L., Akil, H., Carder, B., & Liebeskind, J. C. Analgesia from electrical stimulation in the brainstem of the rat. *Science*, 1971, **174**, 1351–1354.

Meduna, L. von. General discussion of the cardiazol therapy. *Am. J. Psychiat.* (Suppl.), 1938, **94**, 40–50.

Melzak, R., & Wall, P. D. Pain mechanisms: A new theory. *Science*, 1965, **150**, 971–979.

Menninger, W. C. *Bull. Menninger Clinic*, 1948 (Jan.), **12**, 1–25.

Merton, P. A. How we control the contraction of our muscles. *Scientific American*, 1972, **226**, 30–37.

Mettler, F. A. (Ed.) *Selective Partial Ablation of the Frontal Cortex. A Correlative Study of its Effects on Human Psychotic Subjects.* New York: Paul Hoeber, 1949.

Mettler, F. A. (Ed.) *Psychosurgical Problems* (The Columbia Greystone Associates, Second Group). New York: Blakiston, 1952.

Meyers, R. Surgical experiments in therapy of certain "extrapyramidal" diseases: Current evaluation. *Acta Psychiat. Neurol. Suppl.*, 1951, **67**, 1–42.

Miller, N. E. Experiments on motivation. *Science*, 1957, **126**, 1271–1278.

Miller, N. E. Central stimation and other new approaches to motivation and reward. *Am. Psychol.*, 1958, **13**, 100–108.

Miller, N. E. Motivational effects of brain stimulation and drugs. *Fed. Proc.*, 1960, **19**, 846–854.

Miller, N. E. Some motivational effects of electrical and chemical stimulation of the brain. *Electroenceph. Clin. Neurophysiol. Supp.*, 1963, **24**, 247–259.

Miller, N. E. Chemical coding of behavior in the brain. *Science*, 1965, **148**, 328–338.

Miller, N. E. Learning of visceral and glandular responses. *Science*, 1969, **163**, 434–445.

Milner, B. Psychological defects produced by temporal lobe excision. *Res. Publ. Assoc. Res. Nerv. Ment. Dis.*, 1958, **36**, 224–257.

Mirsky, A. F. Studies of the effects of brain lesions on social behavior of Macaca Mulatta: Methodological and theoretical considerations. *Ann. N. Y. Acad. Sci.*, 1960, **85**, 785–794.

Mishkin, M. Cortical visual areas and their interactions. In A. G. Karczmar & J. C. Eccles (Eds.), *Brain and Human Behavior.* New York: Springer Verlag, 1972, pp. 187–208.

Moan, C. E., & Heath, R. G. Septal stimulation and the initiation of heterosexual behavior in a homosexual male. *Behav. Ther. Exp. Psychiat.*, in press.

Mogenson, G. L., & Morgane, C. W. Effects of induced drinking on self-stimulation of the lateral hypothalamus. *Exp. Brain Res.*, 1967, **3**, 111-116.

Mogenson, G. J., & Stevenson, J. A. F. Drinking and self-stimulation with electrical stimulation of the lateral hypothalamus. *Physiol. Behav.*, 1966, **1**, 251-254.

Mogenson, G. J., & Stevenson, J. A. F. Drinking induced by electrical stimulation of the lateral hypothalamus. *Exp. Neurol.*, 1967, **17**, 119-127.

Moniz, E. *Tentatives Opératories dans le Traitement de Certaines Psychoses.* Paris: Masson, 1936.

Moniz, E. Mein Weg zur Leukotomie. *Dtsch. Med. Wochensch.*, 1948, **73**, 581-583.

Moniz, E. How I succeeded in performing the prefontal leukotomy. In A. Sackler, M. Sackler, R. Sackler, & F. Marti-Ibanez (Eds.), *The Great Psychodynamic Therapies in Psychiatry.* New York: Paul Hoeber Med. Div., Harper & Row, 1956, pp. 131-137.

Monroe, R., & Heath, R. G. Psychiatric observations. In R. G. Heath (Ed.), *Studies in Schizophrenia.* Cambridge: Harvard University Press, 1954, pp. 345-386.

Montagu, M. F. A. (Ed.), *Man and Aggression.* London: Oxford University Press, 1968.

Moore, D., & Smithers, B. C. Prefontal leukotomy. *Can. Med. Assoc. J.*, 1970, **102**, 876.

Munk, H. Ueber den Hund ohne Grosshirn. *Arch. Anat. Physiol. Physiol. Abt.*, **1894**, 355-369.

Nakao, H. Emotional behavior produced by hypothalamic stimulation. *Am. J. Physiol.*, 1958, **194**, 411-418.

Narabayashi, H. Stereotaxic amygdalectomy. In B. E. Eleftheriou (Ed.), *The Neurobiology of the Amygdala.* New York: Plenum Press, 1972, pp. 459-483.

Narabayashi, H., & Mizutani, T. Epileptic seizures and the stereotaxic amygdalotomy. *Confin. Neurol.*, 1970, **32**, 289-297.

Narabayashi, H., Nagao, T., Saito, Y., Yoshida, M., & Nagahata, M. Stereotaxic amygdalotomy for behavior disorders. *Arch. Neurol.*, 1963, **9**, 1-16.

Narabayashi, N., & Uno, M. Long range results of stereotaxic amygdalectomy for behavior disorders. *Confin. Neurol.*, 1966, **27**, 168-171.

Nashold, B. S., & Friedman, H. Dorsal column stimulation for control of pain. Preliminary report on 30 patients. *J. Neurosurg.*, 1972, **36**, 590-597.

Nashold, B. S., Friedman, H., Glenn, J. F., Grimes, J. H., Barry, W. F., & Avery, R. Electromicturition in paraplegia. Implantation of a spinal neuroprosthesis. *Arch. Surg.*, 1972, **104**, 195-202.

Nashold, B. S., & Gills, J. P. Chemical stimulation of telencephalon, diencephalon and mesencephalon in unrestrained animals. *J. Neurophathol. exp. Neurol.*, 1960, **19**, 580-590.

Nashold, B. S., & Huber, W. V. (Eds.). The second symposium on Parkinson's disease. *J. Neurosurg.*, 1966, **24**, 118-481. (Supplement)

Nauta, W. J. H. The problem of the frontal lobe: A reinterpretation. *J. Psychiat. Res.*, 1971, **8**, 167-187.

Nielson, H. C., Doty, R. W., & Rutledge, L. T. Motivational and perceptual aspects of subcortical stimulation in cats. *Am. J. Physiol.*, 1958, **194**, 427-432.

Nieto, D., & Escobar, A. Major psychosis. In J. Minckler (Ed.), *Pathology of the Nervous System*, Vol. III. New York: McGraw-Hill, 1972, pp. 2654-2665.

Nivens, L. Death by Ecstasy, in D. A. Wollheim and T. Carr, Eds., *World's Best Science Fiction*, New York: Ace, 1970.

Ojemann, G. A., & Fedio, P. Effect of stimulation of the human thalamus and parietal and temporal white matter on short-term memory. *J. Neurosurg.*, 1968, **29**, 51-59.

Ojemann, G. A., Fedio, P., & van Buren, J. M. Anomia from pulvinar and subcortical parietal stimulation. *Brain*, 1968, **91**, 99-116.

Olds, J. Physiological mechanisms of reward. In M. R. Jones (Ed.), *Nebraska Symposium on Motivation*. Lincoln: University of Nebraska Press, 1955, pp. 73-138.

Olds, J. A physiological study of reward. In D. McClelland (Ed.), *Studies of Motivation*. New York: Appleton, 1955, pp. 134-143.

Olds, J. Runway and maze behavior controlled by basomedial forebrain stimulation in the rat. *J. comp. physiol. Psychol.*, 1956, **49**, 507-512.

Olds, J. Satiation effects in self-stimulation of the brain. *J. comp. physiol. Psychol.*, 1958, **51**, 675-678.

Olds, J. Self-stimulation of the brain. *Science*, 1958, **127**, 315-324.

Olds, J. Approach-avoidance dissociations in rat brain. *Am. J. Physiol.*, 1960, **199**, 965-968.

Olds, J. Hypothalamic substrates of reward. *Physiol. Rev.*, 1962, **42**, 554-604.

Olds, J. Pleasure centers in the brain. *Scientific American*, 1965, **195**, 105-116.

Olds, J. The central nervous system and the reinforcement of behavior. *Am. Psychol.*, 1969, **24**, 114–132.

Olds, J., & Milner, P. Positive reinforcement produced by electrical stimulation of septal area and other regions of rat brain. *J. comp. physiol. Psychol.*, 1954, **47**, 419–427.

Olds, J., & Olds, M. E. the mechanisms of voluntary behavior. In R. G. Heath (Ed.), *The Role of Pleasure in Behavior*. New York: Hoeber Med. Div., Harper & Row, 1964, pp. 23–53.

Olds, M. E., & Olds, J. Approach-escape interactions in rat brain. *Am. J. Physiol.*, 1962, **203**, 803–810.

Oliver, L. *Parkinson's Disease*. Springfield, Ill.: Charles C. Thomas, 1967.

Oliver, W. Account of the effects of camphor in a case of insanity. *London Med. J.*, 1785, **6**, 120–130.

Oliver, W. G. *Electrical Anaesthesia*. Comprising brief history of its discovery, a synopsis of experiments. Also, full directions for its application in surgical and dental operations. Buffalo, N.Y.: Murray, Rockwell & Co., 1858.

Panksepp, J. Aggression elicited by electrical stimulation of the hypothalamus in albino rats. *Physiol Behav.*, 1971, **6**, 321–329.

Papez, J. W. A proposed mechanism of emotion. *Arch. Neurol. Psychiat.*, 1937, **38**, 725–743.

Parkinson's Disease: Present Status and Research Trends. U. S. Public Health Service Publication No. 1491 (Revised 1968). Superintendent of Documents U. S. Government Printing Office, Washington, D. C.

Penfield, W. Functional localization in temporal and deep Sylvian areas. *Res. Publ. Assoc. Res. Nerv. Ment. Dis.*, 1958, **36**, 210–226.

Penfield, W., & Baldwin, M. Temporal lobe seizures and the technic of subtotal temporal lobectomy. *Ann. Surg.*, 1952, **136**, 625–634.

Penfield, W., & Perot, P. The brain's record of auditory and visual experience—A final summary and discussion. *Brain*, 1963, **86**, 595–696.

Persson, N. Self-stimulation in the goat. *Acta Physiol. Scand.*, 1962, **55**, 276–285.

Peterson, M. C., Dodge, H. W., Sem-Jacobsen, C. W., Lazarte, J. A., & Holman, C. B. Clinical results of selective leukotomy based on intracerebral electrography. *J. Am. Med. Assoc.*, 1955, **159**, 774–775.

378 Bibliography

Phillips, A. G., Cox, V. C., Kakolewski, J. W., & Valenstein, E. S. Object-carrying by rats: An approach to the behavior produced by brain stimulation. *Science*, 1969, **166**, 903–905.

Phillips, R. E. "Wildness" in the Mallard duck: Effects of brain lesions and stimulation on "escape behavior" and reproduction. *J. Comp. Neurol.*, 1964, **122**, 139–155.

Pinneo, L. R., Erickson, E. E., & Kinney, R. A. Selective deep brain stimulation with external electrodes. In D. U. Reynolds & A. E. Sjoberg (Eds.), *Neuroelectric Research*. Springfield, Ill.: Charles C Thomas, 1971, pp. 405–425.

Pinneo, L. R., Kaplan, J. N., Elpel, E. A., Reynolds, P. C., & Glick, J. H. Experimental brain prosthesis for stroke. *Stroke*, 1972, **3**, 16–26.

Ploog, D. Social communication among animals. In F. O. Schmitt (Ed.), *The Neurosciences: Second Study Program*. New York: Rockefeller University Press, 1970, pp. 349–360.

Plum, F. Neuropathological findings. In S. S. Kety & S. Matthysse (Eds.), *Prospects for Research on Schizophrenia. Neuroscience Research Program Bull.*, 1972, **10**, 384–388.

Pool, J. L. Topectomy. *Proc. Roy. Soc. Med.*, 1949, **42**, Suppl. 1–3.

Poppen, J. L. Technic of prefrontal lobotomy. *J. Neurosurg.*, 1948, **5**, 514–520.

Poschel, B. P. H. Do biological reinforcers act via the self-stimulation areas of the brain? *Physiol. Behav.*, 1968, **3**, 53–60.

Poschel, B. P. H. Mapping of rat brain for self-stimulation under monoamine oxidase blockade. *Physiol. Behav.*, 1969, **4**, 325–331.

Poschel, B. P. H., & Ninteman, F. W. Norepinephrine: A possible excitatory neuro-hormone of the reward system. *Life Sci.*, 1963, **10**, 782–788.

Poschel, B. P. H., & Ninteman, F. W. Hypothalamic self-stimulation: Its suppression by blockade of norepinephrine biosynthesis and reinstatement by methamphetamine. *Life Sci.*, 1966, **5**, 11–16.

Poschel, B. P. H., & Ninteman, F. W. Excitatory (antidepressant?) effects of monoamine oxidase inhibitors on the reward system of the brain. *Life Sci.*, 1964, **3**, 903–910.

Post, F., Rees, W. L., & Schurr, P. H. An evaluation of bimedial leucotomy. *Br. J. Psychiat.*, 1968, **114**, 1223–1246.

Pribram, K. H. Some physical and pharmacological factors affecting delayed response performance of baboons following frontal lobotomy. *J. Neurophysiol.*, 1950, **13**, 373–382.

Puusepp, L. Alcune considerazioni sugli interventi chirurgici nelle malattie mentali. *Gior. Accad. med. Torino*, 1937, **100**, 3–16.

Rado, S. Emergency behavior. In P. Hoch & J. P. Zubin (Eds.), *Anxiety.* New York: Grune & Stratton, 1950, pp. 150-176.

Ramamurthi, B., Balasurbramaniam, V., Kalyanaraman, S., Arjundas, G., & Jagannathan, K. Stereotaxic ablation of the irritable focus in temporal lobe epilepsy. *Confin. Neurol.*, 1970, **32,** 316-321.

Ramon y Cajal, S. *Studies on the Cerebral Cortex (Limbic Structures)* (L. M. Kraft, Trans.). London: Lloyd-Luke, 1955.

Ramsey, G. V. A short history of psychosurgery. *Am. J. Psychiat.*, 1952, **108,** 813-816.

Ramsey, P. *The Patient as Person, Exploration in Medical Ethics.* New Haven, Conn.: Yale University Press, 1970.

Ranson, S. W. Some functions of the hypothalamus. Harvey Lecture. *Bull. N. Y. Acad. Med.*, 1937, **13,** 241-271.

Ray, O. S. *Drugs, Society, and Human Behavior.* Saint Louis: C. V. Mosby, 1972.

Ray, O. S., Hine, B., & Bivens, L. W. Stability of self-stimulation responding during long test sessions. *Physiol. Behav.*, 1968, **3,** 161-164.

Redfearn, J. W. T., Lippold, O. C. J., & Costain, R. A preliminary account of the clinical effects of polarization of the brain in depressive illness. *Br. J. Psychiat.*, 1964, **110,** 773-785.

Reis, D. J. Central neurotransmitters in aggressive behavior. In W. S. Fields & W. H. Sweet (Eds.), *Neural Bases of Violence and Aggression.* St. Louis: Warren H. Green, In press.

Reynolds, D. V. Surgery in the rat during electrical analgesia induced by focal brain stimulation. *Science*, 1969, **164,** 444-445.

Roberts, W. W. Both rewarding and punishing effects from stimulation of posterior hypothalamus of cat with same electrode at same intensity. *J. comp. physiol. Psychol.*, 1958, **51,** 400-407.

Roberts, W. W. Fear-like behavior elicited from dorsomedial thalamus of cat. *J. comp. physiol. Psychol.*, 1962, **55,** 191-197.

Roberts, W. W., & Carey, R. J. Rewarding effect of performance of gnawing aroused by hypothalamic stimulation in the rat. *J. comp. physiol. Psychol.*, 1965, **59,** 317-324.

Roberts, W. W., & Kiess, H. O. Motivational properties of hypothalamic aggression in cats. *J. comp. physiol. Psychol.*, 1964, **58,** 187-193.

Roberts, W. W., Steinberg, M. L., & Means, L. W. Hypothalamic mechanisms for sexual, aggressive and other motivational behaviors in the opossum (Didelphis virginiana). *J. comp. physiol. Psychol.*, 1967, **64,** 1-15.

Robinson, B. W. Vocalization evoked from forebrain in Macaca mulatta. *Physiol. Behav.*, 1967, **2**, 345–354.

Robinson, B. W. Aggression: Summary and overview. In B. E. Eleftheriou & J. P. Scott (Eds.), *The Physiology of Aggression and Defeat.* New York: Plenum Press, 1971, pp. 291–302.

Robinson, B. W., Alexander, M., & Bowne, G. Dominance reversal resulting from aggressive responses evoked by brain telestimulation. *Physiol. Behav.*, 1969, **4**, 749–752.

Robinson, B. W., & Mishkin, M. Ejaculation evoked by stimulation of the preoptic area in monkey. *Physiol. Behav.*, 1966, **1**, 269–272.

Robinson, B. W., & Mishkin, M. Alimentary responses to forebrain stimulation in monkeys. *Exp. Brain Res.*, 1968, **4**, 330–366.

Roeder, F., & Müller, D. The stereotaxic treatment of paedophillic homosexuality. *German Medical Monthly* (G. R. Graham, editor of English language edition), Stuttgart: Georg Thieme Verlag, 1969, **14**, 265–271.

Roeder, F., Müller, D., & Orthner, H. Stereotaxic treatment of psychoses and neuroses. In W. Umbach (Ed.), *Special Topics in Stereotaxis.* Stuttgart: Hippokrates-Verlag, 1971, pp. 82–105.

Roeder, F., Orthner, H., & Müller, D. The stereotaxic treatment of pedophilic homosexuality and other sexual deviations. In E. Hitchcock, L. Laitinen, & K. Vaernet (Eds.), *Psychosurgery.* Springfield, Ill.: Charles C Thomas, 1972, pp. 87–111.

Romaniuk, A. The formation of defensive conditioned reflexes by direct stimulation of the hypothalamic "flight-points" in cats. *Acta. Biol. Exp. (Warsaw)*, 1964, **24**, 145–151.

Romaniuk, A. Representation of aggression and flight reactions in the hypothalamus of the cat. *Acta Biol. Exp. (Warsaw)*, 1965, **25**, 177–186.

Rorvik, D. Someone to watch over you (for less than 2¢ a day). *Esquire*, 1969, **72**, 164.

Rosenhan, D. L. On being sane. *Science*, 1973, **179**, 250–258.

Rosvold, H. E., Mirsky, A. F., & Pribram, K. H. Influence of amygdalectomy on social behavior in monkeys. *J. comp. physiol. Psychol.*, 1954, **47**, 173–178.

Routtenberg, A., & Lindy, J. Effects of the availability of rewarding septal and hypothalamic stimulation on bar-pressing for food under conditions of deprivation. *J. comp. physiol. Psychol.*, 1965, **60**, 158–161.

Rylander, G. Personality analysis before and after frontal lobotomy. *Assoc. Res. Nerv. Ment. Dis., The Frontal Lobes*, 1948, **27**, 691–705.

Sakel, M. The nature and origin of the hypoglycemic treatment of psychoses. *Am. J. Psychiat.* (Suppl.), 1938, **94**, 24–40.

Sakel, M. J. The classical Sakel shock treatment. In A. Sackler, M. Sackler, R. Sackler, & R. Marti-Ibañez (Eds.), *The Great Physiodynamic Therapies in Psychiatry.* New York: Paul Hoeber Med. Div., Harper & Row, 1956, pp. 13–75.

Sano, K. Sedative neurosurgery. *Neurologia*, 1962, **4**, 112–142.

Sano, K. Sedative stereoencephotomy: Fornicotomy, upper mesencephalic reticulotomy and postero-medial hypothalamotomy. In T. Tokizane & J. P. Schadé (Eds.), *Correlative Neurosciences*, Part B: *Clinical Studies.* New York: Elsevier, 1966, pp. 350–372.

Sano, K., Mayanagi, Y., Sekino, H., Ogashiwa, M., & Ishijima, B. Results of stimulation and destruction of the posterior hypothalamus in man. *J. Neurosurg.*, 1970, **33**, 689–707.

Sano, K., Yoshioka, M., Ogashiva, M., Ishijima, B., & Ohye, C. Posteromedial hypothalatomy in the treatment of aggressive behaviors. *Confin. Neurol.*, 1966, **27**, 164–167.

Sano, K., Yoshioka, M., Ogashiwa, M., Ishijima, B., Ohye, C., Sekino, H., & Mayanagi, Y. Autonomic, somatomotor and electroencephalographic responses upon stimulation of the hypothalamus and the rostral brain stem in man. *Confin. Neurol.*, 1967, **29**, 257–261.

Sawa, M., Yukiharu, U., Masaya, A., & Toshio, H. Preliminary report on the amygdalectomy on the psychotic patients, with interpretation of oral-emotional manifestations in schizophrenics. *Folia Psychiat. Neurol. Jap.*, 1954, **7**, 309–316.

Schaltenbrand, G. The effects of stereotaxic electrical stimulation in the depth of the brain. *Brain*, 1965, **88**, 835–840.

Schiff, M. Untersuchungen über die motorischen Functionen des Grosshirns. (Translated from the Italian by F. Borel.) *Archiv. exp. path. Pharmakol.*, 1875, **3**, 171–179.

Schreiner, L. H., & Kling, A. Behavioral changes following rhinencephalic injury in cat. *J. Neurophysiol.*, 1953, **16**, 643–659.

Schreiner, L. H., & Kling, A. Rhinencephalon and behavior. *Am. J. Physiol.*, 1956, **184**, 486–490.

Schvarcz, J. R., Driollet, R., Rios, E. & Betti, O. Stereotaxic hypothalamotomy for behavior disorders. *J. Neurol. Neurosurg. Psychiat.*, 1972, **35**, 356–359.

Schwartzbaum, J. Changes in reinforcing properties of stimuli following ablation of the amygdaloid complex in monkeys. *J. comp. physiol. Psychol.*, 1960, **53**, 388–395.

Scoville, W. B. Selective cortical undercutting. *Proc. Roy. Soc. Med.*, 1949, **42**, Suppl. 3–8.

Scoville, W. B. Selective cortical undercutting as a means of modifying and studying frontal lobe function in man. *J. Neurosurg.*, 1949, **6**, 65–73.

Scoville, W. B. Recent thoughts on psychosurgery. *Connecticut Medicine*, 1969, **33**, 453–456.

Scoville, W. B. The effect of surgical lesions of the brain on psyche and behavior in man. In A. Winter (Ed.), *The Surgical Control of Behavior. A Symposium.* Springfield, Ill.: Charles C Thomas, 1971, pp. 53–68.

Scoville, W. B. Psychosurgery and other lesions of the brain affecting human behavior. In E. Hitchcock, L. Laitinen, & K. Vaernet (Eds.), *Psychosurgery: Proceedings of the II International Conference on Psychosurgery*, Copenhagen, 1970. Springfield, Ill.: Charles C Thomas, 1973, pp. 5–21.

Scribonius, L. *De compositionibus medicamentorum.* Liber unus. (Joanne Ruellio, Ed.) Paris: Wechel, 1529. 8II., 31 fol. [see fol. 1b, third paragraph].

Sem-Jacobsen, C. W. *Depth-Electrographic Stimulation of the Human Brain and Behavior.* Springfield, Ill.: Charles C Thomas, 1968.

Sem-Jacobsen, C. W., & Torkildsen, A. Depth recording and electrical stimulation in the human brain. In E. R. Ramey & D. S. O'Doherty (Eds.), *Electrical Studies on the Unanesthetized Brain.* New York: Paul B. Hoeber, 1960, pp. 275–290.

Seward, J. P., Uyeda, A., & Olds, J. Resistance to extinction following cranial self-stimulation. *J. comp. physiol. Psychol.*, 1959, **52**, 294–299.

Shealy, C. N., Mortimer, J. T., & Hagfors, N. R. Dorsal column electroanalgesia. *J. Neurosurg.*, 1970, **32**, 560–564.

Shealy, C. N., Mortimer, J. T., & Reswick, J. B. Electrical inhibition of pain by stimulation of the dorsal columns: Preliminary clinical report. *Anesth. Anal.*, 1967, **46**, 489–491.

Sheldon, C. H., Pudenz, R. H., & Bullara, L. Development and clinical capabilities of a new implantable biostimulator. *Am. J. Surg.*, 1972, **124**, 212–216.

Sheldon, C. H., Pudenz, R. H., & Doyle, J. Electrical control of facial pain. *Am. J. Surg.*, 1967, **114**, 209–212.

Sherwood, S. L. Stereotaxic recordings from the frontal and temporal lobes of psychotics and epileptics. In E. R. Ramey & D. S. O'Doherty (Eds.), *Electrical Studies on the Unanesthetized Brain.* New York: Paul B. Hoeber, 1960, pp. 374–401.

Simmons, F. B., Epley, J. M., Lummis, R. C., Guttman, L. S., Frishkopf, L. S., Harmon, L. D., & Zwicker, E. Auditory nerve electrical stimulation in man. *Science*, 1965, **148**, 104–106.

Simonoff, L. N. Die Hemmungsmechanismen der Säugetiere experimentell bewiesen. *Arch. Anat. Physiol.*, Leipsig, 1866, **33**, 545–564.

Smith, A. & Kinder, E. Changes in psychological test performance of brain operated schizophrenics after 8 years. *Science*, 1959, **129**, 149–50.

Smith, W. K. The functional significance of the rostral cingular cortex as revealed by its response to electrical stimulation. *J. Neurophysiol.*, 1945, **8**, 241–255.

Spiegel, E. A. Indications for stereoencephalotomies. A critical assessment. *Confin. Neurol.*, 1969, **31**, 5–10.

Spiegel, E. A., & Wycis, H. T. *1st International Symposium on Stereoencephalotomy*. Basel: Karger, 1962.

Spiegel, E. A., Wycis, H. T., Baird, H. W., III & Szekely, E. G. Physiopathologic observations on the basal ganglia. In E. R. Ramey & D. S. O'Doherty (Eds.), *Electrical Studies on the Unanesthetized Brain*. New York: Paul B. Hoeber, 1960, pp. 192–213.

Spiegel, E. A., Wycis, H. T., & Freed, H. Thalatomy: Neuropsychiatric aspects. *N. Y. State J. Med.*, 1949, **49**, 2273–2274.

Spiegel, E. A., Wycis, H. T., Freed, H., & Orchinik, C. Thalamotomy and hyperthalamotomy for the treatment of psychoses. *Assoc. Res. Nerv. Ment. Dis.*, 1953, **31**, 379–391.

Spiegel, E. A., Wycis, H. T., Marks, M., & Lee, A. J. Stereotaxic apparatus for operations on the human brain. *Science*, 1947, **106**, 349–350.

Stark, P., & Boyd, E. S. Effects of cholinergic drugs on hypothalamic self-stimulation response rates of dogs. *Am. J. Physiol.*, 1963, **205**, 745–748.

Steck, H., & Bovet, H. The results obtained by insulin therapy in Cery from 1929 to 1937. *Am. J. Psychiat.* (Suppl.), 1938, **94**, 166–167.

Stein, L. Inhibitory effects of phenothiazine compounds on self-stimulation of the brain. *Dis. Nerv. Syst., Suppl.*, 1961, **22**, 1–5.

Stein, L. Effects and interactions of imipramine, chlorpromazine, reserpine, and amphetamine on self-stimulation: Possible neurophysiological basis of depression. *Recent Adv. biol. Psychiat.*, 1962, **4**, 288–308.

Stein, L. New methods of evaluating stimulants and antidepressants. In J. H. Nodine & J. H. Moyer (Eds.), *Psychosomatic Medicine,*

384 Bibliography

the First Hahnemann Symposium. Philadelphia: Lee & Febiger, 1962, pp. 297-311.

Stein, L. Self-stimulation of the brain and the central stimulant action of amphetamine. *Fed. Proc.,* 1962, **23,** 836-850.

Stein, L. Psychopharmacological substrates of mental depression. In S. Garattini & M. N. G. Dukes (Eds.), *Antidepressant Drugs.* Amsterdam: Excerpta Medica International Congress Series No. 122, 1966, pp. 130-140.

Stein, L. Chemistry of purposive behavior. In J. Tapp (Ed.), *Reinforcement and Behavior.* New York: Academic Press, 1969, pp. 328-355.

Stein, L. Neurochemistry of reward and punishment: Some implications for the etiology of schizophrenia. *J. Psychiat. Res.,* 1971, **8,** 345-361.

Stein, L., & Ray, O. S. Brain stimulation reward "thresholds" self-determined in rat. *Psychopharmacologia,* 1960, **1,** 251-256.

Stein, L., & Wise, C. C. Possible etiology of schizophrenia: Progressive damage of the noradrenergic reward mechanism by endogenous 6-hydroxydopamine. *Science,* 1971, **171,** 1032-1036.

Stephan, F. K., Valenstein, E. S., & Zucker, I. Copulation and eating during electrical stimulation of the rat hypothalamus. *Physiol. Behav.,* 1971, **7,** 587-593.

Stevens, J. R., Mark, ·V. H., Ervin, F., Pacheco, P., & Suematsu, K. Deep temporal stimulation in man. Long latency, long lasting psychological changes. *Arch. Neurol. (Chicago),* **1969,21,**157-169.

Sweet, W. H., Ervin, F., & Mark, V. H. The relationship of violent behavior to focal cerebral disease. In S. Garattini & E. Sigg (Eds.), *Aggressive Behavior.* New York: John Wiley & Sons, 1969, pp. 336-352.

Talbert, G. A. Ueber Rindenreizung am freilaufendeu Hunde nach. J. R. Ewald. *Arch. Anat. Physiol. (Physiol. Abt.),* 1900, **24,** 195-208.

Tan, E., Marks, I. M., & Marset, P. Bimedial leucotomy in obsessive-compulsive neurosis: A controlled serial enquiry. *Br. J. Psychiat.,* 1971, **118,** 155-164.

Terzian, H. Observations of the clinical symptomatology of bilateral partial or total removal of the temporal lobes in man. In M. Baldwin & P. Bailey (Eds.), *Temporal Lobe Epilepsy.* Springfield, Ill.: Charles C Thomas, 1958, pp. 510-529.

Terzian, H., & Dalle Ore, G. Syndrome of Klüver and Bucy reproduced in many by bilateral removal of the temporal lobes. *Neurology,* 1955, **5,** 373-380.

Teuber, H. L. Unity and diversity of frontal lobe functions. In J. Kornorski, H. L. Teuber, & B. Zernicki (Eds.), *The Frontal Granular Cortex and Behavior. International Symposium.* Acta Neurobiologiae Experimentalis Warsaw, 1972, **32,** 615–656.

Thomas, G. J., Hostetter, G., & Barker, D. J. Behavioral functions of the limbic system. In E. Stellar & J. M. Sprague (Eds.), *Progress in Physiological Psychology,* Vol. II. New York: Academic Press, 1968, pp. 229–311.

Turnbull, C. *The Forest People.* New York: Simon & Schuster, 1961.

Turnbull, F. Neurosurgery in the control of unmanageable affective reactions: A critical review. *Clin. Neurosurg.,* 1969, **16,** 218–233.

Turnbull, I. M. Bilateral cingulumotomy combined with thalotomy or mesencephalic tractotomy for pain. *Surg. Gyn. Obst.,* 1972, **134,** 958–962.

Uchimura, Y., & Narabayashi, H. Stereoencephalotom. *Psychiat. Neurol. Jap.,* 1951, **52,** 65 (Japanese edition).

Umemoto, M., & Kido, R. Feeding responses elicited by the electrical stimulation of lateral hypothalamus in the cat: The effect of methamphetamine. *Jap. Psychol. Res.,* 1967, **9,** 14–19.

Ursin, H. The temporal lobe substrate of fear and anger. *Acta Psychiat. Scand.,* 1960, **35,** 378–396.

Ursin, H. & Kaada, B. R. Functional localization within the amygdaloid complex in the cat. *Electroenceph. Clin. Neurophysiol.,* 1960, **12,** 1–20.

Vaernet, K., & Madsen, A. Stereotaxic amygdalotomy and basofrontal tractotomy in psychotics with aggressive behaviour. *J. neurol. neurosurg. Psychiat.,* 1970, **33,** 858–863.

Valenstein, E. S. Problems of measurement and interpretation with reinforcing brain stimulation. *Psychol. Rev.,* 1964, **71,** 415–437.

Valenstein, E. S. Independence of approach and escape reactions to electrical stimulation of the brain. *J. comp. physiol. Psychol.,* 1965, **60,** 20–31.

Valenstein, E. S. The anatomical locus of reinforcement. In E. Stellar & J. M. Sprague (Eds.), *Progress in Physiological Psychology,* Vol. 1. New York: Academic Press, 1966, pp. 149–190.

Valenstein, E. S. Behavior elicited by hypothalamic stimulation: A prepotency hypothesis. *Brain Behav. Evol.,* 1969, **2,** 296–316.

Valenstein, E. S. (Ed.). Motivation, Emotion and Behavior Elicited by Activation of Central Nervous System Sites. Symposium held at the Convention of the American Psychological Association in Washington, D. C., September 4, 1969. *Brain Behav. Evol.,* 1969, **2** (whole issue), 289–376.

Valenstein, E. S. Stability and plasticity of motivational systems. In F. O. Schmitt (Ed.), *The Neurosciences: Second Study Program.* New York: Rockefeller University Press, 1970, pp. 207–217.

Valenstein, E. S. Channeling of responses elicited by hypothalamic stimulation. *J. Psychiat. Res.*, 1971, **8**, 335–344.

Valenstein, E. S. *Brain Stimulation and Motivation.* Chicago: Scott-Foresman, 1973.

Valenstein, E. S., & Beer, B. Reinforcing brain stimulation in competition with water reward and shock avoidance. *Science*, 1962, **137**, 1052–1054.

Valenstein, E. S., & Beer, B. Continuous opportunity for reinforcing brain stimulation. *J. exp. anal. Behav.*, 1964, **7**, 183–184.

Valenstein, E. S., Cox, V. C., & Kakolewski, J. W. Modification of motivated behavior elicited by electrical stimulation of the hypothalamus. *Science*, 1968, **159**, 1119–1121.

Valenstein, E. S., Cox, V. C., & Kakolewski, J. W. The motivation underlying eating elicited by lateral hypothalamic stimulation. *Physiol. Behav.*, 1968, **3**, 969–971.

Valenstein, E. S., Cox, V. C., & Kakolewski, J. W. The hypothalamus and motivated behavior. In J. Tapp (Ed.), *Reinforcement.* New York: Academic Press, 1969, pp. 242–285.

Valenstein, E. S., Cox, V. C., & Kakolewski, J. K. Reexamination of the role of the hypothalamus in motivation. *Psychol. Rev.*, 1970, **77**, 16–31.

Valenstein, E. S., Kakolewski, J. W., & Cox, V. C. A comparison of stimulus-bound drinking and drinking induced by water deprivation. *Commun. behav. Biol.*, Part A, 1968, **2**, 227–233.

Valenstein, E. S., & Valenstein, T. Interaction of positive and negative neural systems. *Science*, 1964, **145**, 1456–1458.

Van Buren, J. M. Sensory, motor and autonomic effects of mesial temporal stimulation in man. *J. Neurosurg.*, 1961, **18**, 273–288.

Van Buren, J. M. Confusion and disturbance of speech from stimulation in vicinity of the head of the caudate nucleus. *J. Neurosurg.*, 1963, **20**, 148–157.

Van Buren, J. M. The abdominal aura: A study of abnominal sensations occurring in epilepsy and produced by depth stimulation. *Electroenceph. clin. Neurophysiol.*, 1963, **15**, 1–19.

Van Buren, J. M. Incremental coagulation. In E. A. Spiegel, A. Barbeau, & L. J. Doshay (Eds.), *Parkinson's Disease. Trends in Research and Treatment.* New York: Grune & Stratton, 1965, pp. 155–156.

Van Buren, J. M. Evidence regarding a more precise localization of the posterior frontal-caudate arrest response in man. *J. Neurosurg.*, 1966, **24**, 416–417.

Van Buren, J. M. Incremental coagulation in stereotaxic surgery. *J. Neurosurg.* (suppl.), 1966, **24**, 458–462.

Van Buren, J. M. A stereotaxic instrument for man. *Electroenceph. clin. Neurophysiol.*, 1968, **24**, 458–466.

Van Buren, J. M., & Baldwin, M. Comparison of sensations about mouth, face and head-neck elicited by cortical and depth stimulation in man. In J. F. Bosma (Ed.), *Second Symposium on Oral Sensation and Perception.* Springfield, Ill.: Charles C Thomas, 1970, pp. 148–169.

Van Buren, J. M., & Maccubbin, D. A. An outline atlas of the human basal ganglia with estimation of anatomical variants. *J. Neurosurg.*, 1962, **19**, 811–839.

Van Lawick-Goodall, J. The behavior of free-living chimpanzees in the Gombe Stream Reserve. *Anim. Behav. Monogr.*, 1968, **1**, Part III.

Vaughn, E., & Fisher, A. E. Male sexual behavior induced by intracranial electrical stimulation. *Science*, 1962, **137**, 758–760.

Waggoner, K. Psychocivilization or electroligarchy: Dr. Delgado's amazing world of ESB. *Yale Alumni Mag.*, 1970, **33**, 20–25.

Walker, A. E., & Marshall, C. Stimulation and depth recording in man. In D. E. Sheer (Ed.), *Electrical Stimulation of the Brain.* Austin: University of Texas Press, 1961, pp. 498–518.

Walter, G. W., & Crow, H. J. Depth recording from the human brain. *Electroenceph. clin. Neurophysiol.*, 1964, **16**, 68–72.

Ward, A. A., Jr. The anterior cingular gyrus and personality. *Res. Publ. Assoc. Nerv. Ment. Dis.*, 1948, **27**, 438–445.

Wasman, M., & Flynn, J. P. Directed attack elicited from hypothalamus. *Am. Med. Assoc. Arch. Neurol.*, 1962, **6**, 220–227.

Watts, J. W. & Freeman, W. Psychosurgery for the relief of unbearable pain. *J. Int. Coll. Surg.*, 1946, **9**, 679–683.

Weinstein, S. & Teuber, H. L. Effects of penetrating brain injury on intelligence test scores. *Science*, 1957, **127**, 1036–1037.

Werssowetz, O. F. von. *Parkinsonism.* Springfield, Ill.: Charles C Thomas, 1964.

Wetzel, M. C. Self-stimulation after-effects and runway performance in the rat. *J. comp. physiol. Psychol.*, 1963, **56**, 673–678.

Wiener, N. *Time, Communication and The Nervous System.* New York Academy of Sciences Annals, 1948, **50**, 197–220.

388 Bibliography

White, J. C. Autonomic discharge from stimulation of the hypothalamus in man. *Res. Publ. Assoc. Res. Nerv. Ment. Dis.*, 1940, **20**, 854–863.

White, J. C. Modification of frontal leukotomy for relief of pain and suffering in terminal malignant disease. *Ann. Surg.*, 1962, **56**, 394–403.

White, J. C., & Sweet, W. H. *Pain and the Neurosurgeon. A Forty-Year Experience.* Springfield, Ill.: Charles C Thomas, 1969.

Whitty, C. W. M., Duffield, J. E., Tow, P. M., & Cairns, H. Anterior cingulectomy in the treatment of mental disease. *Lancet*, 1952, **262**, 475–481.

Wilkinson, H. A., & Peele, T. L. Modification of intracranial self-stimulation by hunger satiety. *Am. J. Physiol.* 1962, **203**, 537–540.

Wilkinson, H. A., & Peele, T. L. Intracranial self-stimulation in cats. *J. comp. Neurol.*, 1963, **121**, 425–440.

Williams, J. M., & Freeman, W., Evaluation of lobotomy with special reference to children. *Assoc. Res. Nerv. Ment. Dis.*, 1953, **31**, 311–318.

Wilson, I., & Warland, E. H. Pre-frontal leucotomy in 1,000 cases. Great Britian, Board of Control (England and Wales). London, His Majesty's Stationery Office, 1947. 31 pp. (Abstract in *Lancet*, 1947, **252**, 265–266.)

Winkler, F. Die cerebrale Beeinflussung der Schweisskretion. *Arch. ges. physiol.*, 1908, **125**, 584–594.

Woods, J. W. Taming of the wild Norway rat by rhinencephalic lesions. *Nature*, 1956, **170**, 869.

Wycis, H. T., & Spiegel, E. A. Thalamotomy and mesencephalothalamotomy: Neurosurgical aspects (including treatment of pain). *New York J. Med.* 1949, **49**, 2275–2277.

Wyrwicka, W., & Doty, R. W. Feeding induced in cats by electrical stimulation of the brain stem. *Exp. Brain Res.*, 1966, **1**, 152–160.

Yakovlev, P. I. Discussion of: Cassidy, W. L., Ballantine, H. T. & Flanagan, N. B. Frontal cingulotomy for affective disorders. *Pec. Adv. Biol. Psychiat.*, 1965, **8**, 269–275.

Young, P. T. Appetite, palatability and feeding habit: A critical review. *Psychol. Bull.*, 1948, **45**, 289-320.

Zeigarnik, B. V. Relationship between local and general cerebral factors in brain injuries. *Neuropat. psikhiat.*, **1944** (in Russian).

Notes

1. There were early observations that suggested that the cerebral cortex was important for movement. One of these could have led to the identification of the motor area of the cortex almost 200 years before it was discovered. In 1691, Robert Boyle, the Anglo-Irish chemist, described a horseman who suffered from a combined motor and sensory paralysis on one side of his body after being thrown from his horse. When the large spicule of bone which was pressing down on one side of the brain was removed, the young nobleman completely recovered.

2. Elliot S. Valenstein *Brain Stimulation and Motivation,* Scott, Foresman, Glendale, III, 1973.

3. The importance of a prepared mind cannot be overestimated. It is very likely that when Dr. Frederic Gibbs reported in 1936 that some hypothalamic electrodes were able to elicit purring reactions from cats, the electrodes were located in "self-stimulation" sites.

4. The limbic system has connections with structures in the midbrain located in the pons. These structures have been referred to as the "limbic midbrain area" and they also contain part of the "rewarding" and "punishing" neural systems.

5. Drs. Stein and Wise suggested that positive reward is dependent on a neural circuit coded with the neurotransmitter norepinephrine. Extrapolating from the self-stimulation data, Stein and Wise speculated that schizophrenia may be caused by a destruction of norepinephrine synapses as a result of an enzyme deficiency that causes an accumulation of 6-hydroxydopamine, a substance that destroys norepinephrine synapses. They claimed that brain injections of 6-hydroxydopamine permanently eliminate self-stimulation, but recent evidence seems to indicate that self-stimulation returns providing the

animals are given sufficient opportunity to recover from the debilitating effects of the injections. (Antelman et al., 1972.)

6. Dr. Moniz knew of the Jacobsen-Fulton work before he performed his first operation, but in a paper entitled "My Road to Leucotomy" ("Mein Weg zur Leukotomie"), written in 1948, he asserted: "It was no sudden inspiration which caused me to work out the surgical operation which I named *prefrontal leucotomy*. . . . People who suffer from melancholia and are tormented by unhappy compulsive ideas, and for whom a medical treatment, a shock treatment or psychotherapy, is of no use, live in everlasting anguish. . . . These morbid ideas are deeply rooted in the synaptic complex. . . . On these grounds, after two years' of deliberation, I determined to sever the connecting fibers of the neurons in question. . . ." It does seem likely, nevertheless, that the presentations at the International Neurology Congress had a decisive influence on Moniz. In addition to the report of the Jacobsen-Fulton work, Dr. R. M. Brickner (see References) described in great detail the behavior of a patient whose frontal lobes had been radically removed because of a tumor. Although the patient seemed less inhibited and perhaps less capable of complex synthesis of ideas, no general intellectual impairment was found.

7. On August 26, 1943, the Veterans Administration issued a communication encouraging all consulting and staff neurosurgeons at its neuropsychiatric installations to obtain special training in prefrontal lobotomy operations. Cases to be selected for surgery were those "in which apprehension, anxiety, and depression are present, also cases with compulsions and obsessions, with marked emotional tension," where all other forms of therapy including shock therapy had failed. Dr. William C. Menninger has written that of the 15 million men examined prior to admission to the armed forces of the United States during World War II, 12 percent (1,846,000) were rejected for psychiatric reasons. An additional 632,000 were discharged after admission because of "mental breaks." The mental hospitals were so crowded at the end of World War II that very few of those discharged for psychiatric reasons could be admitted. There were 100,000 new admissions to mental hospitals in 1943 and only 67,000 discharges. In 1946 there were 271,209 admissions to mental hospitals. In 1945, $200 million was spent for the care of mental patients, but it has been estimated that if even minimum standards of care and treatment were maintained the cost would have been $700 million. The figure would have to be multiplied several times to adjust for the present dollar value.

8. Stereotaxic instruments do not compensate adequately for individual differences in brain dimensions. The injection of radiopaque dyes into the fluid-filled spaces (ventricles) of the brain makes it

possible to visualize them with X-rays, but for target structures located any distance from the ventricles, these landmarks become increasingly less reliable. It would be most convenient if every brain structure had its own characteristic electrical pattern that could be used as a means of identifying the position of the electrode tip, but unfortunately only a relatively few structures have idiosyncratic patterns that are sufficiently reliable to be useful for this purpose.

9. The critical brain areas involved have not been clearly delineated. There is some evidence that destruction of a portion of the overlying cortex in the temporal lobes, the so-called pyriform cortex, may be critical for the hypersexuality observed. Some investigators have tentatively concluded that the more medially located portions of the amygdala nuclei complex may have to be destroyed to produce the reduction in aggressive behavior in animals.

10. There are also a few reports, such as that of Drs. H. Terzian and G. Dalle Ore of Italy and also one by Dr. M. Sawa and his collaborators in Japan, that much of the Klüver-Bucy syndrome including hypersexuality and increased orality could be observed in patients following bilateral temporal lobe removal. Dr. Yong Kim has observed hypersexuality following amygdalectomy to patients under his care in Berlin. Other investigators report they do not see any signs of increased sexual interests following amygdalectomies or that in the rare instances when it may occur it is short lasting (see discussions on pages 218–219).

11. The term "psychic blindness" had been used during the 1890s by German investigators of cortical function. Dr. H. Munk used the term *Seelenblindheit* and Dr. F. Goltz applied the term *Hirnsehschwache* to refer to a loss of higher integrative visual functions rather than a loss in visual sensitivity.

12. A scruple is an old apothecary measure that dates back to a Roman measure of weight. It is equal to 20 grains or 1/24 of an ounce.

13. The notion that there are physiological mechanisms that are brought into play to combat extreme reactions has been suggested in many forms by a great number of investigators. Cannon described "The Wisdom of the Body" and homeostatic mechanisms that defended the constancy of the internal environment. Pavlov used the concept of "protective inhibition" that was brought into play by very intense stimulation. Earlier, the word *parabiosis* was used in the Russian literature by Wedensky to refer to a state bordering on life and death which triggered defensive reactions.

14. *Tonic* refers to a tight contraction of muscles, which produces an extension of the body. The *clonic* stage consists of an alternation of muscular contractions and relaxation, which produces flailing movements.

15. This is a good example of clinical information leading to animal experimentation rather than the reverse. The fact that electroconvulsive treatment, as well as traumatic head injuries, produces amnesia for recent events has led to a "dual process" hypothesis of memory storage. There is much evidence that information storage involves a relatively short period of *consolidation* during which time the memory trace is judged to be vulnerable because it is subject to disruption. A more permanent storage that follows may be dependent on the synthesis of macromolecules, according to prevailing views (see John, 1967 and Agranoff, 1971).

16. This does not mean that psychiatrists generally believe that most mental disorders have a biological cause or can be completely cured by biological manipulations.

17. One of the first applications of the cathode-ray oscilloscope to neurophysiology was undertaken by Herbert Gasser and Joseph Erlanger of Washington University in St. Louis, who demonstrated that nerves were made up of separate fibers of different diameters and corresponding differences in thresholds, conduction velocities, magnitude of responses, and firing repetition rates. They divided nerve fibers into A, B, and C categories with the A fibers having the largest diameter. In 1944, Erlanger and Gasser received the Nobel Prize "for their discoveries concerning the highly differentiated properties of single nerve fibers."

18. It was very common during this period to use the passage of electric current as a remedy for a great variety of illnesses. Many books on electrotherapeutics appeared during the middle of the nineteenth century.

19. There is no need to be frightened by these anatomical terms, which merely describe the outstanding physical features of the area. Thus the globus pallidus is a round and pale structure, the red nucleus appears red pigmented, and the substantia nigra is the substance with black pigment.

20. The early operations on patients suffering from involuntary movement disorders interrupted the primary pathway that controlled movement. Such operations, which were performed at one of several places between the cerebral cortex and the spinal cord, usually left the patient with a partial paralysis. Following the serendipity resulting from the occlusion of the anterior choroidal artery and some collaborative animal research with Professor Fred Mettler of the Columbia University College of Physicians and Surgeons, Cooper performed planned arterial occlusions in many patients over a period of a few years. The other techniques described in the text replaced the arterial operation.

21. Relatively localized destruction of neural tissue in the depths of the brain can be accomplished by electrolytic coagulation with direct current or radio frequency (RF) energy delivered through electrodes. Tissue can also be destroyed by various chemical means including alcohol injected through cannulae. Specific pharmacological agents that destroy only those neurons which utilize a particular neurotransmitter have recently been used on experimental animals and are likely to be tested on humans. The chemical 6-hydroxydopamine when injected into a brain region primarily destroys the synapses using norepinephrine.

Neural tissue in the depths of the brain can also be destroyed by miniature knives and wire loops that can be withdrawn into a cannula while being inserted to the desired depth and then extruded and rotated. Cryogenic surgery with cooling probes capable of destroying brain tissue by freezing has also been used clinically.

Focused ultrasound waves have been used on a limited scale by Drs. W. Fry and R. Meyers of the University of Illinois to make brain lesions of a very controlled size. The advantage of this method is that by using three or four low-energy beams no brain damage is created by penetration—the damage is restricted to the neural tissue at the point of focus of the beams and blood vessels are said not to be injured. It may also be possible to selectively destroy fiber tracts without damaging nerve cells and to depopulate glandular cells—such as in the pituitary—without disrupting the vascular system. The drawback of the method is that the equipment is very expensive and requires a great amount of space, a large circular bone flap must be removed from the skull (ultrasonic waves cannot be used through the intact skull, but the dura matter covering the brain can be left intact), and the instrument lenses must be immersed in a bath of degassed saline contained within the area of the bone flap.

Dr. Petter Lindstrom, who is affiliated with the University of Pittsburgh and the Veterans Administration Hospital, reported that a single unfocused sonic beam selectively destroys fiber tracts but not nerve cells. As a substitute for lobotomy, Lindstrom has used "prefrontal sonic treatment" as a means of destroying fiber tracts in the frontal lobes for either intractable pain or psychiatric disorders.

Dr. Lars Leksell of the Karolinska Institute in Sweden developed a technique for making well-defined brain lesions without any surgical cutting. The patient's head is positioned inside a specially constructed helmet that can focus several beams of radiation from a cobalt gamma unit on a preselected target within the brain. The size of the lesion depends on the plane of the the intersecting beams and their intensity. Only local anesthesia is necessary and the patient is reported to experience little discomfort. The equipment is very expensive and in spite of the fact that the first human application was undertaken in 1968, the instrument has not been adopted by others.

Dr. Geoffrey Knight of the Royal Postgraduate Medical School in London has described a method of destroying neural tissue by implanting radioactive seeds of the element yttrium in the brain (see pages 290–293).

22. There is a high probability for abnormal foci that trigger seizures to be located in temporal lobe structures. The brain structures below the surface in the temporal region seem to be especially likely to contain such foci since its position in the skull increases its vulnerability to mechanical injury, birth trauma, and blood vessel constrictions. There also seems to be a high susceptibility to infections in this region. Rabies, which often produces paroxysms of rage and terror (the French, German, and Italian words for rabies means rage), is known to cause lesions in the temporal lobe, particularly the hippocampus. Moreover, the linear alignment of the neurons of the hippocampus increases the probability that the cells will fire in synchrony, which is one characteristic of seizures. The amygdala also may have a high seizure propensity; Dr. Sebastian Grossman reported that a single injection of a cholinergic substance into this structure caused abnormal electrical activity and vicious and hypersensitive behavior that persisted until the animals were sacrificed six months later.

23. Dr. Norman Geschwind, Professor of Neurology at the Harvard Medical School, described the common psychiatric picture of the temporal lobe epileptics at the Houston Neurological Symposium, March 10, 1972. According to Dr. Geschwind, it is rare to find either depressed or affectless features in these patients, and there are few trivial events in their lives. These patients frequently lack a sense of humor and reflect a deepening of emotional experience and concern with "cosmic" affairs. There is often a high incidence of religiosity and they tend to be preoccupied (frequently over their depth) with philosophical issues. Many of these patients are involved in writing novels, essays, and treatises.

24. It is possible that the differences in observations following partial amygdalectomies may be attributed to the part of this structure that is destroyed. Elzbieta Fonberg reported that the behavior of dogs after destruction of the medial or lateral parts of the amygdala can be sharply contrasted, and Holger Ursin and B. R. Kaada provided evidence of functional localization within the amygdala of the cat. Unfortunately, the evidence is not consistent between species and there is almost no useful anatomical behavioral data at the human level.

25. Speculation about the therapeutic value of changing the balance between the sympathetic and parasympathetic branches of the autonomic nervous system is not a new idea. Dr. Manfred Sakel, who in-

troduced the insulin treatment for psychiatric disorders in 1927, wrote: "The physiological principle underlying this treatment was that psychiatric disorders of all kinds can be influenced therapeutically by causing an intensification of the tonus of the parasympathetic end of the autonomic nervous system. . . . The overstimulation of the sympathicus seemed to be the predominant cause of the nervous malfunction. . . . The reasoning behind the original experiments. . . was based on the assumption that insulin would act as a sympaticotonal drug which would stimulate the vagus in order to counteract the temporarily overstimulated sympathicus." Later, Dr. Ernest Gellhorn presented a large body of experimental evidence suggesting that the hypothalamus undergoes what he referred to as a "tuning" process to predispose it to respond with either parasympathetic or sympathetic dominance (see pages 151–154).

26.   Dr. Breggin's views were read into the *Congressional Record* (February 24, 1972; Vol. 18 No. 26) by Congressman Cornelius E. Gallagher of New Jersey and were also presented at the Houston Neurological Symposium on Neural Basis of Violence and Aggression (Houston, Texas, March 10, 1972). While sharing some of Dr. Breggin's concerns about the possible dangers of psychosurgery, and past abuses in its practice, I am not at all sympathetic with the numerous distortions of the facts that his crusading and zealous attitude seems to generate. He has made no attempt to evaluate the experimental evidence on the results of psychosurgery. Instead, he searches the literature for any phrase he can use to create the impression that psychosurgery necessarily "mutilates the personality" and "destroys the individual's capacity for autonomy and independence." Breggin does not accurately describe the serious and intractable psychiatric condition of many of the patients on whom psychosurgery has been performed and prefers to convey the impression—often by quoting out of context—that psychosurgery is the result of a casual decision by men of ill will. He is against any form of physical therapy including the use of all drugs and electroconvulsive treatment, but he offers little that would be useful in treating seriously disturbed psychiatric patients. Breggin attempts to create allies for his cause by falsely charging that psychosurgery is particularly aimed at women and the black population. Unfortunately, these charges have been uncritically accepted and repeated by a number of persons who have not taken the trouble to check the accusations.

27.   There are conditions that increase the probability of revealing abnormality in the standard scalp EEG. Abnormalities are more likely to be seen during sleep, after the patient has breathed rapidly and deeply (hyperventilation), during exposure to photic flashes, after administration of cataleptic drugs such as metrazol, or following breathing of

inhalents containing amphetamine or other stimulants. These methods are sometimes referred to as "activated electroencephalography."

28. The tragic conclusion of this fictional account probably reflects Michael Crichton's concern about the psychological consequences of remote brain stimulation. The story actually presents an imaginative description of the psychological breakdown that could result from the use of a "terminal" output of a computer to manipulate a person's moods and emotions. Also worth mentioning is the fact that in later editions of *The Terminal Man,* Crichton added a postcript stating that he was mistaken in his belief that there was a high correlation between psychomotor epilepsy and aggression, he writes: "I am persuaded that the understanding of the relationship between organic brain damage and violent behavior is not so clear as I thought at the time I wrote the book."

29. Many examples could be provided, but one of the more interesting concerns Lenin's brain. In 1924, the Soviet government invited Oskar Vogt of the Kaiser Wilhelm Institute for Brain Research to come to Moscow to study Lenin's brain. The project was extended over two and one-half years and involved the training of several Soviet scientists and contributed to the establishment of the Moscow Brain Institute.

30. These pathologists tend to regard as potentially significant some evidence of diffuse cellular damage in the hypothalamus, thalamus, and limbic structures of senile psychotics. The fact that similar (perhaps less extensive) damage is found in the brains of nonpsychotic senile patients, however, clearly diminishes the impact of the observations.

31. Evidence of pathology may be much more subtle in the nervous system than in other organs. A functional abnormality in a particular brain structure may be caused by the relative contribution of input from other brain areas, where on the nerve cells the incoming (afferent) fibers terminate (see figures 22 and 23), minute physical characteristics of the synapse and the prevailing balance between different neurotransmitters. All of these factors influence the level of activity of nerve cells, but at present they would be extremely difficult to measure.

32. There was some irony in this since Goltz had actually concluded that emotions were regulated subcortically and he publicly debated against David Ferrier, who argued for cortical localization (see figure 5).

33. In the 1930s Puusepp collaborated on 14 prefrontal operations following the psychosurgical procedure introduced by Egas Moniz. Puusepp observed that after the surgery of the patients "became more tranquil and were reacting normally to the environment."

34. This did not occur only in the United States (cf pages 54–55 and footnote 7), but in England, Japan, and other countries as well. Ac-

cording to the Ministry of Health in England, psychosurgical procedures reached their height between 1948 and 1954 with an average exceeding 1100 operations per year. Dr. Sadao Hirose of the Nippon Medical School in Tokyo has indicated that several thousand psychosurgical operations have been performed in Japan. The first operation was done in 1939 by Mizuko Nakata; the Freeman-Watts prefrontal lobotomy technique was introduced in 1942.

35. Chlorpromazine was introduced in 1952.

36. Such dynamic theories of memory would depend on the continuous passage of nerve impulses within a neuronal net. Ralph Gerard and many others have argued that the brain's 10 billion nerve cells do not have adequate power or sufficient number to maintain all our memories in constantly active circuits—one circuit for each memory. The evidence that most memories are retained after the brain's electrical activity is disrupted by cooling, electric shock, and other means also indicates that the storage of information in the brain does not depend on the maintainance of activity in neural nets. It is possible that reverberating circuits play a brief role in consolidating memory "engrams" into a more stable physicochemical change appropriate for long-term storage.

37. Amygdalectomies as well as hypothalamic operations could have logically been discussed in this chapter on psychosurgery. Since they have already been considered in the previous chapter on the surgical control of violence and aggression, however, they will not be stressed here.

38. Those desiring more details on these procedures may want to consult the report of the Second International Conference on Psychosurgery edited by Edward Hitchcock et al (1972).

39. Knight selected the substantia innominata because at this site it is possible to avoid the fibers connecting the thalamus and frontal lobes. He believes, but other disagree, that adverse effects are produced if frontothalamic connections are interrupted.

40. The neurosurgery performed for movement disorders and epilepsy evokes a much less emotional reaction, probably because of the mistaken belief that this surgery is always performed on deranged or diseased tissue. Also involved, however, is the different reaction to brain surgery when it is undertaken for what is regarded as a specific medical problem in contrast to attempts to modify the behavior and mental state of psychiatric patients.

41. In the fifteenth and sixteenth centuries a person who was mentally deranged was commonly said to have "stones in his head." Sometimes as an attempt to produce change by the power of suggestion—and other times out of pure charaltanism—superficial incisions were made

in the scalp and stones, which previously had been palmed, were dropped into a basket in view of the struggling patient. This seems to be an old practice for it is present in the art of Bosch in Amsterdam, Jan Sanders in the Prado, and the etchings of Pieter Brueghel the elder. Later representations tended to be more comical. The seventeenth century paintings of the "stone drawers" by Frans Hals and Jan Steen in the Boiijman Van Beuningen Museum (Rotterdam) are of the latter type. Steen has pictured a screaming fool tied to a chair while an incision is made in the occipital region of the head. An old woman is seen holding a pail into which a giggling boy is throwing stones, one by one.

42. Earlier, Foltz and White's report that following cingulectomy addicted monkeys do not experience the severe visceral changes that normally accompany abrupt opium withdrawal had added support for the position that cingulectomy might benefit patients whose emotional reactions were incapacitating.

43. Drs. Sidney Weinstein and Hans-Lukas Teuber studied a group of former soldiers who had received penetrating brain injuries 10 years earlier in World War II. All the men had been given the Army General Classification Test (AGCT) prior to their injuries. The AGCT is a standardized intelligence test which correlates highly with other tests purported to evaluate "general intelligence." The men with damage to the frontal area of the brain showed little or no change when they were retested on the AGCT. These negative findings may not apply to all tests. Dr. Ward Halstead, for example, studied lobotomized patients on a battery of different subtests, many of his own design, and concluded that the "frontal lobes, long regarded as silent areas, are the portion of the brain most essential to biological intelligence." Drs. Aaron Smith and Elaine Kinder also reported significant deficits in performance on the Wechsler-Bellevue Intelligence Tests 8 years after topectomy. The deficits, which were evident only on certain subtests, were not detected during testing administered only 120 days after surgery.

44. This relationship between the frontal lobes and the ability to delay responses can even be found in the early lineage of primates. Bruce Masterton and L. C. Skeen of Florida State University recently reported that the relative amount of prefrontal cortex in ground-dwelling insectivores (hedgehog), arboreal insectivores (tree shrew), and prosimian primates (bush baby) is a good predictor of performance on the problem-solving tasks involving a delay. The more prefrontal cortex, the better the performance on these tasks.

45. The first report that stimulation of the prefrontal area may evoke autonomic responses was published in 1875 by M. Schiff, who described experiments under way in Florence, Italy, which suggested that this part of the cortex directly activated the heart.

46. It is known that experimental lesions or tumors in the ventromedial hypothalamic area can cause voracious eating and produce extreme obesity. Not uncommonly, atrophy of the testes and ovaries have been reported after this hypothalamic area has been ablated and in females ovulation may be abolished. It has also been shown that following destruction of this region, animals and humans may become very irritable and aggressive. Indeed Sano, who operates on the posterior region of the hypothalamus to calm aggressive patients, has made a point of mentioning his concern about avoiding destruction of the ventromedial nucleus for fear that he might increase rather than decrease aggressive tendencies (see pages 233-236). The effects of unilateral lesions, however, may be much less severe than those produced by bilateral ablations.

In 1953, Spiegel, Wycis, Freed, and Orchinik reported that they made one to three small bilateral electrolytic lesions in the *lateral* hypothalamus in 20 agitated and assaultive schizophrenic patients. Proceding cautiously because of their concern about the vital functions regulated in this brain region, they expressed surprise over how well the patients tolerated the operation. The majority of the patients were said to have become less agitated and more manageable, but they were not cured and remained hospitalized.

47. Dr. F. Roeder and his colleagues at Göttingen note that each year there are 17,000 accusations of sexual crimes committed on juveniles in the German Federal Republic. They comment that the expense of a stereotaxic ventromedial hypothalamic lesion is negligible compared to the high cost of confinement in a prison or hospital for many years.

Index